Additional Praise for The Homeopathic Rev...

"Dana Ullman takes the reader from the origin... century system of medicine into a twenty-fi... ...ence. In this fascinating ride through medical history, he shows us that many of the world's most famous and respected people of the past 200 years have advocated for and appreciated this other approach to medicine. I am personally amazed that so many of my cultural heroes have benefited from this misunderstood science and healing art. Homeopathy deserves a definitive place in health care today."

— Leonard A. Wisneski, MD, FACP, endocrinologist and Clinical Professor of Medicine at George Washington University Medical Center; adjunct faculty in the Department of Physiology and Biophysics at Georgetown University; and author of *The Scientific Basis of Integrative Medicine*

"A tour-de-force of individuals interested in homeopathy around the world and through history! This book should be of interest to all who use alternative medicine."

— Wayne B. Jonas, MD, president and chief executive officer of the Samueli Institute

"Drawing upon the extensive use of homeopathy by historical figures, founders of modern medicine, and current celebrities, *The Homeopathic Revolution* documents the long-standing efficacy of homeopathy. Given the research breakthroughs in the biological and clinical effects of nanopharmacology, it is a certainty that homeopathy has an evolving scientific foundation in the integrative medicine of the future."

— Kenneth R. Pelletier, PhD, MD, Clinical Professor of Medicine, University of Arizona, and author of *The Best Alternative Medicine: What Works? What Does Not?*

"As the interest in alternative approaches to medicine continues to multiply, Dana Ullman's *The Homeopathic Revolution* provides an absolutely compelling case for the past, present, and future of this potent approach to health and healing."

— Ken Dychtwald, PhD, author of *The Power Years, Bodymind, Age Wave, Age Power,* and *Healthy Aging*

"This book shows that wise people know homeopathy is really effective.... So many of the renowned scientists and inventors have always been spiritual; it is only their less-renowned fellow scientists who want to reduce reality to matter."

— Jan Scholten, MD, author of *Homeopathy and Minerals* and *Homeopathy and the Elements*

Other Books by Dana Ullman

Everybody's Guide to Homeopathic Medicines (with Stephen Cummings)

The One Minute (Or So) Healer: 500 Simple Ways to Heal Yourself Naturally

The Steps to Healing: Wisdom from the Sages, the Rosemarys, and the Times

Essential Homeopathy: What It Is and What It Can Do for You

Homeopathy A-Z

The Consumer's Guide to Homeopathy

Discovering Homeopathy: Your Introduction to the Science and Art of Homeopathic Medicine

Homeopathic Medicines for Children and Infants

THE HOMEOPATHIC REVOLUTION

Why Famous People and Cultural Heroes Choose Homeopathy

DANA ULLMAN, MPH

Foreword by
DR. PETER FISHER

North Atlantic Books
Berkeley, California

Copyright © 2007 by Dana Ullman. All rights reserved. No portion of this book, except for brief review, may be reproduced, stored in a retrieval system, or transmitted in any form or by any means—electronic, mechanical, photocopying, recording, or otherwise—without the written permission of the publisher. For information contact North Atlantic Books.

Published by
North Atlantic Books
P.O. Box 12327
Berkeley, California 94712

and
Homeopathic Educational Services
2036 Blake St.
Berkeley, California 94704

Cover and book design © Ayelet Maida, A/M Studios
Printed in the United States of America

The Homeopathic Revolution: Why Famous People and Cultural Heroes Choose Homeopathy is sponsored by the Society for the Study of Native Arts and Sciences, a nonprofit educational corporation whose goals are to develop an educational and crosscultural perspective linking various scientific, social, and artistic fields; to nurture a holistic view of arts, sciences, humanities, and healing; and to publish and distribute literature on the relationship of mind, body, and nature.

North Atlantic Books' publications are available through most bookstores. For further information, call 800-733-3000 or visit our website at www.northatlanticbooks.com.

Library of Congress Cataloging-in-Publication Data
Ullman, Dana.
The homeopathic revolution : why famous people and cultural heroes choose homeopathy / by Dana Ullman.
    p. ; cm.
Includes bibliographical references and index. Summary: "Focuses on some of the most famous and respected people and cultural heroes of the last two centuries—literary greats, sports stars, scientists, film and TV stars, artists, and politicians—and how they have chosen homeopathy to treat themselves and/or their families" —Provided by publisher.
ISBN-13: 978-1-55643-671-0
ISBN-10: 1-55643-671-8
1. Homeopathy—Miscellanea. 2. Celebrities—Health and hygiene. I. Title.
[DNLM: 1. Homeopathy—history. 2. Famous Persons. 3. History, 19th Century. 4. History, 20th Century. WB 930 U41hr 2007] RX72.U44 2007
615.5'32—dc22
2007020325

2 3 4 5 6 7 8 9 10 11 12 UNITED 14 13 12 11 10 09 08

Contents

Acknowledgments... XI
Foreword by Dr. Peter Fisher, Physician to Her Majesty Queen
   Elizabeth II XVII

Introduction 1
   The Real Limitations of Conventional Medicine............ 6
   How Scientific Is Modern Medicine?...................... 10
   Understanding and Rewriting History 13

CHAPTER 1. Why Homeopathy Makes Sense and Works:
   Nanopharmacology at Its Best........................... 17
   Understanding Homeopathy 17
   The Wisdom of Symptoms—The Underlying Basis of
      Modern Physiology and Homeopathy 19
   Medicines That Respect the Wisdom of the Body 21
   Treating Syndromes, Not Diseases 22
   Homeopathic Medicine—Nanodoses, with Powerful
      Results 24
   The Clinical Evidence for Homeopathy................... 28
   Possible Explanations for Nanodoses..................... 32
   Quantum Medicine 35

CHAPTER 2. Why Homeopathy Is Hated and Vilified.................. 39
   Attacks against American Homeopaths in the Nineteenth
      Century 43
   Attacks against European Homeopaths in the Nineteenth
      Century 45
   Attacks against Asian Homeopaths in the Nineteenth
      Century 48
   Oliver Wendell Holmes and His Attack on Homeopathy 50
   Modern-Day Attacks on Homeopathy.................... 53
   The Evolution of Science and Medicine 57
   My "I Have a Dream" Speech 58

CHAPTER 3. Literary Greats: Write On, Homeopathy! 63
Henry David Thoreau, Henry Wadsworth Longfellow, Harriet Beecher Stowe, Louisa May Alcott, Emily Dickinson, Henry James, William James, Nathaniel Hawthorne, William Cullen Bryant, Washington Irving, Mark Twain, Johann Wolfgang von Goethe, Fyodor Dostoevsky, Anton Chekhov, Charles Dickens, W. B. Yeats, William Makepeace Thackeray, George Bernard Shaw, Sir Arthur Conan Doyle, Alfred, Lord Tennyson, Rabindranath Tagore, Norman Cousins, Barbara Cartland, J. D. Salinger, Gabriel García Márquez

    American Writers..63
    European Literary Greats 74
    An Eastern Advocate 82
    Modern Literary Greats..................................82

CHAPTER 4. Sports Superstars: Scoring with Homeopathy 89
David Beckham, Martina Navratilova, Boris Becker, José Maria Olazábal, Paul O'Neill, Kelly Slater, Arnie Kander, David Moncoutié, Nancy Lopez, Hermann Maier, Misty Hyman, Marie-Hélène Prémont, Elvis Stojko

CHAPTER 5. Physicians and Scientists: Coming Out of the Medicine Closet 99
Samuel Hahnemann, Charles Darwin, Sir John Forbes, Sir William Osler, Emil Adolph von Behring, Sidney Ringer, Charles Frederick Menninger, August Bier, Royal S. Copeland, Grant Selfridge, William J. Mayo and Charles H. Mayo, C. Everett Koop, Brian Josephson

    Samuel Hahnemann, MD 101
    Charles Darwin..104
    Sir John Forbes, MD 114
    Sir William Osler, MD 116
    Emil Adolph von Behring, MD......................116
    Sydney Ringer, MD 119
    Mary Everest Boole 119
    August Bier, MD..120
    Emil Grubbe, MD.......................................122
    Harold Randall Griffith, MD........................122
    Charles Frederick Menninger, MD.................124
    Grant L. Selfridge, MD................................126
    Royal S. Copeland, MD 126
    William J. Mayo, MD, and Charles H. Mayo ...128
    Charles Best, MD 129
    C. Everett Koop, MD 130
    Brian Josephson, PhD 130

CHAPTER 6. Stage, Film, and Television Celebrities: Starring in Homeopathy 137
Edwin Booth, Sarah Bernhardt, Douglas Fairbanks, Jr., Marlene Dietrich, John Wayne, Catherine Zeta-Jones, Lesley Ann Warren, Pamela Anderson, Jane Seymour, Suzanne Somers, Lindsay Wagner, Michael Caine, Julia Sawalha and Nadia Sawalha, Louise Jameson, Susan Hampshire, Priscilla Presley and Lisa Marie Presley, Ben Vereen, Ashley Judd, Naomi Watts, Jennifer Aniston, Tobey Maguire, Orlando Bloom

CHAPTER 7. Musicians: Singing Out for Homeopathy 153
Ludwig van Beethoven, Nicolo Paganini, Frédéric Chopin, Robert Schumann, Samuel Barber, Sir Yehudi Menuhin, Cher, Tina Turner, Paul McCartney, George Harrison, Ravi Shankar, Pete Townshend, Bob Weir, Paul Rodgers, Annie Lennox, Axl Rose, Jon Faddis, Dizzy Gillespie, Shirley Verrett

CHAPTER 8. Artists and Fashionistas: Homeopathy in Style 173
Vincent van Gogh, Camille Pissarro, Claude Monet, Pierre-Auguste Renoir, Paul Gauguin, Jackson Pollock, Antoni Gaudi, Karl Lagerfeld, Vidal Sassoon, Jerry Hall, Jade Jagger, Cindy Crawford

CHAPTER 9. Politicians and Peacemakers: Voting with Their Lives and Health 183
U.S. Presidents Lincoln, Tyler, Hayes, Garfield, Arthur, Harrison, McKinley, Harding, Coolidge, Hoover, and Clinton; William Lloyd Garrison; Jacob H. Gallinger; Mark A. Hanna; José de San Martin; Benjamin Disraeli; Mahatma Gandhi; Muhammad Ayub Khan; Tony Blair

Abraham Lincoln 183
William Lloyd Garrison 187
John Tyler 188
Rutherford B. Hayes 188
James Garfield 188
Chester A. Arthur 190
Benjamin Harrison 191
Jacob H. Gallinger, MD 191
William McKinley 192
Mark A. Hanna 194
Warren G. Harding 194
Calvin Coolidge 197
Herbert Hoover 198
José Francisco de San Martín 199
Benjamin Disraeli 199

Mexican Politicians.. 201
Political and Spiritual Leaders of India 201
Adolf Hitler... 203
Muhammad Ayub Khan 207
Karl Carstens.. 207
William Jefferson Clinton 208
Thorbjørn Jagland 208
Tony Blair 209

CHAPTER 10. **Women's Rights Leaders and Suffragists: Pro-Homeopathy** 213

Elizabeth Cady Stanton, Florence Nightingale, Mary Coffin Ware Dennett, Susan B. Anthony, Clara Barton, Lydia Folger Fowler, Melanie d'Hervilly Hahnemann, Clemence Sophia Lozier, Julia Ward Howe, Lucretia Mott, Julia Holmes Smith, Rebecca Lee Crumpler, Susan Smith McKinney, Florence Nightingale Ward, Coretta Scott King

The First Women Physicians 217

CHAPTER 11. **Corporate Leaders' and Philanthropists' Support for Homeopathy: A Rich Tradition** 229

John D. Rockefeller, Hiram Sibley, George Eastman, Charles F. Kettering; Robert Bosch

John D. Rockefeller, Sr.. 230
Hiram Sibley 240
George Eastman 240
Charles F. Kettering 240
George Worthington 243
The Rich and Powerful in Four Key American Cities...... 244
Other Americans 249
European Patrons... 251
Robert Bosch.. 254
Where Did the Money Go? 255
Modern-Day Corporate Leaders and Philanthropists....... 265

CHAPTER 12. **The Royal Medicine: Monarchs' Longtime Love for Homeopathy** 271

Queen Adelaide of England, Queen Mary and King George V of England, King Leopold I of Belgium, Emperors Napoleon I and III of France, Grand Duke Constantine P. Romanov of Russia, Queen Olga of Württemberg, Czar Alexander II of Russia, Princess Wilhelmina Auersberg of Bohemia, King Vittorio Emmanuel of Sardinia, Queen Isabelle of Spain, King Friedrich Wilhelm IV of Prussia, King Kalakaua and Queen Liliuokalani of Hawaii, Prince Charles of England

British Monarchs	271
Other European Monarchs	274
Other Monarchs	291
Attacks on Royal Support for Homeopathy	292
Royal Homeopathy Today	294

CHAPTER 13. Clergy and Spiritual Leaders: More than Prayer for Homeopathy 301

Popes Leo XII, Gregory XVI, Pius IX, Pius XII, and Paul VI; Father Augustus Muller; Rev. Thomas Everest; Archbishop of Dublin; Toussaint Rapous and Pierre-August Rapous; Father J. M. Veith; Rev. Johannes Helfrich; Theodore Dwight Held; Theodore Parker; Henry Ward Beecher; Right Reverend Charles Perry; Rabbi Menachem Mendel Schneerson; Rabbi Shlomo Carlebach; Mirza Tahir Ahmad; Sir Syed Ahmed Khan Bahadur; Ramakrishna Paramahamsa; Swami Vivekananda; Meher Baba; Swami Muktananda; Mary Baker Eddy; Mother Teresa; Emanuel Swedenborg

Biblical References to Homeopathic Principles	302
Vatican Support for Homeopathy	304
European Support from Leading Clergymen	308
American Clergy	317
Australian and Asian Clergy	320
Jewish Support	321
Muslim Clerics' Support	324
Eastern Spiritual Leaders	325
Colleges and Hospitals	333
Mary Baker Eddy	335
Mother Teresa	338
Emanuel Swedenborg	339

Homeopathic Resources	345
Homeopathic Organizations	345
Homeopathic Internet Sites	345
Suggested Reading	347
Notes	349
Index	369
About the Author	387

I believe what prevents men from accepting the homeopathic principles is ignorance, but ignorance is criminal when human lives are at stake. No honest man faced with the facts of homeopathy can refuse to accept it. He has no choice. When I had to face it, I had to become a follower. There was no choice if I were to continue to be an honest man. ... Truth always demands adherence and offers no alternative.

– Sir John Weir, physician to six monarchs,
including four generations of British monarchs

Acknowledgments

I stand on the shoulders of every homeopathic practitioner and every homeopathic patient before me. And because there have been hundreds of thousand of homeopaths and tens of millions of patients, I am standing tall.

A great amount of the information in this book was obtained from the people who benefited from homeopathy themselves. When one considers how much a person's health influences his or her life, it is amazing how many biographies and autobiographies have little or no information about the health care the person received. Yet, it is also impressive how many famous people and cultural heroes have publicly announced the special benefits they have received from homeopathic medicines.

Often the people who recorded these experiences are formally trained historians or biographers, others are clinicians or fellow patients, and still others are friends or family. This book is evidence that we are all historians. Anyone who writes or speaks about his or her experiences creates a record, and sometimes, someone picks up one thread and another to weave together a pattern.

The pattern that history provides on the use of homeopathic medicines by many of the most famous and respected heroes of the past 200 years remained relatively unrecognized until now. Although I had been a serious student and appreciator of homeopathy since 1972, I still did not have a sense of the depth or breadth of experience with homeopathic medicines until I began research on this project. And then, magic began to happen. Whenever I began to investigate a certain person or topic, someone would contact me or connect me to the precise information I needed.

The magic that I have personally witnessed imbues my experience in writing this book with an aura of wonderment. Michel de Montaigne, the sixteenth-century French literary great, said, "No wind blows on a ship with no port of destination." Indeed, once I decided on writing this book, I began to feel a wind at my back taking me places that I needed to go.

I want to express special appreciation to and for www.wikipedia.org as well as Homéopathe International at www.homeoint.org. Both of these websites are impressive treasure troves of information.

I also want to thank the Taubman Medical Library Homeopathy Collection at the University of Michigan (www.hti.umich.edu/h/homeop/). And I express profound appreciation for the various libraries at the University of California at Berkeley, as well as the Berkeley Public Library.

Speaking of libraries, I have a profound appreciation for the library in my own computer, thanks to the truly magnificent homeopathic software programs, RADAR and Kent Homeopathic Associates. Both of these programs contain information from hundreds of homeopathic books and journals, and doing various searches in these programs makes a researcher's (or a clinician's) efforts much easier.

Many people alerted me to certain people who should be included in this book or provided some specific and helpful feedback on at least one chapter. This long list includes: David Anick, MD, PhD, Fredrik Lid Annaniassen, Debby Applegate, Barbara Armstrong, Reed Asplundh, Melissa Assilem, RSHom, Josh Baran, Jhane Barnes, Yaakov Bar-Nahman, Julie Bernard, Jane Ramsey Best, Steve Blendell, Derek Briggs, Jennifer Brost, Rowlee Brown, Jennifer Buhl, Cathie Caccia, Miranda Castro, RSHom, Becky Crabtree, Dr. Anita Davies, Carol-Ann Galego, Chris Gillen, German Guajardo, MD, George Guess, MD, DHt, Nancy Herrick, PA, Milton F. Heller, Jr. (son-in-law to Joel T. Boone, MD), Ifeoma Ikenze, MD, Diana Jones, Ted Jordon, DO, Tauseef Khan Ahmad, Fredi Kronenberg, PhD, Muthu Kumar, Liz Lalor, Martha Libster, PhD, RN, Leilanae Lifton, Dale Moss, Lynn MacDonald, PhD, Francois Mai, PhD, Dr. Robert Mathie (of the Homeopathic Trust, in the UK), Kayla Moonwatcher, ND, Suki Munsell, Alain Naude, Francesco Negro, MD, Jennifer Nieves (archivist at Dittrick Medical History Center, Case Western University), Jeff Opt (NCR Archivist for Dayton History), Leonard Pitt, Michael

Quinn, RPh, N. Rehmatullah, MD (National Vice-President, Ahmadiyya Muslim Community, USA), Dor Remsen, Barry Rosen, Ruth Rosen, PhD, Barbara Seaman, Fran Sheffield, Nancy Siciliana, Dhrub Kumar Singh, Jan Stiles, APRN, MA, DHM, Lauren Tessier, Dr Trevor Thompson, Karl F. Volkmar, Neal White, PhD, Cyrus Wood-Thomas, DC, Janet Zand, OMD, and Roger Van Zandvoort.

I also want to thank some of the people who translated into English select articles or chapters, including Lucy de Pieri, Teresa Kramer, Tanya Marquette, and Nancy Siciliana. (A special high-potency thanks to Nancy, who went above and beyond my call for assistance.) My assistants, Angela Nusbaum and Jesse Motito, did many little things to make my life easier, and I am blessed to have them on the team.

I also wish to thank Alissa Gould for sending me a packet of articles with references to at least a dozen people mentioned in this book, Amanda Rubin for helping me make contacts for a potential film about this book, Teresa Kramer for helping to translate important information about Beethoven and Napoleon and who provided me helpful editing feedback on a couple of chapters, and Barbara Dossey, PhD, for her referral to an important but little known reference to Florence Nightingale.

Some people provided particularly expert feedback and/or detailed editing on one or more chapters. These include: James Bowman, MD, ND, Ludwig M. Deppisch, MD, Robert Juette, PhD, Dianna Medea, CCH, MA, and Christopher Phillips, CCH.

I truly appreciate the supportive and enthusiastic quotations this book has received from a diverse group of physicians, professors, authors, and cultural heroes. These quotations grace the back cover, inside the book, and the book's website. Coming "out of the medicine closet" to express support for homeopathy takes some courage. I thank them for having this courage and commitment to healing.

A big shout-out to Doug Hoff, my webmaster, who has designed and supervised the website for this book (www.HomeopathicRevolution.com) as well as my main website (www.homeopathic.com). His commitment to homeopathy and to my work is greatly appreciated.

Jeanine and Guy Saperstein, Anna Cox, and Janice Carter have not simply shown their support for this book but have provided support for my work in the past.

I give a special thanks to Francis Treuherz of London. Francis is one of the few people in the world who has a larger personal collection of homeopathic books and journals than I do, and his generosity of time, energy, and friendship has been significant. Begabati Lennihan, RN, was not only generous with her time, energy, and wisdom, but she was kind enough to grant a scholarship to her school (Teleosis in Boston) to Lauren Tessier in partial exchange for library reference work for portions of this book.

I give deep thanks to Harris L. Coulter, PhD (the leading homeopathic historian of the twentieth century), one of the very few historians who has written about medical history without a bias against homeopathy, and to the late Julian Winston (a lay historian of homeopathy), whose books provide important details about homeopaths and their literature that are not easily accessible. (His CD-ROM, *American Homoeopaths 1825–1963*, Great Auk Publishing, New Zealand, provides birth and death records of seemingly every American homeopath, their school and year of graduation, and their memberships in key homeopathic organizations.) Thank you also to the late Jacques Baur, MD, who sent me a packet of articles in 1985 about Napoleon I and Napoleon III.

It is essential to express appreciation to Richard Grossinger, my publisher, whose handshake is as good as any legal document. His longtime commitment to homeopathy and his intellectual muscle for esoteric and exoteric worldviews are inspiring. Winn Kalmon was masterful in her editing, and I was blessed to have her expertise working on the final version of this book.

Living in the San Francisco Bay Area, I am blessed with a community of friends and colleagues who are deeply committed to creating a healthier and more peaceful planet. They continually inspire me. A special thank you to: David Surrenda (consultant to CEOs, godfather to my son, and generous spirit), Lisa Rafel (a chanteuse and soul sister), Patrice Wynne (enthusiastic goddess, avid reader, and former bookseller), Devi Jacobs (a diva, a connector, and a co-conspirator), Daniel and Patricia Ellsberg (inspirations to truth-telling and to looking at the Big Picture), Dr. Adam Duhan and Eve Contente (power couple and humble and playful souls), Marybeth Love and Michael Russom (integrators of hearts and minds), Russ and Suki Munsell (a polymath and a polyheart), Dorothy and Jim Fadiman (livers of life on the cutting edge and conscious conscientiousness), Michael Parenti (a political analyst and historian who knows that history is no mystery), Brett Weinstein (teacher of the art of friendship and fellow dancer), to my in-laws who remind me that I am just me, and to my first cousins who prove that this is so.

Sanford Ullman, MD, was not just my father; he was my pediatrician, my family doctor, my editor (of previous books), and my greatest supporter, only matched by my mother, Estelle Ullman, who consistently had faith in and love for me. I simply wish that they were still around to see this book in print. I am blessed to have a sister, Dyan, and her family, to continually confirm that blood isn't just thicker than water—it runs deeper too.

Finally, the biggest thanks go to my wife, Clare, who has endured my life commitment to homeopathy. Clare didn't simply marry a man—she also married homeopathy. And a thank you to our son, Jake, who has regularly shown me the real benefits of homeopathic medicine and who at age 13 either innocently or intuitively has promised to carry on my work for homeopathy.

Foreword

In the pages of this book, Dana Ullman paints a vivid historical and geographical panorama of homeopathy through the remarkable range of famous people and cultural heroes who have used and supported it: from Mahatma Gandhi to the French 1998 World Soccer champions; from Chopin to Cher, Charles Darwin, J. D. Rockefeller, and Pope John Paul II; several generations of the British royal family and eleven U.S. presidents over 150 years, to mention but a few. Quite a selection! But homeopathy isn't the preserve of the rich and famous. It is also widely used by ordinary people: in modern India alone there are more than 200,000 trained homeopathic practitioners.

But despite its popularity and durability homeopathy has been, and continues to be, the subject of fierce polemical attacks from the scientific and medical establishment. In 2005, the leading medical journal *The Lancet* proclaimed in an anonymous editorial the "End of Homeopathy." This reminded me of the famous telegram sent by Mark Twain (another enthusiast for homeopathy): "Reports of my death are greatly exaggerated."

Of course, the fact that the extraordinary range of talented, intelligent, and independent-minded people depicted in this book benefited from homeopathy does not represent a scientific argument, but it is a strong "no smoke without fire" argument. Homeopathy is accused of being "implausible" because of its use of extremely dilute medicines. But is it not at least equally implausible that such a diverse group of remarkable individuals would have espoused it, over such a long period, if its effects were imaginary? Meanwhile, the evidence that it has real and valuable therapeutic effects, and the scientific understanding of how those effects might be mediated, is steadily accumulating.

There is a sinister side to the story, too. As Ullman shows, in the early years of the twentieth century U.S. homeopathy was all but destroyed by a murky cocktail of money and self-interest: the Flexner Report of 1910 led to the closure of nineteen of the twenty-two homeopathic medical colleges—including five of the seven black schools and all but one of the womens' medical colleges. The result was fewer but richer doctors, with greater homogeneity of race (white) and gender (male), and style of practice (drug-based).

But homeopathy is remarkably resilient. Ullman recounts, for instance, how it bounced back from a ban imposed by the Austro-Hungarian emperor in the nineteenth century. Likewise, in recent years it has staged a strong comeback in America, with an astonishing 500 percent growth in use between 1990 and 1997. But history teaches us not to be complacent. The forces that led to its sharp decline in the early twentieth century have not disappeared. It continues to be viewed with great skepticism by many in the medical establishment who cannot comprehend how the very high dilutions used in homeopathic medicines could possibly have any effects. But history also teaches us that the opinions of professors, no matter how distinguished, are a very poor guide to what subsequent generations will discover.

Homeopathy will ultimately convince the medical and scientific world of what the many remarkable individuals sketched by Dana Ullman have long known: homeopathy is a therapeutic art and science of unique potential.

Dr. Peter Fisher,
Clinical Director,
Royal London Homoeopathic Hospital
Physician to Her Majesty Queen Elizabeth II

Introduction

Galileo Galilei has been called the father of astronomy, of modern physics, and even of science. Despite his many significant contributions, Church officials considered his ideas heretical and insisted that he recant his assertions. Galileo encouraged Church officials simply to look through his telescope to verify what he was saying about the sun, not the earth, being the center of our solar system. Still, the Church officials refused to even look through his telescope.

Galileo was imprisoned, though his sentence was later commuted to house arrest for the remaining years of his life. Publication of his previous or future works was formally forbidden, though, lucky for us all, this censorship was not strictly enforced.

Just as Church officials refused to look through Galileo's telescope, many medical doctors have refused to try homeopathic medicines. Typically, they insist that homeopathic medicines do not work, and they have asserted that homeopaths and their patients are misguided.

Surprisingly, conventional physicians and their organizations have had an unscientific attitude toward homeopathy—rarely taking homeopathy seriously, rarely reading the several hundred clinical studies that have tested these medicines, rarely reviewing the several hundred basic science studies that have verified biological activity, and rarely, if ever, taking or prescribing a homeopathic medicine. In the nineteenth century, American and European physicians were reprimanded by medical organizations for even consulting with a homeopathic physician. It is ironic that conventional physicians who assume the mantle of defenders of science have maintained such an ill-informed and antagonistic attitude toward homeopathy. The old saying "competition breeds contempt" seems to express the contempt that conventional physicians hold for homeopathy.

And yet, despite the significant skepticism from many conventional physicians and despite the 200 years of savage attacks against homeopathy and homeopaths by conventional medical organizations and institutions, homeopathy has survived—and, today, is thriving throughout Europe, India, and South America.

Homeopathy has survived because millions of people have benefited from it. Whether for common minor ailments, chronic complaints, or life-threatening conditions, homeopathic medicines have been used by many famous people and cultural heroes from every walk of life. This use of homeopathic medicines by the cultural heroes mentioned in this book doesn't necessarily mean that everyone used only these natural medicines, but the majority of the people highlighted in this book sought out homeopathic treatment as a first resort.

In the light of the most famous words of Hippocrates, the father of medicine, "First, do no harm," the people covered here were smart to use safer methods to heal before more risky and more dangerous conventional methods. It is therefore apt to refer to homeopathy as "first medicine."

To clarify, it must be said upfront that most skeptics tend to assume incorrectly that advocates for homeopathy are antagonistic to conventional medical treatments. This overly simplistic perspective inaccurately portrays a flawed, black-and-white attitude. Advocates of homeopathy may have a strong critique of many conventional medical treatments, but this doesn't mean that they oppose the appropriate use of antibiotics, painkillers, surgical procedures, and/or many other drug treatments that provide blessed temporary relief.

Although scientific medicine may verify that a drug treatment reduces or eliminates a symptom, many educated people know that there is a significant difference between symptomatic relief and real cure of disease. In fact, modern physiology now supports the long-held assumption behind homeopathic and natural medicine that many symptoms actually represent important defenses of the body. Therefore, when "scientific medicine" prides itself for providing symptomatic relief or cure, this benefit rarely stands the test of time. Very few prescription drugs today have proven themselves successful for more than thirty years, let alone 200 years. Moreover, history and clinical experience frequently find decreasing long-term efficacy of drugs and increasing side effects over time.

This book provides details about cultural heroes and their stories relative to choosing homeopathic care. The real-life cases of people over decades of time and in the treatment of a great variety of diseases and syndromes provide a different and important lens to view efficacy of treatment. The people highlighted in this Introduction are described in greater depth in the chapter on cultural elements with which they are associated.

For instance, it is improbable that the naturalist and scientist **Charles Darwin** could have completed his seminal book, *Origin of Species,* if not for the homeopathic treatment that he received a decade before the book's publication. For twelve years Darwin was often incapacitated by episodes of stomach pains, vomiting, severe boils, heart palpitations, and trembling, and then he experienced two years of fainting spells and seeing spots before his eyes. In just six weeks of treatment by a homeopath, Dr. James Gully, he improved dramatically.

In part inspired by the small doses used in homeopathy, Darwin conducted some little-known experiments on plants using extremely small doses of substances and noticing dramatic effects. He was actually embarrassed to report his findings, and in part due to the highly emotional and antagonistic attitude toward homeopathy from mainstream scientists, Darwin avoided using the words "homeopathic doses."

Darwin's own letters confirm that he had great admiration for his homeopathic doctor and his treatments, though these facts are scandalously missing from the history of medicine and science (Darwin, 1903). This omission is but one more example of how history tends to ignore subjects that don't fit or support the dominant worldview.

Even many of the most respected physicians of the past 200 years expressed interest in and appreciation for homeopathy, including **Sir William Osler, Emil Adolph von Behring, August Bier, Charles Frederick Menninger,** and **C. Everett Koop.**

Corporate leaders such as **J. D. Rockefeller** and **Charles Kettering** appreciated the homeopathic care that they received throughout their adult life. Rockefeller called homeopathy "an aggressive and progressive step in medicine," and he lived to age 97 (outliving his homeopath, who lived only to 93). Kettering encouraged two major American corporations (National Cash Register and General Motors) to establish medical clinics for their employees that utilized care from homeopathic physicians. Kettering himself relied upon the care given him by his homeopathic physician, T. A. McCann, MD.

With Kettering's help, Ohio State University started a college of homeopathic medicine in 1914. Kettering also gave $1 million to Ohio State University in 1920 to help create a research laboratory for the homeopathic medical school. However, shortly after this contribution, representatives from the AMA strongly encouraged the school's president to close down the homeopathic school and warned him that teaching homeopathic medicine could result in loss of medical accreditation (Roberts, 1986). Shortly after this meeting, the university returned Kettering's entire contribution and closed down the school of homeopathic medicine.

At least eleven American presidents used or supported homeopathic medicines, as did two British Prime Ministers and past and present heads of state throughout the world. **Joel T. Boone, MD**, was the homeopathic physician to three American presidents—**Harding, Coolidge,** and **Hoover**. No other physician in American history has had this longevity in the treatment of presidents.

Homeopathy also has a long history of support from many of the world's human rights leaders and others who advocated for freedom from colonial rule. **Mahatma Gandhi**, as well as many leaders for India's movement for independence from England, also advocated for homeopathy, as did **José de San Martín**, who led the independence movement in several South American countries. A large number of people who opposed slavery were equally strong in their advocacy for homeopathy, including **William Lloyd Garrison, Daniel Webster**, and **Henry Ward Beecher**. And the vast majority of the early women's rights leaders in the United States, including **Susan B. Anthony, Elizabeth Cady Stanton,** and **Lucretia Mott**, considered homeopathic medicine to be an integral part of social reform that was necessary for the public good.

Numerous leading artists and musicians of the nineteenth and twentieth centuries developed a fine appreciation for homeopathy. Impressionist painter **Camille Pissarro** insisted that his friends and fellow artists seek homeopathic treatment, including **Vincent van Gogh, Claude Monet, Pierre-Auguste Renoir**, and **Edgar Degas**. And if they chose to not go to homeopaths themselves, Pissarro sometimes provided homeopathic treatment himself.

The nineteenth-century musical geniuses **Ludwig van Beethoven, Nicolo Paganini, Frédéric Chopin,** and **Richard Wagner** generated interest in and use of homeopathic medicine that has been followed through by more modern musical greats **Yehudi Menuhin, Dizzy Gillespie, Tina Turner, Cher, Paul McCartney**, and **George Harrison**, among many others. Beethoven dedicated two canons to his homeopathic physician and Tina Turner acknowledged that homeopathic treatment helped her recover from tuberculosis.

The leading stage and early silver-screen actress **Sarah Bernhardt** loved homeopathy so much that she insisted upon homeopathic treatment for herself and the entire cast wherever she acted. More recently, **Catherine Zeta-Jones** bragged that her new "love interest" is homeopathic *Arnica,* because it was was so helpful to her during the filming of the song-and-dance musical *Chicago,* treating her sprains and strains of overexertion.

Homeopathy became so popular among religious leaders that seven popes and scores of bishops and other leading clergy honored homeopathic physicians for the special care they provided, and many of these became homeopaths themselves. Even **Mary Baker Eddy**, founder of Christian Science, received training in homeopathy and was a regular prescriber of homeopathic medicines. Staid institutions like the Russian Orthodox Church actually encouraged their clergy to learn to prescribe homeopathic medicines because such treatment not only provided real health benefits but also led to an increased number of people converting to the faith. Many Jewish rabbis and Muslim clerics have either sought out homeopathic treatment or learned to provide it themselves.

Homeopathy was so popular among the nineteenth-century literary greats that, despite the diversity of subject matters, one thing in common was their use of and appreciation for homeopathic medicine. **Thoreau, Emerson, Longfellow, Stowe, James, Alcott, Hawthorne, Irving, Twain, Goethe, Dostoevsky, Doyle, Shaw, Dickens,** and **Tennyson** were all advocates for homeopathy.

Athletes need a special competitive edge at whatever level they perform, and because injuries can have serious implications for their career, many superstar athletes have used homeopathic medicines. **David Beckham, Martina Navratilova, Boris Becker, José Maria Olazábal,** and a dozen or so Olympic medalists have publicly expressed appreciation for homeopathy. It is indeed special when athletes share their secrets to establishing and maintaining their world-class physical abilities, and, increasingly, the secret use of homeopathic medicines is coming out of the sports closet.

Obviously, kings and queens can choose whatever health and medical care they want, and it is remarkable that so many monarchs during the past 200 years have chosen homeopathic medicine as their primary method of treatment. Some ill-informed skeptics suggest that homeopathy is some type of "new age," experimental healing system, but the the widespread support for homeopathy from various monarchs suggests that homeopathy is both "old world" and "tried-and-true."

Ultimately, while the vast majority of people have utilized the conventional medicine of their day, many notable members of society have consistently sought out and used homeopathic medicines as an integral part of their health care.

The Real Limitations of Conventional Medicine

Conventional medicine adherents have consistently asserted that its methods are scientifically verified, and they have ridiculed other methods that are suggested to have therapeutic or curative effects. In fact, conventional physicians have consistently worked to disallow competitors, even viciously attacking those in their own profession who have questioned conventional treatments or provided alternative modalities.

And yet, strangely enough, whatever has been in vogue in conventional medicine in one decade has been declared ineffective, dangerous, and sometimes barbaric in the ensuing decades. Surprisingly, despite this pattern in history, proponents and defenders of "scientific medicine" tend to have little or no humility, continually asserting that today's cure is truly effective.

The good news about conventional medicine and one of its remarkable features for which it should be honored is its history of consistently and repeatedly disproving its own treatments. The fact that only a handful of conventional drugs have survived thirty or more years is strong testament to the fact that conventional medicine is honorable enough to acknowledge its mistakes.

Medical history uncovers an obvious pattern in the discovery and application of drug treatments. Initially, there is great excitement about a new drug's discovery. Research has seemingly proven its safety and efficacy and leads to widespread appreciation for the drug's ability to provide relief. Over time, there are minor concerns about the drug's side effects, until more research and clinical practice uncover more serious concerns about its side effects. Then, more research and clinical experience lead to more serious questions about the drug's real safety and efficacy, until there is general acknowledgment that the drug doesn't work as well as previously assumed, and there is recognition of an increasingly long list of serious side effects over time. However, these problems are not really problems because a new drug emerges, with short-term research that suggests it is a better drug after all. That is, until new research confirms that it is neither as effective nor as safe as previously thought. And the cycle has continued like this for a century or more.

Like the fashion industry with its regular changes in style, the drug industry makes its profits on the newest drugs rather than on the older ones—and not just any profits, but sickeningly high profits.

In 2002, the combined profits ($35.9 billion) of the ten largest drug companies in the Fortune 500 were more than the combined profits ($33.7 billion) of the remaining 490 companies together (Angell, 2004, 11).[1] The only reason these drug companies did not maintain this shocking financial advantage is that the oil companies' profits have increased considerably with the Iraq War, thus raising the 490 non-drug companies' profits slightly higher. But then again, one would assume that the profits of 490 of the largest companies in the world would be substantially more than just ten companies in one commercial field.

This economic information is important, even essential, because *learning how to separate the "science" of medicine from the business of medicine has never been more difficult.* The combined efforts of the drug companies and the medical profession, which together may be called the "medical-industrial complex," have been wonderfully effective in convincing consumers worldwide that modern medicine is the most scientific discipline that has ever existed. Before discussing homeopathy, it is important, if not necessary, to raise basic questions about what "scientific" medicine is—and is not.

Physicians today rarely run drug companies. Instead, businessmen run them. It is, therefore, not surprising that Marcia Angell, MD, a Harvard professor of medicine and former editor of the famed *New England Journal of Medicine,* wrote:

> Over the past two decades the pharmaceutical industry has moved very far from its original high purpose of discovering and producing useful new drugs. . . . Now primarily a marketing machine to sell drugs of dubious benefit, this industry uses its wealth and power to co-opt every institution that might stand in its way, including the U.S. Congress, the FDA, academic medical centers, and the medical profession itself. (Levi, 2006)

There is big big money to be made in drug sales, and brilliant marketing has led too many of us to ignore or excuse this bully side of medicine.

Yes, a gorilla is in the house, but anyone who refers to him as a gorilla is usually called a quack or a crank. This gorilla was not born yesterday; he has been growing for generations. A part of his self-defense propensities is to eliminate competing forces, whether the other side seeks cooperation or not. Any competitive force is frequently and soundly attacked. The history of homeopathy shows this side of medicine, for from 1860 to the early twentieth century, the AMA had a consultation clause in its code of ethics that members were not allowed to consult with a medical doctor who practiced homeopathy and weren't even allowed to treat a homeopath's patients. At a time in medical history when doctors bloodlet their patients to death and regularly prescribed mercury and various caustic agents to sick people, the only action that the AMA considered reprehensible and actionable was the "crime" of consulting with a homeopath.

In fact, the entire Medical Society of New York was kicked out of the AMA in 1881 simply because this state's medical organization admitted into its membership any medical doctors who utilized homeopathic medicines, no matter what their academic credentials were. They only rejoined the AMA twenty-five years later (Walsh, 1907, 207).

This King Kong, however, is not a monster to everyone. In fact, this big gorilla is wonderfully generous to executives, to large sales and marketing forces, to supportive politicians , and to the media from whom he buys substantial amounts of advertising (and thus, an incredible amount of positive media coverage). And this gorilla is wonderfully generous to stockholders. While it may seem inappropriate to criticize profits, it is important and appropriate to do so when profits are unbelievably excessive, when long-term efficacy hasn't stood the test of time, and when common use of more than one drug at a time is rarely if ever scientifically tested for efficacy.

Although these observations just mentioned may seem harsh and offensive to some people, they are made with the concurrent acknowledgment that most of us know someone whose life was saved or at least whose health was significantly restored by conventional medical treatments. I myself am the son of a fabulous father who was a physician and insulin-dependent diabetic. In other words, I would not be alive today if it were not for some important conventional medical discoveries such as insulin.

We should not "throw the baby out with the bathwater," nor do we want to ignore the bathwater in which we place our babies. Most of us also know someone whose health has been seriously hurt, or whose life was cut short, by modern medical treatments.

Drug companies defend their large profits by asserting that they spend tremendous amounts of money on research and development, but they tend to hide the fact that they spend approximately three times more money on marketing and administration. And the obscenely high profits of the drug companies take into account all known expenses. Ultimately, drug companies are wonderfully creative in convincing us all that their drug treatments are "scientific," and too many of us actually believe them.

It is therefore important to understand what is truly meant when drug companies and the media assert that drugs are "scientifically proven."

How Scientific Is Modern Medicine?

Mahatma Gandhi was once asked by a reporter what he thought about Western civilization, and in light of the uncivilized treatment by the British government of his nonviolent actions, he immediately replied, "Western civilization? Yes, it is a good idea." Likewise, if he were asked what he thought about "scientific medicine," he would probably have replied in a similar manner.

The idea of scientific medicine is a great one, but is modern medicine truly, or even adequately, "scientific"?

Modern medicine uses the double-blind and placebo-controlled trial as the gold standard by which effectiveness of a treatment is determined.[2] On the surface, this scientific method is very reasonable. However, serious problems in these studies are widely acknowledged by academics but remain unknown to the general public. Fundamental questions about the meaning of the word "efficacy" are rarely, if ever, raised.

For instance, just because a drug treatment seems to eliminate a specific symptom doesn't necessarily mean that it is "effective." In fact, getting rid of a specific symptom can be the bad news. Aspirin may lower your fever, but physiologists recognize that fever is an important defense of the body in its efforts to fight infection. Painkilling drugs may eliminate the acute pain in the short term, but because these drugs do not influence the underlying cause of the discomfort, they do not really heal the person, and worse, they can lead to physical and psychological dependency, addiction, tolerance, and increased heart disease. Sleep-inducing drugs may lead you to fall asleep, but they do not lead to refreshed sleep, and these drugs ultimately tend to aggravate the cycle of insomnia and fatigue. Uncertainty remains for the long-term safety and efficacy of many modern drugs for common ailments, despite the high hopes and sincere expectations from the medical community and the rest of us for greater certainty.

The bottom line to scientific research is that a scientist can set up a study that shows the guise of efficacy. In other words, a drug may be effective for a very limited period of time and afterwards cause various serious symptoms. For example, a very popular anti-anxiety drug called Xanax was shown to reduce panic attacks during a two-month experiment, but once the person tries to reduce or stop the medication, panic attacks can increase 300–400 percent (*Consumer Reports,* 1993). Would as many patients take this drug if they knew this fact, and based on what standard can anyone honestly say that this drug is "effective"?

To get FDA approval to market a drug, most of the studies for psychiatric conditions last only six weeks (Angell, 2004, 112). In view of the fact that most people take anti-depressant or anti-anxiety medicines for many years, how can anyone consider these short-term studies scientifically valid? What is so little known and so sobering is that research to date has found that placebos were 80 percent as effective as the drugs—with fewer side effects (Angell, 2004, 113).

Marcia Angell, MD, author of the powerful book *The Truth about Drug Companies,* said it plainly and directly: "Trials can be rigged in a dozen ways, and it happens all the time" (Angell, 2004, 95).

Conventional drugs used today are so new that there is very little long-term research on them. There are good reasons why the vast majority of modern drugs that were used just a couple of decades ago are not prescribed any more: They don't work as well as previously assumed, and/or they cause more harm than good.

Sadly and strangely, physicians do not see that there is something fundamentally wrong with the present medical model. Instead, once an old drug is found to be ineffective or dangerous, doctors and drug companies simply assert the "scientifically proven" efficacy of a new drug. Despite this recurrent pattern, doctors are prescribing drugs at record-breaking rates:

- In 2005 the volume of prescription drugs sold in the U.S. was equal to 12.3 drugs for every man, woman, and child in that year alone (compared to 1994, when 7.9 prescription drugs per year were on average purchased by every American). (Kaiser Family Foundation, 2006)
- According to a 2005 study, 44 percent of all Americans take at least one prescription drug and 17 percent take three or more prescription drugs (This number increased 40 percent between 1994 and 2000). (*Medscape*, 2005)

The extremely high numbers listed above are considerably higher if one adds in the over-the-counter drugs that doctors recommend or that patients take on their own. When a patient takes more than one drug at a time, the research conducted on each of the drugs individually becomes virtually meaningless. Considering how many people take two or more drugs together raises serious doubts about the scientific ground on which physicians stand (except in those few instances when a multiple-drug protocol has been tested, as has occurred with some drugs in the treatment of people with AIDS).

One might hope that the American public would greatly benefit from receiving the "best" and certainly most expensive care that modern medicine has to offer. However, this simply isn't true. In fact, the following statistics powerfully state the real limitations of what the "best" medical care provides:

- According to 2006 data, the infant mortality rate in the United States was ranked twenty-first in the world, worse than South Korea and Greece and only slightly better than Poland.

- Data from 2006 also showed that the life expectancy rate in the United States was ranked seventeenth in the world, tied with Cyprus and only slightly ahead of Albania. (InfoPlease, 2007)

One of the largest drug companies in the world is GlaxoSmithKline. It was therefore a bit shocking, but not surprising, when Allen Roses, worldwide vice-president of genetics, acknowledged that "The vast majority of drugs—more than 90 percent—only work in 30 percent or 50 percent of the people" (Connor, 2003). The public is not frequently given this degree of honesty.

Understanding and Rewriting History

Who controls the past controls the future:
who controls the present controls the past.
– George Orwell, author of *1984*

History provides us with a tremendously diverse body of evidence about our past, but ultimately, only a small portion of history is told in our history books. The interpretation of our past and the select use of certain historical facts and figures taint our understanding of what really happened.

Historians commonly remark that whichever country wins a war or whichever worldview dominates another, the history is told through that country's perspective or that dominant point of view. This is certainly true in the history of medicine. For instance, medical historians commonly have portrayed conventional medical practice of the past as barbaric, dangerous, and old-fashioned, and yet they have asserted that today's medical care is at the apex of "scientific medicine." The assertion that today's medical care is "proven" is a consistently repeated mantra.

History also tends to portray those who lose a war and who represent a minority point of view as having less than positive attributes. For instance, those physicians practicing medicine differently than the orthodox medical practice might be called cranks, crackpots, and quacks. Such name-calling is a wonderfully clever way to trivialize potentially valuable contributions, whether or not one understands what these contributions really are.

Besides name-calling, practitioners of the conventional and dominating paradigm often spin facts to make the strong and solid features of a minority practice into something strange and weird. The fact that homeopaths use smaller doses than used in orthodox medicine has been portrayed as homeopathy using "wimpy" doses that theoretically could not have any physiological effect. Accusations that homeopathic medicines could not possibly have any effect are made without knowledge, experience, or humility, and such accusations simply become evidence of the accuser's unscientific attitude and his or her ignorance of the diverse body of basic scientific work on the effects of nanodoses of certain substances in specific situations.

The fact that homeopaths have used their medicines for more than 200 years is spun as evidence that this system of medicine has not "progressed." Another interpretation here is that the same homeopathic medicines used 200 years ago are still used today, along with hundreds of new ones, primarily because the old ones still work. The art of using homeopathic medicines is that they are not prescribed for a localized disease but for a syndrome or pattern of symptoms of which the localized disease is a part.

The fact that homeopaths interview a patient to discover his or her unique symptoms has been spun to make homeopathy seem like a quirky system that revels in inane facts about a patient. However, the detailed symptoms and characteristics of the patient that homeopaths collect may seem inane only to people who are not familiar with the unique and critical nature of these individualizing features of each person. Homeopathy provides a sophisticated method by which a patient's characteristics are applied to selecting and prescribing the most effective homeopathic medicine.

In light of the fact that history tends to be written by the victors, this writer predicts that history will soon be rewritten.

References
Angell, M. *The Truth about Drug Companies.* New York: Random House, 2004.
Connor, S. Glaxo Chief: Our Drugs Do Not Work on Most Patients, *The Independent* (UK), December 8, 2003.

Introduction

Consumer Reports, High Anxiety. January 1993, 19–24.

Darwin, F. (ed.). *The Life and Letters of Charles Darwin.* New York, D. Appleton & Co., 1903.

Kaiser Family Foundation, *Prescription Drug Trends,* June 2006. http://www.kff.org/rxdrugs/upload/3057-05.pdf

InfoPlease.com. www.infoplease.com/ipa/A0004393.html, 2007.

Levi, R. Science Is for Sale, *Skeptical Inquirer,* July/August 2006, 30:4, 44–46.

Medscape, More Americans Take Prescription Medication. May 3, 2005. www.medscape.com/viewarticle/500164

Roberts, W. H. Orthodoxy vs. homeopathy: Ironic developments following the Flexner Report at the Ohio State University, *Bulletin on the History of Medicine,* Spring 1986, 60:1, 73–87.

Walsh, J. J. *History of the Medical Society of the State of New York.* New York: Medical Society of the State of New York, 1907.

CHAPTER 1

Why Homeopathy Makes Sense and Works: Nanopharmacology at Its Best

Despite its significant popularity throughout the world, homeopathy is commonly misunderstood, condemned, or simply unknown.

This book is full of personal experiences from people who claim that homeopathic medicines provided great benefit to them, but no single experience provides real "proof" of the value of homeopathy. However, when a large body of experience is verified and a body of scientific studies provides additional evidence of the value of using homeopathic medicines, one can and should have a better sense of the important role that homeopathy has played in the past and will play in the future of health care.

Winston Churchill once asserted, "The longer you can look back, the further you can look forward." Although this book will primarily discuss the experiences of people during the past 200 years, there is also ample evidence of the use of certain homeopathic principles since the earliest recorded human history. This longer view of time provides a large lens through which to understand history and predict the future.

Understanding Homeopathy

The word *homeopathy* is derived from two Greek words: *homoios* meaning similar, and *pathos* meaning suffering. Homeopathy's basic premise, the principle of similars, refers to the recurrent observation and experience that whatever syndrome of symptoms a substance causes in overdose in healthy people will elicit a healing response when given in specially prepared *nanodoses* (very small doses) to people whose disease has this similar syndrome of symptoms.

Let's look at a specific example. Exposure to an onion's juices is known to cause tears from the eyes and a fluid nasal discharge that may even burn the upper lip. People with allergies or with common cold symptoms who exhibit these and other similar symptoms that onion causes will benefit from taking homeopathic doses of an onion.

Because symptoms represent the best efforts of our body in its defense against infection or stress, it makes sense to utilize medicines that help mimic these defense processes rather than inhibit or suppress them. The beauty of the homeopathic principle of similars is that a respect for the body's wisdom is inherent within it, thereby utilizing and optimizing the significant self-healing and self-regulating powers of the body.

It is important to note that immunizations and allergy treatments are two of the very few applications in modern medicine today that actually stimulate the body's own defenses in the prevention or treatment of specific diseases. It is not simply a coincidence that both of these treatments are derived from the homeopathic principle of similars.

Homeopathic medicine is so widely practiced by physicians in Europe that it is no longer considered "alternative medicine" there. Approximately 30 percent of French doctors and 20 percent of German doctors use homeopathic medicines regularly, while more than 40 percent of British physicians refer patients to homeopathic doctors (Fisher and Ward, 1994), and almost half of Dutch physicians consider homeopathic medicines to be effective (Kleijnen, Knipschild, and Riet, 1991).

Homeopathic medicine also once had a major presence in American medical care. In the early twentieth century there were twenty-two homeopathic medical schools in the United States, including Boston University, University of Michigan, New York Medical College, Ohio State University, Hahnemann Medical College, University of Minnesota, and even the University of Iowa. Further, many of America's cultural elite were homeopathy's strongest advocates.

In his Pulitzer Prize-winning book *The Social Transformation of American Medicine,* Paul Starr noted, "Because homeopathy was simultaneously philosophical and experimental, it seemed to many people to be more rather than less scientific than orthodox medicine."

This chapter presents a case for homeopathy in light of the most recent developments in science and medicine. Readers interested in learning more about the scientific experimentation on homeopathy would benefit from other published works in the field, referenced in this chapter.

I apologize to those readers who have an open mind about homeopathy but who have been introduced to it by individuals who have not adequately explained this art and science in a clear or convincing fashion. It is hoped that both skeptics *and* those open-minded but inadequately informed people will benefit from the following overview of the homeopathic system.

The Wisdom of Symptoms—The Underlying Basis of Modern Physiology and Homeopathy

The underlying principle of homeopathy is also at the heart of modern physiology. It is commonly understood in medicine today that symptoms are not just something "wrong" with the body, but, rather, they represent the efforts of the body to defend and heal itself from a variety of infective agents and/or stresses. The body creates fever, inflammation, pain, discharge, or whatever is necessary in order to defend and heal itself. While these symptoms represent the body's best efforts to heal, they are not always successful in doing so.

Medical science today is increasingly recognizing symptoms as adaptive responses of the body. Standard texts of pathology define the process of inflammation as the manner in which the body seeks to wall off, heat up, and burn out infective agents or foreign matter. The cough has long been known as a protective mechanism for clearing breathing passages. Diarrhea has been shown to be a defensive effort of the body to remove pathogens or irritants more quickly from the colon. Discharges are understood as the body's way of ridding itself of dead bacteria, viruses, and cells. Even high blood pressure is an important defense and adaptation to the internal and external stresses that a person experiences.

The derivation of the word *symptom* is helpful to better understanding of the disease process and the healing process. The word symptom comes from a Greek root and means "something that falls together with something else." Symptoms are a sign or signal of something else, and treating them doesn't necessarily change that something else. Just because a drug gets rid of a symptom does not mean that the person is cured. In fact, drugs that suppress or inhibit a symptom tend to provide only a guise of success and sometimes drive the disease deeper into the body, leading to more serious illness. Using drugs to suppress symptoms is akin to pulling the plug on your car's oil pressure warning light. Just because the light is turned off doesn't mean that your car's oil pressure problem is "cured." In fact, ignoring that light may lead to your car's breakdown.

It should be noted that people often incorrectly assume that conventional drugs have side effects. Actually, in purely pharmacological terms, drugs do not have side effects; drugs only have effects, and physicians arbitrarily differentiate between those effects that they like as the effects of the drug, while they call those symptoms that they don't like "side effects." One would not say that a bomb that destroys buildings and kills people has one or the other as a side effect. One cannot truly separate out one effect from the other. Both are effects of a bomb.

According to homeopathic philosophy, the reason that drugs create effects that are often worse than the original disease is that these drugs tend to suppress the symptoms the sick person is experiencing and push them deeper into the body. When a drug is given that prevents the body from creating its initial defensive response to an infection or a stress, the body is forced to develop a less effective or efficient way to re-establish its dynamic health. Many homeopaths believe that this observation about symptom and disease suppression may explain why people today are experiencing more serious chronic illnesses at earlier and earlier ages and why there is such an epidemic of mental illness (physical disease is suppressed deeply enough that the disease is pushed into the psyche).

Once one recognizes that symptoms are important and useful defenses of the body, it makes less sense to use drugs that inhibit or suppress this wisdom of the body. Instead of using drugs to suppress symptoms, it makes sense to use medicines to strengthen the body's own defense system so that the body can more effectively heal itself. Like the increasingly popular field of *biomimicry* (Benyus, 1997), in which scientists seek to mimic the wisdom of nature to create new and sustainable technologies, homeopaths seek to find a medicine that will mimic the wisdom of the body to initiate real healing, not just symptom suppression.

Medicines That Respect the Wisdom of the Body

The use of the principle of similars in healing actually has ancient roots (Coulter, 1975). In the fourth century BC, Hippocrates is known to have said, "Through the like, disease is produced, and through the application of the like it is cured." The famed Delphic Oracle in Greece proclaimed the value of the law of similars, stating, "That which makes sick shall heal." Paracelsus, a well-known sixteenth-century physician and alchemist, used the law of similars extensively in practice and referred to it in writings. His formulation of the "Doctrine of Signatures" spoke directly of the value in using similars in healing. He affirmed, "You there bring together the same anatomy of the herbs and the same anatomy of the illness into one order. This simile gives you understanding of the way in which you shall heal."

Using a substance to treat the similar symptoms that it causes is also present in conventional medicine, with immunizations being the most obvious example—small doses of a "weakened" pathogen are used to prevent what larger doses cause. None other than the originator of immunology, Dr. Emil Adolph von Behring (1905), directly pointed to the origins of immunizations when he asserted, "By what technical term could we more appropriately speak of this influence than by Hahnemann's word 'homeopathy.'"[3] Modern allergy treatment, likewise, utilizes the homeopathic approach by the use of small doses of allergens in order to create an antibody response.

Conventional medicine also uses homeopathy's principle of similars in choosing radiation to treat people with cancer (radiation causes cancer), digitalis for heart conditions (digitalis creates heart conditions), and Ritalin for hyperactive children (Ritalin is an amphetamine-like drug that normally causes hyperactivity). Other examples are the use of nitroglycerine for heart conditions, gold salts for arthritis, and colchicine for gout.[4]

It should be acknowledged that although the conventional medical treatments mentioned above may be homeopathic-like, they do not follow other fundamental principles of homeopathy. Immunizations and allergy treatments are given to prevent or cure special ailments, while homeopathic medicines are substances individually prescribed based on the overall syndrome of body and mind symptoms the person is experiencing, and therefore a homeopathic medicine is thought to strengthen the person's overall body-mind constitution, not just to prevent or treat a specific illness. Also, these conventional medical treatments are not individually prescribed to the high degree of selectivity that is common in homeopathy, and they are not prescribed in as small or as safe a dose.

And speaking of dose, this subject is vital. Homeopaths have uncovered an amazing and initially confusing power of the human organism—sick people develop hypersensitivity to substances that cause the similar symptoms that they are experiencing. Further, by giving very small doses of this substance, a person can and will experience an immunological and therapeutic benefit without a toxic burden.

To differentiate homeopathy from conventional medical treatments, Hahnemann coined the words *allopathy* and *allopathic medicine.* Whereas homeopathic prescriptions were based on a specific principle of similars, allopathic treatments were mostly based on the use of opposites (such as the use of laxative drugs for constipation, and constipating drugs for treating diarrhea).[5] Hahnemann asserted that treatments that were not based on the principle of similars didn't cure the person but primarily suppressed symptoms, providing only temporary relief and pushing the disease deeper inside.

Treating Syndromes, Not Diseases

There is a very common tendency for Western physicians to diagnose specific diseased states, and there is a similar desire among patients for this determination. However, conventional medical diagnosis tends to assume that most disease is localized to a specific part of the body. Heart disease is considered to be a heart problem, headaches are in the head, ear infections are in the ear, and so on.

Although there is an obvious tendency by modern physicians to understand the more complex disease state of each disease, the bottom line is that the vast majority of medical treatments tend to be directed at a specific symptom, a localized condition, or a single physiological process. Homeopaths, in comparison, do not consider any disease to be local or restricted to a single physical process. They consider all disease to be a syndrome, of which the local symptom represents only a part of the person's disease.

The homeopaths' appreciation for understanding and treating the more complex syndrome of the person explains why homeopaths assert that there is rarely a single medicine that can cure everyone with a specific disease. Thus, when one asks a homeopath what the treatment is for this or that disease, the usual answer is neither simple nor direct. Instead, homeopaths emphasize that treatment is individualized according to a person's overall syndrome, though sometimes just to make the conversation easier to understand, homeopaths sometimes inform the person of some of the more commonly indicated medicines for people with specific syndromes that include certain diseased states.

For some 200 years, hundreds of thousands of homeopaths throughout the world have carefully catalogued (and now computerized) the idiosyncratic physical, emotional, and mental symptoms that thousands of substances have caused in healthy people. Homeopaths have thereby created the most extensive body of toxicological information available today, though this information focuses on the symptoms that these substances cause, not on the doses in which they cause them. Homeopaths have found and verified that whatever symptoms a substance has been found to cause, it can also cure in specially prepared homeopathic doses.

Thousands of substances have undergone toxicological studies, which homeopaths call *provings*. These experiments are conducted on human subjects, not animals, to determine what *syndrome of symptoms* various substances from the plant, mineral, animal, or chemical kingdoms cause in overdose. Homeopaths have found that these experiments lay the foundation for learning which symptoms and syndromes each substance causes in overdose, and thus, what affinity each substance has to the human body. This is medicine at its most complex and precise.

When homeopaths see patients, they obtain the unique and detailed health history of each patient, and they then seek to find the specific plant, mineral, animal, or chemical substance that would cause the *similar syndrome of symptoms* that the patient is experiencing. It is not surprising that homeopaths throughout the world today use sophisticated expert software to help them individualize medicinal substances to their patients.[6]

After finding a match between a substance's toxicology and the patient's specific symptom pattern, the homeopath gives a specially prepared nanodose of this medicinal agent.

Homeopathic Medicine— Nanodoses, with Powerful Results

Homeopathic medicine presents a significantly different pharmacological approach to treating sick people. Instead of using strong and powerful doses of medicinal agents that have a broad-spectrum effect on a wide variety of people with a similar disease, homeopaths use extremely small doses of medicinal substances that are highly individualized to a person's physical and psychological syndrome of disease.

Homeopathic medicines are so small in dose that it is appropriate to refer to them as a part of the newly defined field of nanopharmacology. (The prefix *nano* derives from Latin and means dwarf; today, the prefix is used in nanotechnology or the nanosciences, which explore the use of extremely small technologies or processes, at least one-billionth of a unit, designated as 10-9, though our use of the word nanopharmacology and nanodose draws from its modern usage, suggesting "very small and very powerful.") To understand the nature and the degree of homeopathy's nanopharmacology, it is important to know how homeopathic medicines are made.

Making Homeopathic Medicines

Most homeopathic medicines are made by diluting a medicinal substance in double-distilled water. It should be noted that physicists who study the properties of water commonly acknowledge that water has many mysterious and amazing properties. Homeopathic manufacturers use double-distilled water, which is highly purified, enabling the medicinal substance to infiltrate the water and change its structure (Roy, et al., 2005). A significant body of research by chemists and physicists has shown that homeopathic water may be different than simply double-distilled water (Chaplin, 2007; Elia, 1999; Elia, et al., 2004).

Each substance is diluted, most commonly, 1 part of the original medicinal agent to 9 or 99 parts double-distilled water. The mixture is then vigorously shaken by a process called *succussion*. The solution is then diluted again 1:9 or 1:99 and vigorously shaken. This process of consecutive diluting and shaking is repeated 3, 6, 12, 30, 200, 1,000, or even 1,000,000 times. Simply diluting the medicines without vigorously succussing them doesn't activate the medicinal effects.

Ever since the beginning of homeopathy in the early 1800s, homeopathic medicines have been made in glass bottles. Homeopathy's founder, Samuel Hahnemann, MD, was one of the leading chemists of his day, and like all chemists of that time, he assumed that glass was inert, thus not contaminating the medicines. Very recent research, however, has shed new light on the specific role that glass vials have in the making of homeopathic medicines. (See "Possible Explanations for Nanodoses" later in this chapter.)

More than 200 years of experience have shown that the more a substance undergoes potentization (the process of sequential dilution with vigorous shaking), the more powerful the medicine becomes, the longer it acts, and the fewer doses are generally needed. Because of these observations and experiences, homeopaths refer to medicines that have been potentized 200 times or more as high potencies and those that have been potentized 12 times or fewer as low potencies.

In this light, homeopaths assert that their medicines are *not* simply extremely small doses. Instead, they affirm that the double-distilled water is changed and becomes imprinted and activated. If you chemically analyzed and compared a blank CD with a CD containing 1,000 books or 1,000 songs, both CDs would be composed of the same chemistry. A CD may have information encoded on it that cannot be differentiated by chemistry. Likewise, water is a medium that becomes encoded with the medicines and its structure changed (Roy, et al., 2005), even though normal chemical analysis of the water in which homeopathic medicines are made will not find obvious differences.

Homeopaths will be the first to acknowledge that their medicines will not have any effect at all, unless the person taking them has a hypersensitivity to the specific medicine taken. People will have this hypersensitivity if and when they exhibit the syndrome of symptoms that the substance has previously been found to cause.

It is admittedly difficult to accept the possibility that such nanopharmacological doses can have any effect at all. And yet, some highly respected basic scientific research as well as clinical studies have begun to verify the claims that homeopaths and their patients have made since the 1800s.

Principle and Power of Resonance
The principle of similars can be understood in light of the physics of music. For example, whenever a C note is played on a piano (or any instrument), all C notes reverberate, while other notes are not affected at all. Even when one instrument is relatively far away from another, its C strings will reverberate when a C note is played. The important observation here is that hypersensitivity exists when there is *resonance.*

Ultimately, homeopathy is a medical system based on resonance. Two hundred years of experience by hundreds of thousands of homeopaths have consistently discovered that specially prepared, extremely small doses of medicine can powerfully augment a person's healing response when there is a *similarity* between the toxicology of the medicine and the symptom complex of the sick person. When a patient is given a homeopathic medicine that does not match his or her symptoms, nothing happens. But when there is a match, the patient experiences significant improvement in overall health.

Other Evidence of the Power of Nanodoses
A significant body of conventional scientific research has verified the powerful biochemical effects of extremely low concentrations of biological agents. Chemicals in the brain called beta-endorphins are known to

modulate natural killer cell activity in dilutions of 10-18 (this expression means that a substance was diluted 1:10 eighteen times). Interleukin 1, an important part of our immune system, has been found to exhibit increased T-cell clone proliferation at 10-19. Pheromones (hormones emitted externally by various animals and insects) will result in hypersensitive reaction when as little as a single molecule is received.[7]

In addition to the repeated observations that the human body has its demonstrated hypersensitivity to certain chemicals, there is also a very large body of scientific evidence showing a "biphasic" (two phases) response pattern to chemicals. More specifically, extremely small doses of a substance exhibit different and sometimes opposite effects than what they cause in high concentrations. For instance, it is widely recognized that normal medical doses of atropine block the parasympathetic nerves, causing mucous membranes to dry up, while exceedingly small doses of atropine cause increased secretions to mucous membranes (Goodman and Gilman, 2001).

The fact that drugs can have two phases of action, depending upon their concentration, is a little known but consistently observed phenomenon. In fact, many medical and scientific dictionaries refer to *hormesis* or "the Arndt-Schulz law" as the observations that weak concentrations of biological agents stimulate physiological activity, medium concentrations of agents depress physiological activity, and large concentrations halt physiological activity.

Hundreds of studies have been done on hormesis by conventional scientists, none of which even mention homeopathy (Stebbing, 1982; Oberbaum and Cambar, 1994; Calabrese, 2005; Calabrese and Blain, 2005). The research journal *Science* asserted that hormesis, "a concept once discredited in scientific circles, is making a surprising comeback" (Kaiser, 2003, 378).

Those skeptics of homeopathy who question the efficacy of homeopathic high-potency medicines should not question the potential benefits of the low-potency homeopathic doses. In fact, the vast majority of homeopathic medicines sold directly to consumers in the U.S. and Europe through pharmacies and health food stores are the low-potency medicines that have trace amounts of the medicines. The homeopathic medicines used in high potencies (which generally do not have molecular traces of the original medicinal substance) are primarily prescribed by professional homeopaths who know how to individually select these more powerfully potentized medicines for which the person will be hypersensitive.

Just as humankind went west to explore new frontiers and is now exploring the frontier of space, today scientists and physicians are exploring nanotechnologies and nanopharmacologies. It is only a matter of time before scientists and physicians learn that homeopathic medicine presents a fertile ground for exploring and exploiting the power of nanodoses.

The Clinical Evidence for Homeopathy

It is perplexing that some physicians and journalists have actually asserted that there is "no research" confirming the efficacy of homeopathic medicine. Such statements represent misinformation efforts against homeopathy and result from simple ignorance of the scientific literature or prejudice against homeopathy. These attitudes have no place in discussions of scientific medicine, and those who say or suggest that homeopathy is "disproven" are simply incorrect and misinformed.

By reading this section, you will have a sense of the scientific evidence for homeopathy. And there are always new studies. You can access information about new research via some of the resources described below.

Before discussing the recent well-controlled and double-blind clinical trials, it is important to make reference to earlier research on homeopathic medicines. Homeopathy first developed popularity in Europe and the United States primarily because of the astounding successes it experienced in treating people suffering from the various infectious disease epidemics in the nineteenth century. The recorded death rates in the homeopathic hospitals from cholera, scarlet fever, typhoid, yellow fever, pneumonia, and others was typically one-half to even one-eighth of conventional medical hospitals (Bradford, 1900; Coulter, 1973). Similar results were also carefully recorded in mental institutions and prisons under the care of homeopathic physicians, compared to those under the care of conventional doctors (Homeopathy in Public Institutions, 1893).[8] It is unlikely that these consistent and significant results in treating people suffering from infectious disease epidemics could be attributed to a placebo effect.

It is important to note that some of the earliest placebo-controlled and double-blind studies ever performed were actually conducted by homeopathic physicians. For a detailed history of the nineteenth-century and early twentieth-century studies, see *The Trials of Homeopathy* by Dr. Michael Emmans Dean.[9] For an excellent summary of this history as well as a comprehensive review of modern clinical research on homeopathic medicines, see my e-book, *Homeopathic Family Medicine.* Another resource on modern basic science and clinical research on homeopathic medicine is the Samueli Institute (www.siib.org).

A summary of some of the high-quality modern placebo-controlled and double-blind studies is outlined here.

An independent group of physicians and scientists evaluated homeopathic clinical research prior to October 1995 (Linde, et al., 1997). They reviewed 186 studies, 89 of which met their pre-defined criteria for their meta-analysis. They found that on average patients given a homeopathic medicine were 2.45 times more likely to have experienced a clinically beneficial effect than those given a placebo.[10]

The most important question that good scientists pose about any clinical research is whether there have been replications of clinical studies by independent researchers. When at least three independent researchers verify the efficacy of a treatment, it is considered to be valid and effective.

Three separate groups of researchers have conducted clinical trials in the use of a homeopathic medicine (*Oscillococcinum* 200C) in the treatment of influenza-like syndromes (Ferley, et al., 1989; Casanova and Gerard, 1992; Papp, et al., 1998). Each of these trials was relatively large in the number of subjects (487, 300, and 372), and all were multi-centered, placebo-controlled, and double-blinded (two of the three trials were also randomized). These trials showed statistically significant results in the homeopathic treatment of the flu.

One very significant study of homeopathic medicine was conducted at the University of Vienna Hospital in the treatment of people with chronic obstructive pulmonary disease (COPD). COPD is a general term for a group of respiratory ailments, including chronic bronchitis and emphysema, and is the fourth leading cause of death in the U.S.

A randomized, double-blind, placebo-controlled study was performed to assess the influence of the homeopathic medicine *Kali bichromicum* (potassium dichromate) 30C on the amount of tenacious, stringy secretions from the throat in critically ill patients with a history of tobacco use and COPD (Frass, et al., 2005). In this study, fifty patients received either *Kali bichromicum* 30C globules (group 1) or placebo (group 2). Doses were administered twice daily at intervals of twelve hours. The amount of tracheal (throat) secretions on day two after the start of the study as well as the time for the length of stay in the ICU (intensive care unit) and the successful removal of obstructive mucus from the lung with a tube (extubation) were recorded. The amount of tracheal secretions was reduced very significantly in patients given the homeopathic medicine ($P = <0.0001$). Also, extubation could be performed significantly earlier in patients given homeopathy ($P = <0.0001$), and their length of stay in the hospital was significantly shorter (4.2 days for homeopathic patients and 7.4 days for patients given a placebo).

Another clinical study that has been consistently recognized as some of the highest-quality scientific research was conducted by a group of researchers at the University of Glasgow and Glasgow Homeopathic Hospital. They conducted four studies on people suffering from various respiratory allergies (hay fever, asthma, and perennial allergic rhinitis) (Taylor, et al., 2000). They treated 253 patients and found a 28 percent improvement in visual analogue scores in those given a homeopathic medicine, as compared to a 3 percent improvement in patients given a placebo ($P = 0.0007$).[11]

In the hay fever study, homeopathic doses of various hay-fever-inducing flowers were prescribed, and in the other studies, the researchers conducted conventional allergy testing to assess to which substance each person was most allergic. The researchers then prescribed the 30C (100-30 dosage) of this allergic substance (*House dust mite* 30C was the most commonly prescribed homeopathic medicine).

The researchers called this type of prescribing "homeopathic immunotherapy," and they concluded from their research that either homeopathic medicines work or controlled clinical trials do not.

Three studies of children with diarrhea were also conducted and published in peer-review scientific journals (Jacobs, et al., 2003). A meta-analysis of the 242 children involved in these three studies showed that the children prescribed a homeopathic medicine experienced a highly significant reduction in the duration of diarrhea, as compared with the children given a placebo (P = 0.008, indicating a 99.2 percent chance that this positive result was not simply due to chance). The World Health Organization has deemed that childhood diarrhea is one of the most serious public health problems today, with several million children dying each year as a result of dehydration from diarrhea. The fact that homeopathy is not included in the standard of care for diarrhea in children may one day be considered malpractice.

One unusual study tested homeopathic medicines in the treatment of fifty-three patients with fibromyalgia, a newly recognized syndrome that includes musculoskeletal symptoms, fatigue, and insomnia (Bell, et al., 2004). Participants given individually chosen homeopathic treatment showed significantly greater improvements in tender point count and tender point pain, quality of life, and global health, and a trend toward less depression, compared with those patients who underwent the same homeopathic interview process but were given a placebo. "Helpfulness from treatment" in homeopathic patients as compared to those given a placebo was very significant (P = 0.004).

What is also extremely interesting about this study was that the researchers found that people on homeopathic treatment also experienced changes in EEG readings (a measure of brain electrical activity). Not only did subjects given a homeopathic medicine experience improved health, they were shown to experience changes in brain wave activity. This evidence of clinical benefits and objective physiological action from homeopathic medicines in people with chronic symptoms constitutes very strong evidence that these nanodoses can have observable effects.

The above body of evidence should be adequate for verifying that homeopathic medicines do have therapeutic benefits, but there is even evidence that these nanodoses can have significant biological activity. One important study was led by a professor of chemistry who was formerly a skeptic of homeopathy (Dr. Madeleine Ennis) but who now recognizes that these medicines have significant effects (Belon, et al., 2004). Four independent laboratories, each associated with a university, conducted a series of 3,674 experiments using dilutions of histamine beyond Avogadro's number, by which we mean the dose in which there should be in all probability no remaining molecules of the original substance remaining (the fifteenth through nineteenth centesimal dilution, that is, 100-15 to 100–19). The researchers found inhibitory effects of histamine dilutions on a type of white blood cell called basophils. The overall effects were substantially significant (P = <0.0001). The test solutions were made in independent laboratories, the participants were blinded to the content of the test solutions, and the data analysis was performed by a biostatistician who was not involved in any other part of the trial.[12]

Still further, the website of the *New Scientist,* one of the world's most respected popular science magazines, regularly reports on homeopathy and homeopathic research from renowned physicists, chemists, physicians, biologists, and other scientists. Not all of the research reported in the *New Scientist* is positive toward homeopathy, though to date, the majority of its reporting has been (for details, go to www.newscientist.com).

Possible Explanations for Nanodoses

Precisely how homeopathic medicines work remains a mystery, and yet, nature is replete with mysteries and with numerous striking examples of the power of extremely small doses.

For instance, it is commonly known that a certain species of moth can smell pheromones of its own species up to two miles away. It is no simple coincidence that species only sense pheromones from those in the same species who emit them (akin to the homeopathic principle of similars), as though they have developed exquisite and specific receptor sites for what they need to propagate their species. Likewise, sharks are known to sense blood in the water at distances, and when one considers the volume of water in the ocean, it becomes obvious that sharks, like all living creatures, develop extreme hypersensitivity for whatever will help ensure their survival.

That living organisms have some truly remarkable sensitivities is no controversy. The challenging question that remains is: How does the medicine become imprinted into the water and how does the homeopathic process of dilution with succussion increase the medicine's power? Although we do not know precisely the answer to this question, some new research may help point the way.

The newest and most intriguing way to explain how homeopathic medicines may work derives from some sophisticated modern technology. Scientists at several universities and hospitals in France and Belgium have discovered that the vigorous shaking of the water in glass bottles causes extremely small amounts of silica fragments or chips to fall into the water (Demangeat, et al., 2004). Perhaps these silica chips may help to store the information in the water, with each medicine that is initially placed in the water creating its own pharmacological effect.

Further, the micro-bubbles and the nano-bubbles that are caused by the shaking may burst and thereby produce microenvironments of higher temperature and pressure. Several studies by chemists and physicists have revealed increased release of heat from water in which homeopathic medicines are prepared, even when the repeated process of dilutions should suggest that there are no molecules remaining of the original medicinal substance (Elia and Niccoli, 1999; Elia, et al., 2004; Rey, 2003).

Also, a group of highly respected scientists have confirmed that the vigorous shaking involved with making homeopathic medicines changes the pressure in the water, akin to water being at 10,000 feet in altitude (Roy, et al., 2005). These scientists have shown how the homeopathic process of using double-distilled water and then diluting and shaking the medicine in a sequential fashion changes the structure of water.[13]

One metaphor that may help us understand how and why extremely small doses of medicinal agents may work derives from present knowledge of modern submarine radio communications. Normal radio waves simply do not penetrate water, so submarines must use an extremely low-frequency radio wave. The radio waves used by submarines to penetrate water are so low that a single wavelength is typically several miles long!

If one considers that the human body is 70–80 percent water, perhaps the best way to provide pharmacological information to the body and into intercellular fluids is with nanodoses. Like the extremely low-frequency radio waves, it may be necessary to use extremely low (and activated) doses for a person to receive the medicinal effect.

It is important to understand that nanopharmacological doses will not have any effect unless the person is hypersensitive to the specific medicinal substance. Hypersensitivity is created when there is some type of resonance between the medicine and the person. Because the system of homeopathy bases its selection of the medicine on its ability to cause in overdose the similar symptoms that the sick person is experiencing, homeopathy's principle of similars is simply a practical method of finding the substance to which a person is hypersensitive.

The homeopathic principle of similars makes further sense when one considers that modern physiologists and pathologists recognize that disease is not simply the result of breakdown or surrender of the body but that symptoms are instead representative of the body's efforts to fight infection or adapt to stress.

Using a nanodose that is able to penetrate deeply into the body and that is specifically chosen for its ability to mimic the symptoms helps to initiate a profound healing process. It is also important to highlight the fact that a homeopathic medicine is not simply chosen for its ability to cause a similar disease but for its ability to cause a similar syndrome of symptoms of disease, of which the specific localized disease is a part. By understanding that the human body is a complex organism that creates a wide variety of physical and psychological symptoms, homeopaths acknowledge biological complexity and have a system of treatment to address it effectively.

Although no one knows precisely how homeopathic medicines initiate the healing process, we have more than 200 years of evidence from hundreds of thousands of clinicians and tens of millions of patients that these medicines have powerful effects. One cannot help but anticipate the veritable treasure trove of knowledge that further research in homeopathy and nanopharmacology will bring.

Quantum Medicine

Quantum physics does not disprove Newtonian physics; quantum physics simply extends our understanding of extremely small and extremely large systems. Likewise, homeopathy does not disprove conventional pharmacology; instead, it extends our understanding of extremely small doses of medicinal agents.

The founder of homeopathic medicine, Samuel Hahnemann, MD, rewrote and updated his seminal work on the subject five times in his lifetime, each time refining his observations. Homeopaths continue to refine this system of nanopharmacology. While there is not always agreement on the best ways to select the correct remedy or the best nanopharmacological dose to use, the system of homeopathic medicine provides a solid foundation from which clinicians and researchers exploring nanopharmacologies can and should investigate.

References

Behring, E. A. von. *Modern Phthisia-Genetic and Phthisia-Therapeutic Problems in Historical Illumination.* New York, 1905.

Bell, I. R., Lewis, D. A., Brooks, A. J., et al. Improved clinical status in fibromyalgia patients treated with individualized homeopathic remedies versus placebo, *Rheumatology* 2004:1111–1115.

Bellavite, P., and Signorini, A. *Emerging Science of Homeopathy: Complexity, Biodynamics, and Nanopharmacology.* Berkeley: North Atlantic Books, 2002.

Belon, P., Cumps, J., Ennis, M., Mannaioni, P. F., Roberfroid, M., Ste-Laudy, J., and Wiegant, F. A. C. Histamine dilutions modulate basophil activity, *Inflammation Research*, 2004, 53:181–188.

Benyus, J. M. *Biomimicry: Innovation Inspired by Nature.* New York: Quill, 1997.

Bradford, T. L. *The Logic of Figures or Comparative Results of Homoeopathic and Other Treatments.* Philadelphia: Boericke and Tafel, 1900.

Calabrese, E. J. Hormetic Dose-Response Relationships in Immunology: Occurrence, Quantitative Features of the Dose Response, Mechanistic Foundations and Clinical Implications, *Critical Reviews in Toxicology,* 2005, 35:89–295.

Calabrese, E. J., and Blain, R. The Occurrence of Hormetic Dose Responses in the Toxicological Literature, the Hormesis Database: An Overview, *Toxicology and Applied Pharmacology*, 2005, 202:289–301.

Casanova, P. *Multi-centric study involving 100 patients*. Centre de Recherche et de Documentation Technique, University of Marseilles, France, 1983.

Casanova, P., and Gerard, R. *Bilan de 3 annees d'etudes randomisees multicentriques oscillococcinum/placebo, oscillococcinum rassegna della letterature internationale*. Milan: Laboratoires Boiron, 1992.

Chaplin, M. www.lsbu.ac.uk/water/chaplin.html. 2007.

Connelly, B. How Homeopathy Works, *Simillimum*, March 2002, 33–53. www.y2khealthanddetox.com/homeoworks.html.

Coulter, H. L. *Divided Legacy: The Conflict Between Homeopathy and the American Medical Association*. Berkeley: North Atlantic Books, 1973, 302.

Coulter, H. L. *Divided Legacy: The Patterns Emerge—Hippocrates to Paracelsus*. Berkeley: North Atlantic Books, 1975.

Coulter, H. L. *Homeopathic Influences in Nineteenth Century Allopathic Therapeutics*. St. Louis: Formur, 1973.

Dean, M. E. *The Trials of Homeopathy*. Essen, Germany: KVC, 2004.

Demangeat, J.-L., Gries, P., Poitevin, B., Droesbeke J.-J., Zahaf, T., Maton, F., Pierart, C., and Muller, R. N. Low-Field NMR Water Proton Longitudinal Relaxation in Ultrahighly Diluted Aqueous Solutions of Silica-Lactose Prepared in Glass Material for Pharmaceutical Use, *Applied Magnetic Resonance*, 2004, 26:465–481.

Elia, V., and Niccoli, M. Thermodynamics of Extremely Diluted Aqueous Solutions, *Annals of the New York Academy of Sciences*, 1999, 879:241–248.

Elia, V., Baiano, S., Duro, I., Napoli, E., Niccoli, M., and Nonatelli, L. Permanent Physio-chemical Properties of Extremely Diluted Aqueous Solutions of Homeopathic Medicines, *Homeopathy*, 2004, 93:144–150.

Eskinazi, D. Homeopathy Re-revisited: Is Homeopathy Compatible with Biomedical Observations? *Archives in Internal Medicine*, Sept 27, 1999, 159:1981–1987.

Ferley, J. P., et al. A Controlled Evaluation of a Homeopathic Preparation in the Treatment of Influenza-like Syndrome, *British Journal of Clinical Pharmacology*, March 1989, 27:329–335.

Fisher, P., and Ward, A. Medicine in Europe: Complementary Medicine in Europe, *British Medical Journal (BMJ)*, July 9, 1994, 309:107–111.

Frass, M., Dielacher, C., Linkesch, M., Endler, C., Muchitsch, I., Schuster, E., and Kaye, A. Influence of Potassium Dichromate on Tracheal Secretions in Critically Ill Patients, *Chest*, March 2005.

Goodman, L., and Gilman, A. *The Pharmacological Basis of Therapeutics*. Fifth edition. New York: Macmillan, 2001.

Homeopathy in Public Institutions: Saves Life, Time, and Taxes. *Medical and Surgical Record*, V2, February 1893:8–14.

Jacobs, J, Jonas, W. B., Jimenez-Perez, B., and Crothers, D. Homeopathy for Childhood Diarrhea: Combined Results and Meta-analysis from Three Randomized, Controlled Clinical Trials, *Pediatric Infectious Disease Journal*, 2003, 22:229–234.

Josephson, B. Molecule Memories, *New Scientist*, November 1, 1997, 66.

Kaiser, J. Hormesis: A Healthful Dab of Radiation? *Science,* October 2003, vol. 17, no. 5644.

Kleijnen, J., Knipschild, P., and ter Riet, G., Trials of Homoeopathy, *BMJ [British Medical Journal],* February 9, 1991:316–323.

Linde, K., Clausius, N., Ramirez, G., et al. Are the Clinical Effects of Homoeopathy Placebo Effects? A Meta-analysis of Placebo-Controlled Trials, *The Lancet,* September 20, 1997, 350:834–843.

Oberbaum, M., and Cambar, J. Hormesis: Dose Dependent Reverse Effects of Low and Very Low Doses, in P. C. Endler and J. Schulte (eds.), *Ultra High Dilutions.* Dordrecht: Kluwer Academic, 1994.

Papp, R., Schuback, G., Beck, E., et al. Oscilloccinum in Patients with Influenza-like Syndromes: A Placebo-Controlled Double-Blind Evaluation, *British Homeopathic Journal,* April 1998, 87:69–76.

Rey, L. Thermoluminescence of Ultra-High Dilutions of Lithium Chloride and Sodium Chloride. *Physica A,* 2003, 323:67–74.

Roy, R., Tiller, W. A., Bell, I., and Hoover, M. R. The Structure of Liquid Water: Novel Insights From Materials Research; Potential Relevance to Homeopathy, *Materials Research Innovations,* December 2005, 9:4.

Stebbing, A. Hormesis: The Stimulation of Growth by Low Levels of Inhibitors, *Science of the Total Environment,* 1982, 22: 213–234.

Taylor, M. A., Reilly, D., Llewellyn-Jones, R. H., et al. Randomised Controlled Trial of Homoeopathy versus Placebo in Perennial Allergic Rhinitis with Overview of Four Trial Series, *BMJ,* August 19, 2000, 321:471–476.

Ullman, D. *Homeopathic Family Medicine* (an ebook). Berkeley: Homeopathic Educational Services (updated every three months at www.homeopathic.com).

Wiesenauer, M., and Ludtke, R. A Meta-analysis of the Homeopathic Treatment of Pollinosis with Galphimia glauca, *Forsch Komplementarmed,* 1996, 3:230–234.

CHAPTER 2

Why Homeopathy Is Hated and Vilified

On the tombstone of homeopathy's founder, Dr. Samuel Hahnemann, are the Latin words *Aude sapere,* which translate as "dare to be wise, to experience, to taste." Hahnemann's challenge to conventional doctors then and now was to simply try homeopathy and judge for themselves. Sadly, however, most doctors did not honor this simple challenge. In fact, most physicians have maintained a prejudiced and unscientific attitude toward the subject. In other words, they didn't know much about homeopathy, and they never tried it, but they didn't like it.

In the nineteenth century many physicians chose to try homeopathy and were surprised and impressed by the therapeutic results, even in the treatment of the infectious disease epidemics that raged during that time. In response to the growing popularity of this "new" medicine, homeopathic medical schools were created to teach basic medical sciences as well as how to prescribe homeopathic medicines. Boston University, New York Homeopathic Medical College, Hahnemann Medical College (of Philadelphia), and several others in the United States were founded to educate a new breed of physician.

Homeopaths did something else that was never done before. For the first time in history, a large and growing group of medical doctors began to criticize publicly the way "regular" medicine was practiced. Further, homeopathic physicians asserted that orthodox medical care did more harm than good.

Before this time, physicians maintained a certain gentlemanly attitude toward each other. Although there have always been differences of opinion within medical practice, the emergence of homeopathy and the development of homeopathic medical schools created a stronger and more sustentative analysis and critique of conventional medicine. Increasingly, the threat of homeopathic medicine was that it attracted the most respected literary elite, many of the leading members of the clergy, a large number of the human rights advocates, well-placed politicians, and many of the richest families in America. Homeopathy was emerging as a viable competitor to conventional medicine of the day.

From the origins of homeopathy in Germany in the early 1800s, Dr. Hahnemann and his colleagues sharply criticized the regular doctors' use of high doses of mercury, antimony, arsenic, lead, and other poisons. Conventional physicians of the day also regularly performed bloodletting on their patients by using a knife (called a lancet) to open a vein and release blood in order to get rid of what was considered stagnant or excess blood. Even the use of leeches was common until the mid-1800s.[14] Until the mid-1800s physicians who did not bloodlet their patients were thought to be "quacks."

When any physician publicly criticized another, this was considered a serious offense, but when large numbers of homeopaths were actively asserting that regular medicine was dangerous, this created a war against homeopathy and homeopaths.

A leading medical historian noted that conventional physicians were not offended or threatened when fellow physicians prescribed homeopathic medicines, but when these fellow physicians expressed antagonism to conventional medical practices (as homeopathic physicians did), these actions were unforgivable and led to an all-out war against the homeopaths (King, 1983).

Hahnemann and his fellow homeopaths were not just critical of doctors prescribing dangerous drugs; homeopaths also attacked the prescription of multiple drugs concurrently. The homeopaths asserted that "polypharmacy" (the use of many drugs together) is unscientific because research rarely tests the efficacy of using multiple drugs together. Hahnemann and other homeopaths asserted that the mixing of drugs together created a new combined drug with completely unknown effects upon the human body. Ultimately, homeopaths were seriously questioning how scientific "scientific medicine" really was.

The antagonism against homeopathy and homeopaths among orthodox physicians was significant, but the antagonism among the pharmacists (called apothecaries in the nineteenth century) was even more significant. At that time, it was illegal for physicians to make their own medicines. Instead, physicians were required to write a prescription to be filled at a local apothecary. Commonly, orthodox physicians prescribed four to eight different drugs for a patient, most of which would be prescribed in large and commonly toxic doses.

In comparison, homeopathic physicians generally prescribed only *one* drug per patient and recommended an extremely small dose of it. At the time, the apothecaries were required to charge for their drugs based on the amount of the specific medicine. Needless to say, they could not charge much for homeopathic medicines, and to make things worse, homeopathic medicines require labor-intensive manufacturing.

Due to these important economic factors, apothecaries disliked homeopathy and homeopaths intensely. And in response, homeopaths didn't trust apothecaries to make their medicines properly. In fact, there is a long history of homeopaths questioning the authenticity of the manufacturing of homeopathic medicines from regular apothecaries.

To test the amount of fraud, some German homeopaths in the 1880s made up fictitious names of homeopathic medicines and had patients go to various apothecaries to have them filled.[15] Of the eighty-nine drug stores, only twelve refused to fill these fictitious prescriptions, and many of those stores that didn't fill the prescription did so because they openly said that they didn't sell *any* homeopathic drugs (Homeopathic Pharmacies, 1899). Even after the apothecaries were informed about the fraudulent prescriptions, other tests of these stores found that fraudulent prescriptions were still handed out to customers.

Another reason that homeopathy and homeopaths were vilified was that homeopathy represented a different system of medicine with decidedly different assumptions about health, disease, and the healing process. Conventional practitioners tended to believe that symptoms represented something wrong with the body that needed to be suppressed, inhibited, or controlled, and they used powerful treatments to do this. They categorized different diseases and lumped together those patients with seemingly similar conditions.

In contrast, homeopaths tended to believe that symptoms are not simply something wrong with the person, but rather, represent the person's best internal efforts to defend against infection and/or stress and are the organism's most effective way to re-establish health. Respect for this inner wisdom of the human organism translated further into treatment by using very small, individually chosen medicines that had the capability to cause, if given in overdose, the similar symptoms that the person was experiencing. Because symptoms are understood as defenses of the body, it made sense to homeopaths to mimic this wisdom. Medicines were not prescribed based simply on the disease the patient had but on the entire syndrome of physical and psychological symptoms that each patient experienced.

Homeopathy was also hated and vilified for prescribing extremely small doses of medicines to patients. In the nineteenth century during the initial stages of the Industrial Revolution, there was a strong cultural assumption that the use of larger and more powerful drugs defined "progress." Skeptics of homeopathy insisted that homeopathic drugs were "unmanly" and were simply placebos. The vast majority of conventional physicians of that time (and even today) refused to believe that homeopathic medicines could have any effect, let alone a curative effect.

During the Industrial Revolution, there was also a strong cultural appreciation for the new assembly line, and conventional medicine's orientation of treating everyone who had the same disease with the same drug treatment. Even though patients may have had vastly different symptoms of a specific disease as well as different causative factors, the conventional medical treatment regimens had no method to adapt to these individualizing characteristics. Still, conventional medicine of the day gave people the sense of progress, and that itself provided some therapeutic benefit.

Attacks against American Homeopaths in the Nineteenth Century

A Danish physician, Hans Burch Gram, MD, first introduced homeopathy to America in 1825. Homeopathy grew wildly shortly after it was first introduced, and by 1844, the first national medical society in the U.S. was founded—the American Institute of Homeopathy. Two years later, a rival organization was founded in part to stop the growth of the homeopaths; this organization called itself the American Medical Association (AMA).

At a time in medical history when physicians were rarely if ever reprimanded for practicing dangerous medicine or for any ethical violations, the AMA decided in 1855 to add one rule to its code of ethics, disallowing consultations with homeopathic doctors or other "irregular practitioners." Called the consultation clause, this ethics code even disallowed members of the AMA to treat patients of homeopaths.[16] Further, some medical schools actually revoked the diplomas of alumni who began to practice with homeopathic medicines, suspended students who simply associated with homeopaths, and refused to allow students who apprenticed with homeopaths to attend lectures (Warner, 1999).

The antagonism against homeopathy and homeopaths even created a religious rather than scientific furor. One president of the AMA asserted, "Next to the holy scriptures, and the grace of God, it [the consultation clause] would serve most effectually to guard him [a member physician] from evil" (Warner, 1999, 55).

Astonishingly, the consultation clause was one of the few ethical codes the AMA ever enforced (Coulter, 1975, 208). One AMA member got kicked out of his local medical society for consulting with a homeopath who also happened to be his wife. A New York physician was found guilty of practicing homeopathy (he admitted his own guilt) and was convicted but was fined less than one cent. The jury was so sympathetic to the doctor and his cause that they donated their own fees for jury duty to the local homeopathic society (Rothstein, 1972, 169).

Getting kicked out of the AMA was a serious problem in the 1850s and 1860s, because losing membership in one's local medical society also meant that the physician could lose his right to practice medicine, and it meant that any other physician who consulted with or referred patients to the punished physician could also get kicked out of the local medical society.[17]

In 1867, the AMA made it the duty of every member to report to the Committee on Ethics any consultation with a homeopath or an abortionist. Shortly after this, Dr. A. K. Gardner, one of the founders of the venerable New York Academy of Medicine, was suspended for consulting with a homeopath. While the medical press supported this penalty, the *New York Times* and the *New York Tribune* sharply criticized it (Coulter, 1975, 314).

In 1868, the AMA declared it unethical to consult with doctors who did not graduate from "regular" medical schools. However, because many homeopathic doctors had graduated from these colleges, the AMA's action created more confusion than clarity.

But the proverbial **** really hit the fan in 1881 when a committee of the Medical Society of New York recommended changes in its own consultation clause. In 1883, a new code was adopted that allowed "regular" doctors to consult with "homeopathic doctors." Because this bylaw change differed from the AMA's, the AMA formally tossed the entire Medical Society of New York out of the AMA! In 1884, a new New York medical society was formed called the New York State Medical Association. Two competing conventional medical associations existed until 1906 (Walsh, 1907, 207).

The *New York Times* editorialized, "The AMA says that if a patient's life cannot be saved except by such a consultation, then the patient must die, and no doctor who will allow a homeopathist to help him can be recognized by the Association" (Coulter, 1975, 314).

One of the leaders of the movement in New York to allow consultation with homeopaths was Abraham Jacobi, MD (1830–1919). Dr. Jacobi opened the first children's clinic in the United States and is considered the father of pediatrics.[18] Although Jacobi was branded a traitor to the AMA, shortly after the AMA itself got rid of the consultation clause in 1903, he was voted the AMA's president (Warner, 1999).

Austin Flint, MD (1812–1886), a heart specialist who was a stalwart

AMA member, was a leader of the new organization with its rabid anti-homeopathy policies. He asserted that what really bothered the medical profession was not homeopathic practice but the homeopaths' public opposition to and critique of conventional medical practice (King, 1983). As it turns out, medical historians today acknowledge that conventional medicine of that day was both ineffective and dangerous. The homeopaths' analysis and critique of conventional medicine was indeed accurate.

Ironically, Flint was known to assert that "the only solid basis of therapeutics is clinical experience," and yet, it seems that only his own and his fellow conventional doctors' experiences were valid, not the clinical experiences of thousands of homeopathic doctors (Warner, 1999, 61).

As arrogant as it was for the AMA to kick out the entire New York medical society, other similar stories show the fear and loathing that conventional physicians had for homeopathy and homeopaths. Ultimately, these actions show the degree of threat that homeopathy posed for conventional doctors.

Perhaps the most important reason that conventional physicians disliked homeopathy and homeopaths was well expressed at an AMA meeting by one of the more respected orthodox physicians: "*We must admit that we never fought the homeopath on matters of principles; we fought him because he came into the community and got the business*" (Kaufman, 1971, 158). Although most physicians, past or present, won't as easily admit it, economic issues play a major role in what is practiced and what is allowed to be practiced.

Attacks against European Homeopaths in the Nineteenth Century

Similar economic issues were at play in Europe as well. A French medical student was expelled from a medical school for simply expressing interest in homeopathy. J. P. Tessier, a respected conventional French physician, evaluated the results of homeopathic treatment of patients with pneumonia at the Hospital Ste. Marguerite. Pneumonia was chosen for evaluation because it was a common, well known, and unambiguous disease with a clear diagnosis and prognosis. In order to reduce bias, he arranged for evaluation of the results of treatment by two conventional physicians. Based on results from other studies of his day in the treatment of pneumonia, he expected a mortality rate of 33 percent. However, Tessier found that the patients in this study experienced a 7.5 percent mortality rate (Dean, 2004, 118–120).

When he announced to the Paris Academy that the results were favorable toward homeopathy, he aroused a significant furor. No conventional medical journal would publish his research, so he sent the study to a homeopathic journal. He was summarily expelled from the French medical society for this "crime."

A similar situation occurred in England. The General Board of Health was an agency of the British government. In 1854, Sir Benjamin Hall, a member of England's Parliament, administered the board, and his first act was to set up a General Medical Council of clinicians to conduct a major epidemiological survey of the cholera epidemic, a serious public health problem in that year. The council's report showed that 51.9 percent of patients treated for cholera as in-patients or out-patients in London hospitals had died and that all types of treatment were deemed useless.

The London HomoeopathicHospital in Golden Square had just established a charitable foundation in 1849 and opened its doors in 1850. During the 1854 cholera epidemic, the thirty-bed hospital was devoted to the treatment of the "indigent poor" of the area. The homeopathic hospital, like all other hospitals in London, submitted its records to the council for its report on cholera treatment, but the homeopathic mortality statistics were not listed in the report. The homeopathic hospital experienced a mortality rate of only 16.4 percent of patients.

When Hall asked the council to explain this omission, the reply was:

> That by introducing the returns of homeopathic practitioners, they would not only compromise the value and utility of their averages of cure, as deduced from the operation of known remedies, but they would give an unjustifiable sanction to an empirical practice alike opposed to the maintenance of truth and to the progress of science. (Nichols, 1988, 145–146)

In other words, the statistics from the homeopathic hospital were not listed because their listing would suggest that homeopathic medicines provide a superior treatment for cholera.

Skeptics may wonder how valid the homeopathic hospitals statistics were. It is therefore important to note that the inspector appointed to the district of London refused to visit the homeopathic hospital, so another inspector reluctantly agreed to do so. In a letter to the Homeopathic Hospital on February 22, 1855, he wrote:

> You are aware that I went to your hospital prepossessed against the homeopathic system; that you had in me, in your camp, an enemy rather than a friend, and that I must therefore have seen some cogent reason there, the first day I went, to come away so favourably disposed as to advise a friend to send a subscription to your charitable fund. (Dean, 2004, 127)

In 1858, the conventional physicians sought to have homeopathic practice outlawed. Despite some vitriolic lobbying, this law was not passed, in part because of the evidence of homeopathy's successes in treating the recent cholera epidemic. Still, the British Medical Association passed internal rules that forbade their members from practicing homeopathy or even consulting with a homeopath in the care of any patient. The British doctors even required medical students to sign a pledge that they would never become a homeopath, and they actually failed any student who refused to sign this pledge (Baumann, 1857).

Homeopaths in England continued to seek comparative trials but were always turned down. Even an offer of 5,000 pounds (the equivalent to 1 million pounds today—or $2 million!) was offered by Major Vaughan Morgan in the 1860s to establish a homeopathic ward in a conventional London hospital, and this offer was turned down by every hospital in London due to the real fear that involvement with homeopathy or homeopaths in any way would cause orthodox physicians to leave the hospital and never refer patients there.

If these actions against homeopathy and homeopaths were not enough, the conventional physicians also sought manslaughter charges against homeopaths if and when any patients died under their care. All doctors have some patients who pass away, but the conventional physicians did all they could to make practicing homeopathy difficult or impossible.[19] Despite the much more frequent deaths that occurred under the care of conventional physicians, there is no similar pattern of manslaughter charges against them by homeopaths.

At other times, legal actions were brought against homeopathic physicians for medical malpractice because they didn't utilize bloodletting on their patients nor apply powerful (and dangerous) purgative/laxative drugs. It is ironic that physicians who were practicing such ineffective and dangerous medical practices would seek legal action against those physicians who practiced differently, but such attacks were common in the nineteenth century, even though courts consistently supported the rights of physicians to practice homeopathy.

In 1829, Dr. Karl Friedrich Trinks (1800–1868), one of the leading homeopaths in northern Germany, was the victim of legal actions, suggesting that even the most highly respected homeopathic doctors were not immune to attacks (Jütte, 1998, 79).

Attacks against Asian Homeopaths in the Nineteenth Century

Discussion of the attacks against homeopaths and homeopathy in Asia are of interest because they verify that this experience was not simply a Western anomaly. In fact, homeopathy posed a philosophical, medical, scientific, and economic threat all over the world.

The story of Mahendra Lal Sarkar, MD (1833–1904), is representative of the experience of homeopaths in India. Dr. Sarkar was a conventionally trained physician and scientist. He lived during a time in which cholera killed millions of people, including his mother, who died at the young age of 32. Conventional medical treatments for cholera were ineffective, and many assumed that they did more harm than good.

In the mid-1800s the London Missionary Society and other European immigrants began to introduce homeopathy to the people of India. Doctors at the General Military Hospital in Bombay began to use homeopathic medicines in the treatment of cholera.

Dr. Sarkar began experimenting with homeopathic medicines with some significant successes. He decided to deliver a speech, "On the supposed uncertainty in medical science and on the relationship between disease and the Remedial Agents," before the Bengal branch of the British Medical Association in 1867 (Singh, 2005). As a result of this lecture, he was expelled from the association of which he was the founding secretary. He had become a quack overnight. Orthodox journals like the *Indian Medical Gazette* printed slanderous accusations against him. Sarkar replied in protest, but none of his protest letters were published.

In 1868, Sarkar decided to confront the orthodoxy of the dominant medicine and started the *Calcutta Journal of Medicine* on "catholic principles." He purposefully did not call this journal homeopathic; his first editorial, entitled "Our Creed," stated that "cures [were] effected in diverse ways" (Singh, 2005).

Dr. Sarkar also founded the Indian Association for the Cultivation of Science, the first national science association in India. This organization is still active and highly regarded today (http://www.iacs.res.in).

Although Hahnemann and many European homeopaths were extremely critical of conventional Western medicine of that day, Dr. Sarkar was considerably more diplomatic. He insisted that there was no one single method that cures everyone. Despite this diplomacy, he was either ignored or attacked by conventional physicians in India.

Historians today recognize that homeopathic treatment was one of the effective treatments for cholera in the nineteenth century (Bradford, 1900). For further evidence and stories about the use of homeopathic medicines for cholera, see Chapter 13, Clergy and Spiritual Leaders.

Despite the significant obstacles placed before homeopathy and homeopaths in India, this system of medicine is flourishing there. There are more than 100 homeopathic medical schools and more than 100,000 homeopathic doctors.

Oliver Wendell Holmes and His Attack on Homeopathy

The most famous anti-homeopathy book written in the nineteenth century was by Oliver Wendell Holmes, MD (1809–1894).[20] Called *Homoeopathy and Its Kindred Delusions,* this book was written just six years after Dr. Holmes graduated from medical school. Before Holmes went to medical school, he authored a famous poem in 1830 called "Old Ironside" as well as two articles in 1832 and 1833 entitled "Autocrat at the Breakfast Table" (published in *The Atlantic Monthly*), which gave him a national reputation as a leading American writer and scholar.

Although Holmes had become a professor at Harvard Medical School and although he was a respected poet and author, he actually had very little direct experience practicing medicine before he wrote his attack on homeopathy. Dr. Holmes's essay on homeopathy gained a lot of attention, and today is commonly referred to as a strong critique of homeopathy. However, Holmes's book should actually have been a significant embarrassment to its author and others antagonistic toward homeopathy because it is so full of obvious errors, which authors today still quote as though the book was factual.

It is amazing to note, first, that Dr. Holmes wrote that the one physician who typifies the American medical thinking and practice of that time was Benjamin Rush, MD (1745–1813), a signer of the Declaration of Independence and the surgeon general of the Continental Army.[21] Dr. Rush was one of the leading advocates of "heroic medicine," that is, the frequent and aggressive use of including bloodletting, intestinal purging (with mercury), vomiting (with the caustic agent tartar emetic), and blistering of the skin.

Dr. Rush recommended bloodletting for virtually every patient, and he considered it quackery if a physician did not bloodlet his patients. He even once boasted that he had drawn enough blood to float a seventy-four-gun man-of-war ship (Transactions, 1882).

Rush was also an advocate of forced psychiatric treatment, which in part explains why his portrait is on the emblem of the American Psychiatric Association. One of Rush's favorite methods of treatment was to tie a patient to a wooden board and rapidly spin it so blood flowed to the head. He placed his own son in one of his insane asylum hospitals for twenty-seven years, until he died. Rush also believed that being black was a hereditary illness which he referred to as "negroidism."

In addition to Dr. Holmes's glorification of Dr. Rush's heroic medicine, Holmes had the audacity to call homeopathic medicine "barbaric" because it uses various snake venoms (Holmes, 1891, x).[22] This statement is especially ironic when you consider that one of Dr. Holmes's most famous quotes (from an 1860 article) was his own critique of conventional medical drugs: "I firmly believe that if the whole *materia medica* (materials of medicine), as now used, could be sunk to the bottom of the sea, it would be all the better for mankind—and all the worse for the fishes" (Holmes, 1891).

Dr. Holmes's primary attack was on the extremely small doses that are used in homeopathic medicine. However, Dr. Holmes had seemingly never read a single book on homeopathy or had any meaningful dialogue with a homeopath because he committed a classic error of calculation. When a homeopathic pharmacist makes a medicine, he dilutes one part of the original substance in 9 or 99 parts water (thus, a 1:10 or 1:100 dilution); the glass bottle is then vigorously shaken approximately 40 times, and then the medicinal solution is again diluted 1:10 or 1:100. Ultimately, to make a homeopathic medicine to the 30X or 30C (X being the Roman numeral for 10, and C for 100, the letter referring to the type of dilution), the total amount of water needed is 30 test tubes of water (considerably less than a gallon of water).

However, Dr. Holmes got his calculations confused, and he incorrectly assumed that the homeopathic manufacturer had to have 10 times or 100 times more water than in the previous dilution. Dr. Holmes estimated that the ninth dilution would require ten billion gallons of water and the seventeenth dilution required a quantity equal to 10,000 Adriatic Seas. Dr. Holmes could have easily corrected his error if he had simply gone into one homeopathic pharmacy or had a short conversation with a homeopath. Sadly and strangely, Dr. Holmes and other conventional doctors of that era prided themselves on never talking with a homeopath.

What is even more ironic is that Dr. Holmes arranged for the reprinting of this article in various books from 1842 to 1891 without changing a single word, despite this and numerous other errors.

Dr. Holmes explained in his book that the growth of homeopathy was primarily because conventional physicians tended to overmedicate their patients, even though Holmes later wrote that the public itself "insists on being poisoned" (Holmes, 1891, 186).

Dr. Holmes also attempted to "prove" that homeopathic medicines do not work by quoting a "scientific study." To do this, Holmes referenced in an 1842 article a study by a Dr. Gabriel Andral, professor of medicine in the School of Paris. Holmes referred to Andral as "a man of great kindness of character ... of unquestioned integrity." Holmes reported on Andral's experiment on 130–140 patients using homeopathic medicines, and Holmes quoted Andral saying that on "not one of them did it have the slightest influence" (Holmes, 1891, 80).

Although Dr. Holmes and others have asserted that Andral's experiment provided strong evidence for disproving homeopathy, it must be noted that later in his life, Andral himself acknowledged the serious problems in his study. Although Andral claimed to have used Hahnemann's *Materia Medica Pura* as his guide, he neglected to mention at the time that the book was in German and that he could not read German. One other book by Hahnemann was translated into French at the time of this study, but Andral did not prescribe any of the twenty-two homeopathic medicines in this book for any patients in his study. Even Andral's assistant for this study acknowledged that Andral did not know how to select homeopathic medicines for patients and that he "excuses his ignorance by saying it was unavoidable" (Dean, 2004, 112).

Additional evidence of Andral's complete ignorance of homeopathy was revealed in a review of each of his prescriptions and his use of dosages. He never prescribed any homeopathic medicines for any patient's unique syndrome of symptoms. Instead, he selected a single symptom of his own idiosyncratic choosing and then guessed at the medicine for it. For instance, his prescriptions of *Arnica* for one woman with painful menstruation and for one man with tuberculosis were guesses that were not based on any homeopathic textbook. Further, 75 percent of the patients were given just one dose of one remedy without any follow-up remedy (Irvine, 1844). If patients were not immediately cured by this one dose, he considered homeopathy a failure and then referred the patient for conventional medical treatment.

Andral later asserted that he had never formally granted anyone permission to publish his report on homeopathy, and further, by 1852 he had changed his mind about homeopathy and asserted that it deserved close examination by every physician (Dean, 2004, 112). Despite these facts, Dr. Holmes never changed a word of his essay on homeopathy.

When you consider that Dr. Holmes's book was considered the best critique of homeopathy written in the nineteenth century, one must rightfully acknowledge that serious or sophisticated criticism of homeopathy at this time was neither rational nor accurate.

In 1861, Dr. Holmes finally confessed that homeopathy "has taught us a lesson of the healing faculty of Nature which was needed, and for which many of us have made proper acknowledgements" (Holmes, 1891, x, xiii–xiv). However, he still never instructed his publisher to change a word of his previous writings on homeopathy.

Modern-Day Attacks on Homeopathy

It is difficult to understand adequately the implications of the nineteenth-century attacks against homeopathy and homeopaths, and many people may insist that these types of actions would never happen today. While it may be true that such actions may not happen again (hopefully!), this doesn't mean that the present antagonism against homeopathy and homeopaths isn't similarly insidious and even ruthless. This is a harsh statement, but the following stories are but the tip of the iceberg of the present-day attacks against homeopathy and homeopaths.

In 2005, representatives of World Health Organization (WHO) were working on a report on homeopathic medicine, and one of the skeptics of homeopathy asked to review this report complained bitterly that it was too positive toward homeopathy. He then leaked it to other skeptics and to *The Lancet,* a usually highly respected British medical journal. In response to the potentially positive report on homeopathy from WHO, *The Lancet* published an article attacking the report, which had not even been completed or published (McCarty, 2005), and further, *The Lancet* rushed to publication a comparative study of homeopathic and conventional medical treatment (Shang, et al., 2005).

The idea for comparing clinical studies of homeopathic and conventional medicine is certainly a good one, but actually doing so in a fair and accurate way is more challenging than it may seem. The lead author of this comparative study, however, was not the ideal physician or scientist to evaluate homeopathy objectively—Dr. M. Egger, a Swiss physician who is notoriously and actively anti-homeopathy. Before he completed his study, he informed the editors at *The Lancet* that he had planned to submit his study to them and that he fully expected the results to show that homeopathic medicines didn't work.[23]

Egger and his team first found 110 placebo-controlled trials evaluating the efficacy of homeopathic medicine. Next, they selected 110 "matched" placebo-controlled trials. Finding "matched" trials usually means finding experiments that sought to treat people with a similar disease, in a similar population, and who were treated for a similar period of time, but the researchers never explained how or why they included or excluded any of the conventional medical trials. And needless to say, finding matched experiments is much more difficult than it sounds. Although it is easy to question if these researchers found matched experiments or not, let's give them the benefit of the doubt and say that they were successful in doing so.

Next, the researchers evaluated the quality of research design and how each trial was conducted. The researchers determined that only twenty-one of the homeopathic studies were high-quality, and only nine of the conventional medical studies were of a similar high quality.[24] Then, without adequate explanation, the researchers only evaluated those studies that were both high-quality and had large numbers of patients in each trial. They found eight homeopathic studies that fit these characteristics and only six conventional medical studies. Only two of the eight homeopathic studies used homeopathic medicines that were individualized to each patient, with the remaining studies giving the same medicine to everyone. (This method may make research easier, but it is not necessarily a good test of the homeopathic methodology.)

The eight homeopathic studies and six conventional medical studies were not matched in any way. How or why the researchers would or could claim that these studies were comparable requires some creative thinking. Further, the researchers never provided the analysis of the results of the twenty-one high-quality homeopathic studies as compared with the nine conventional studies.

What is also interesting is the fact that the researchers acknowledged that eight of the homeopathic studies in the treatment of people with acute respiratory tract infections found "substantial beneficial effect" and that this effect was "robust." However, without adequate evidence or explanation, the researchers asserted that these studies could not be trusted and that eight trials is simply not enough for adequate analysis. And yet, these same researchers evaluated eight other homeopathic trials and concluded that they showed no obvious better treatment than the six conventional studies.

If the above concerns were not enough to lead readers to the conclusion that this is "garbage in, garbage out" type of comparative research, there are still even more concerns about this study. For instance, the researchers did not even reveal which studies were selected until many months later. And when the studies were finally announced, it was shocking to note that they had selected a study testing a single homeopathic medicine in the treatment of weight loss (bordering on preposterous because homeopaths assert that there is no one single remedy to augment weight loss), and another study evaluating the use of a homeopathic formula in the prevention of influenza. (There have been at least three large studies verifying the efficacy of homeopathic medicines in the *treatment* of influenza, but only one of these was selected, while the study that evaluated its *prevention* was selected even though it was simply an exploratory investigation, not one that homeopaths expected to have a positive outcome.)

Mark Twain once asserted, "There are lies, damn lies, and statistics."

One must be careful in reading and understanding "scientific" studies because it is easy to get fooled. And when one considers the philosophical, scientific, and economic challenges that homeopathy creates for conventional medicine, it is not surprising that defenders of the medical industrial complex will do all they can to trivialize homeopathy or try to play tricks with statistics to "disprove" it.

Another classic tale about attacks against homeopaths is the case of George Guess, MD (1947–). Dr. Guess graduated from the Medical College of Virginia in 1973 and completed a family practice residency at Southern Illinois University in 1976. Dr. Guess has served on the Board of Directors of the National Center for Homeopathy and as convener for the Council for Homeopathic Education (accrediting body for homeopathic educational courses). Since 1992 he has been the editor of the *American Journal of Homeopathic Medicine,* the journal of the American Institute of Homeopathy, which was founded in 1844, two years before the American Medical Association.

While practicing homeopathy in North Carolina in 1985, the state's medical board deemed that Dr. Guess was not "conforming to the acceptable and prevailing standards of medical practice" and ordered him to cease and desist from practicing homeopathy. Even though not a single patient or consumer had complained to the medical board and even though the board acknowledged that Dr. Guess was a good and safe doctor, the medical board determined that he was not adhering to prevailing standards of medical practice.

Dr. Guess appealed the medical board's decision, and the state Superior Court determined that the medical board's action against Dr. Guess were "arbitrary and capricious" and unsubstantiated by the evidence. The medical board appealed this decision to the North Carolina Board of Appeals, and this court also sided with Dr. Guess. The medical board then appealed this decision to the state's Supreme Court, and this court determined that the medical board possesses sweeping powers to suppress any therapy which it deems nonconformist and that the safety or efficacy of any unconventional medical treatment was irrelevant.

This judicial decision outraged the people of North Carolina, and within a couple of years, their legislature had passed a law that allowed any medical doctor to practice unorthodox therapies as long as the treatments were basically safe. Sadly, however, by the time this law was passed, Dr. Guess had moved to Virginia and established a thriving homeopathic practice there. Since this time, at least five other states in the United States have enacted medical freedom-of-choice laws that allow physicians and non-physicians to practice various natural or alternative therapies.[25]

The Evolution of Science and Medicine

The words "science" and "medicine" are changing and evolving terms. And yet, there is a seemingly innate tendency for physicians and scientists of any era to be resistant to whatever changes are occurring in medicine and science.

While it is certainly appropriate to maintain a certain healthy skepticism about various phenomena, especially those phenomena that seem especially peculiar or unpredictable, all too often physicians and scientists have maintained a closed-minded skepticism that has fostered unscientific thinking and actions.

Nearly fifty years after William Harvey (1578–1657) announced to the world his great discovery about the heart's role in circulating blood throughout the body, the Paris Royal Society of Medicine determined that such action was impossible. Even when Harvey's ideas were accepted into medical and scientific thought, they had little effect on clinical medicine of that time or for the next 200 years.

The Royal College of Physicians of Great Britain greeted Benjamin Franklin with shouts of laughter when he declared the identity of lightning with other electrical phenomena. When the members of the French Academy of Science witnessed a demonstration of Thomas Edison's new invention, the phonograph, one famous professor of medicine literally jumped up and declared: "We have checked and found that it is a matter of ventriloquist hoax, for it is impossible to have a human voice speak from a roller."

This resistance to change is not simply a problem in medicine and science but in virtually every field of human endeavor. The most determined opponents of church reform usually have been bishops and clergy. Even when Jesus lived, his ideas about God, life, and love were not eagerly accepted. In fact, as we all know, he died for his ideas and his actions.

A short story about Johannes Kepler (1571–1630) may be instructive here. Kepler was a highly respected German astronomer who lived in Austria during the last twenty years of his life. However, due to religious persecution for his Protestant beliefs, Kepler, his family, and friends left Austria. When the king of Austria heard that Kepler had left his country, the king sent horsemen to ask that he return. Kepler said, "If I go back, my friends will have to return with me!" And when he was asked how he could wait so long and so patiently for his theories to be accepted, he responded, "The Lord has waited a long time for people to understand the harmony of His creation! Why should I be impatient?"

Science and medicine have a long history of resistance to change. Because part of a healthy scientific attitude includes objectivity and humility, a true, healthy scientific attitude would replace the present name-calling, head-in-the-sand refusal to understand or investigate alternatives.

Abraham Lincoln once asserted, "I am a firm believer in the people. If given the truth, they can be depended upon.... The great point is to bring them the facts." One way to keep people from the facts about homeopathy is to cut off communication to them and from them. Another way to keep people from the facts about homeopathy is to disallow conventional physicians from consulting with homeopathic physicians or their patients. Another way to keep people from the facts about homeopathy is to play games with statistics so that it seems that homeopathic medicines are ineffective.

And yet, as science fiction writer H. G. Wells once asserted, "Kings and empires die; great ideas, once they are born, never die."

My "I Have a Dream" Speech

I have a dream that the world will soon wake up to the practical value of and deep appreciation for the nanodoses of homeopathic medicines.

I have a dream that the homeopathic principle of similars, which has long been utilized in vaccination and allergy treatments, will be appreciated for its power in augmenting immuno-competence.

I have a dream that augmenting the body-mind's own immune and defense system will be a primary goal of medical treatment.

I have a dream that Hippocrates's wisdom of "First, do no harm" will be operationalized by the inclusion of homeopathic medicines in primary care.

I have a dream that a diverse body of scientists will soon explore the dimensions of and potential for the nanodose phenomenon, not only for medical applications but for varied technologies that will help create a healthier, sustainable planet.

I have a dream that even homeopathy's biggest critics will apologize for continuing a history of antagonism that should never have started in the first place.

I have a dream that homeopathy's history of success in treating many infectious epidemic diseases will help us reduce antibiotic use and provide a safer tool for treating people with infections.

I have a dream that people will understand that all disease is a part of a syndrome and can and must be understood in this more complex process.

I have a dream that people will become aware of the real problems that result from using conventional drugs that suppress symptoms, thereby disrupting the body's defensive efforts and pushing the disease deeper into the organism.

I have a dream that people will appreciate the multi-factorial nature to most disease processes and that people will no longer be fooled by over-simplified single-causational factors to disease.

I have a dream that people will *really* respect the wisdom of our body-mind and realize that our symptoms are our organism's best effort to respond to stress or infection.

Let health and freedom ring from the clinic to the hospital.

Let health and freedom ring from the pharmacy to the health food store.

Let health and freedom ring from doctors, from patients, and from insurance companies.

Let health and freedom ring from drug companies, drug regulators, and health policy experts.

Let health and freedom ring from the media and from the Internet.

I have a dream today. Any other dreamers out there?

References

Baumann, J. *The Old and New Therapy with/of Medicine According to the Writings of Others and According to Personal Experience for the Thinking Public.* Remmingen: Oscar Belsenfelder. 1857.

Bradford, T. L. *The Logic of Figures or Comparative Results of Homoeopathic and Other Treatments.* Philadelphia: Boericke and Tafel, 1900.

Coulter, H. L. *Divided Legacy: The Conflict Between Homoeopathy and the American Medical Association.* Volume III. Berkeley: North Atlantic Books, 1973.

Dean, M. E., *The Trials of Homeopathy.* Essen, Germany: KVC, 2004. (This book is a truly excellent book on the history of scientific studies testing homeopathic medicines. Readers will be impressed to learn that some of the earliest double-blind and placebo-controlled trials were in the testing of homeopathic medicines.)

EHM News Bureau. Condemnation for *The Lancet*'s Stance on Homeopathy. *Express Pharma Pulse,* October 6, 2005.

Holmes, O. W. *Medical Essays (1842–1882).* Boston: Houghton, Mifflin and Company, 1891.

Homeopathic Pharmacies in Germany, *Homeopathic Recorder,* 1899, 14:24–29.

Irvine, F. W. M. Andral's Homoeopathic Experiments at La Pitie, *British Journal of Homoeopathy,* 1844.

Jütte, R. *The Paradox of Professionalism, in Culture, Knowledge, and Healing: Historical Perspectives of Homeopathic Medicine in Europe and North America,* eds. R. Jütte, G. B. Risse, and J. Woodward. Sheffield: EAHMHP, 1998.

Kaufman, M. *Homeopathy in America: The Rise and Fall of a Medical Heresy.* Baltimore, Johns Hopkins, 1971.

King, L. S. The AMA Gets a New Code of Ethics, *JAMA,* March 11, 1983, 249(10): 1338–1342.

McCarty, M. Critics Slam Draft of WHO Report on Homoeopathy, *The Lancet,* August 27, 2005, 366:705–706.

Nichols, P. A. *Homoeopathy and the Medical Profession.* London: Croom Helm, 1988.

Rothstein, W. *Physicians in the Nineteenth Century.* Baltimore: Johns Hopkins University Press, 1972.

Shang, A. Huwiler-Muntener, K., Nartey, L., et al. Are the Clinical Effects of Homoeopathy Placebo Effects? Comparative Study of Placebo-Controlled Trials of Homoeopathy and Allopathy, *The Lancet,* 2005, 366:726–732.

Singh, D. K. Choleraic Times and Mahendra Lal Sarkar: The Quest of Homoeopathy as "Cultivation of Science" in Nineteenth Century India, *Med Ges Gesch.* 2005, 24:207–242.

Transactions of the American Institute of Homeopathy, Proceedings of the 35th Session, 1882, 25.

Treuherz, F. The Origins of Kent's Homeopathy, *Journal of the American Institute of Homeopathy,* December 1984, 77(4):130–149.

Ullman, D. *Discovering Homeopathy.* Berkeley: North Atlantic Books, 1991.

Walsh, J. J. *History of the Medical Society of the State of New York.* New York: Medical Society of the State of New York, 1907.

Warner, J. H. The 1880s Rebellion Against the AMA Code of Ethics, in *The American Medical Ethics Revolution,* eds. R. B. Baker, A. L. Caplan, L. L. Emanuel, et al. Baltimore: Johns Hopkins University Press, 1999.

CHAPTER 3

Literary Greats:
Write On, Homeopathy!

American Writers

An often quoted dialogue between Henry David Thoreau and Ralph Waldo Emerson, two nineteenth-century American literary greats, took place on the subject of education. Thoreau was thoroughly disgusted at the state of education in American universities and condemned them *in toto*. Emerson expressed surprise at Thoreau's harsh words, saying, "I would not be so sweeping in my condemnation of the colleges. After all, they instruct in most of the branches of knowledge." Thoreau replied, "That's just the trouble; they teach all of the branches and none of the roots."

A similar critique could be made of medical schools of the nineteenth century as well as those of our present day. And in response to this state of medical education, there grew to be twenty-two homeopathic medical schools in the late 1800s (including Boston University, University of Michigan, Hahnemann Medical College, and New York Homeopathic Medicine College). These homeopathic medical schools not only taught the basic medical sciences with detailed instruction on diagnosis and pathology; they also taught how to treat the whole patient and his or her overall syndrome (not just the disease).

Although conventional medical societies were successful in forcing the closing of the homeopathic medical schools in the twentieth century,[26] homeopathy has always attracted the most educated people in society, and many of the world's literary elite have been some of homeopathy's strongest proponents.

The esteemed medical historian William Rothstein acknowledged that "early American homeopaths were all well educated and cultured physicians ... and manifested an erudition rarely found in regular medical journals of the period" (Rothstein, 1972, 160). He continued, quoting the editor of a leading conventional medical journal who begrudgingly admitted that many homeopaths were "persons of the highest respectability and moral worth."

It is not surprising to learn that many of America's leading literary figures in the nineteenth century were also advocates of this "new medicine," including Henry David Thoreau, Ralph Waldo Emerson, Henry Wadsworth Longfellow, Nathaniel Hawthorne,[27] Harriet Beecher Stowe, Louisa May Alcott, Henry James, and William James. Likewise, several renowned European literary greats were also homeopathic supporters, including Johann Wolfgang von Goethe, Fyodor Dostoevsky, Charles Dickens, W. B. Yeats, William Makepeace Thackeray, and George Bernard Shaw.

In the mid-1800s American transcendentalism became quite popular, initially as a means toward religious reform but then also as a philosophical and literary movement.[28] One of the earliest centers for the New England transcendentalists was a library and bookstore called The Foreign Library, founded in 1839 by **Elizabeth Palmer Peabody** (1804–1894). Her entire family was intimately connected to leaders in the homeopathic and transcendental movements.[29]

One part of the store was allocated to her father, Nathaniel Peabody, for the sale of homeopathic medicines (Perrin-Wilson, 1999).[30] Elizabeth's brother, Nathaniel, was an expert on homeopathy too and was known to make some of his own medicines. Sophia, Elizabeth's youngest sister, married Nathaniel Hawthorne (author of *The Scarlet Letter*), while Mary, her other sister, married Horace Mann (considered the father of American education and the first president of Antioch College). Many decades later **Henry James** (1843–1916) portrayed Sophia Peabody in his book *The Bostonians* (1886), with the character Miss Birdseye, the grand dame of the women's rights movement who also had a deep appreciation for homeopathy (she was played by the famed actress Jessica Tandy in the 1984 movie of this classic novel).

At one point in the book (and the movie), Miss Birdseye is talking with Basil Ransome (played by the late Christopher Reeve) with the following dialogue:

> Ransome: You must tell me how much you take. One spoonful?
> Birdseye: I guess this time, I'll take two. It's homeopathic.
> Ransome: Oh, I have no doubt of that. I presume you wouldn't have anything else.
> Birdseye: Well, it's generally admitted now to be the true system.

Transcendentalism and homeopathy had much in common. Both embodied a deep respect for nature and acknowledged a special wisdom that derived from it. Transcendentalism, like other romantic movements, proposed that the essential nature of human beings is good, while homeopathy recognized that symptoms of illness, despite their discomfort, actually represented positive efforts of a person's entire body to defend itself and to heal, even if it wasn't always successful in effecting a cure.

Transcendentalism and homeopathy also were both influenced by a highly respected Swedish scientist, inventor, and mystic named Emanuel Swedenborg.[31] The first and primary translator of Swedenborg's works into English was a British-born physician who lived in Boston, John James Garth Wilkinson, MD. Wilkinson had trained at the famed homeopathic school, the Hahnemann Medical College in Philadelphia, and he was a very close friend of Henry James, Sr. (1811–1882), whose sons were Henry James and William James. Henry James, Sr. credited Wilkinson with introducing him to the ideas of Swedenborg (see Chapter 13, Clergy and Spiritual Leaders, for more detailed information about Swedenborg), while Wilkinson credited James with introducing him to homeopathy (Treuherz, 1984).

Wilkinson and other homeopaths were particularly intrigued by Swedenborg's law of correspondences, which embodies the Hermetic axiom "as above, so below." The concept of the microcosm being a part of the macrocosm and vice versa and that physical symptoms and mental symptoms are interconnected helped link homeopathic and Swedenborgian religious and medical philosophies.

Ralph Waldo Emerson (1803–1882) was also an appreciator of both homeopathic medicine and Swedenborgian philosophy, and he held great admiration for Wilkinson (Treuherz, 1984). He characterized Wilkinson's style of speaking and writing as being "like the armory of the invincible knights of old." He asserted that Wilkinson "has brought to metaphysics and to physiology a native vigor" and that Wilkinson is an important "champion of Hahnemann" (Emerson, 1856).

Emerson went an eloquent step further in the following statement about the Greek mythological god, Tantalus. According to Greek mythology, Tantalus, a son of Zeus and the nymph Plouto (who was the personification of wealth), was known for having been welcomed to Zeus's table in Olympus, from which he stole nectar and ambrosia to take back to his people, and revealed to them the secrets of the gods. Emerson's reference to 'T is a reference to Tantalus:

> One of the illusions is that the present hour is not the critical, decisive hour. Write it on your heart that every day is the best day in the year. No man has learned anything rightly until he knows that every day is Doomsday. 'T is the old secret of the gods that they come in low disguises. 'T is the vulgar great who come dizened with gold and jewels. Real kings hide away their crowns in their wardrobes, and affect a plain and poor exterior.... So, in our history, Jesus is born in a barn, and his twelve peers are fishermen. 'T is the very principle of science that Nature shows herself best in leasts; it was the maxim of Aristotle and Lucretius; and, in modern times, of Swedenborg and of Hahnemann. The order of changes in the egg determines the age of fossil strata. So it was the rule of our poets, in the legends of fairy lore, that the fairies largest in power were the least in size. (Emerson, 1870)

William James (1842–1910), who attended Harvard Medical School and became an eminent psychologist and philosopher, was another advocate for homeopathy. Although trained as a medical doctor, he never practiced medicine and had a serious disdain for it (Richardson, 2006, 401). In speaking to the Massachusetts legislature in response to a bill that would outlaw anyone except medical doctors from diagnosing or treating for any physical or mental ailment, he asserted, "An enormous mass of experience, both of homeopathic doctors and their patients, is invoked in favor of the efficacy of these remedies and doses" (James, 1898). James wrote to a friend that his work against this bill required the greatest moral effort of his life (Coulter, 1973, III, 467a).

And in a letter to a friend who had complained about persistent abdominal distress, James wrote: "I always believe that homeopathy should get a fair trial in obstinate chronic cases. I *know* that homeopathic remedies are not inert, as orthodox medicine insists they necessarily must be" (James, 1903).

Louisa May Alcott (1832–1888), author of *Little Women,* was another longtime homeopathic patient and appreciator of this new medicine. Besides being a leading author, she was also a nurse. At one dramatic point in *Little Women,* one of the daughters, Beth (played by Claire Danes in the movie), is ill with scarlet fever, and the oldest daughter, Jo (played by Winona Ryder), prescribes homeopathic *Belladonna* to treat her. Later, Jo finds Beth looking through their mother's medicine cabinet where she finds a bottle of camphor and takes it into bed with her. This action provides some sophisticated foreshadowing because camphor is known as an antidote to homeopathic medicines, and thus, it is sad but not surprising when Beth succumbs to the disease.

There are two other references to homeopathy in *Little Women.* The first incident occurs early in the book when Jo hurts her ankle so she chooses to "Bound up her foot with arnica" (in Chapter 3). *Arnica* is a well-known homeopathic remedy for sprains and strains. The second incident occurs shortly after Beth's scarlet fever episode when Jo gets a severe head cold and then takes *Arsenicum* (homeopathic dose of arsenic).

During her childhood, Alcott's family physician was Conrad Wesselhoeft, MD, a Harvard Medical School graduate and a famous Boston homeopath, and she dedicated her last novel, *Jo's Boys,* to him. In this book, its lead character, Nan, is portrayed as a bright, scientifically minded, young girl who is able to keep calm in a crisis. Nan becomes a homeopathic physician who is also dedicated to women's equality. In Chapter 1, some of the early dialogue includes:

> "You knew it. How is your throat?" asked Nan in her professional tone, which was always a quencher to undue raptures.
> "Throat? Oh, ah! yes, I remember. It is well. The effect of that prescription was wonderful. I'll never call homoeopathy a humbug again."

Alcott and many other dedicated homeopathic patients maintained their conviction for homeopathy, not only because they found it effective but because it was an integral part of new scientific thinking and medical reform.

Louisa May Alcott's father, **Amos Bronson Alcott** (1799–1888), was also an advocate for homeopathy. Active in the American transcendental movement, he was a teacher and writer who pioneered "democratic schooling," which encouraged students to get involved in their own education. He was also known for founding a utopian community known as Fruitlands.

Elizabeth Stuart Phelps (1844–1911) was a less known but still popular and respected author of numerous books, including a novel, *Dr. Zay,* which tells the story of a homeopath who attended the New York Medical College and Hospital for Women (for more details about this college, see Chapter 10, Women's Rights Leaders and Suffragists). Phelps described Dr. Zay as a strong and capable woman who is equally committed to homeopathic medicine and social reform.

Emily Dickinson (1830–1886) is considered, with Walt Whitman, as one of the two great American poets of the nineteenth century. Between 1846 and 1852, Emily Dickinson experienced serious problems with her health, specifically a chronic cough, fatigue, and significant weight loss.

Extracting clinical clues from her correspondence, some historians have suggested that she was suffering from tuberculosis (Hirschhorn, 1999).

Tuberculosis was and is a very serious disease, and epidemics of it have erupted at various times in human history. In 1851 it was the cause of one-third of all deaths in Boston, and Emily had many relatives who had died from it. That year, Emily sought treatment with a highly respected homeopath, Dr. William Wesselhoeft[32] in Boston (St. John, n.d.; Hirschhorn, 1999). Emily wrote that he prescribed two homeopathic medicines for her. She didn't think that the medicines were effective, but her older and more practical sister, Lavina, thought otherwise. Lavina (who originally referred Emily and their brother Austin to Dr. Wesselhoeft because he was her homeopath) asserted just two weeks after homeopathic treatment: "I think Emily may be very much improved. She has really grown fat." Because Emily was always extremely thin, this statement of her gaining weight suggests some health improvements. Her brother Austin wrote Emily's closest friend, Susan Gilbert: "He [their father] says Emily is *better* than for years since she returned from Boston" (Thomas, 1988, 219). And lending further support to the real benefits from the homeopathic treatment, within several months, she no longer complained about the chronic cough that she had experienced for five years.

Other biographers of Emily Dickinson said that Wesselhoeft's treatment "brought not only a noticeable improvement in her health but a certain buoyancy of spirit as well" (Bingham, 1955, 175).

Despite the serious health problems that Emily Dickinson experienced in the 1840s and early 1850s, she lived considerably beyond these decades. She died in 1886.

William Cullen Bryant (1794–1878) was another American literary figure who was an ardent advocate for homeopathy. Although trained as a lawyer, he became a poet and then editor of the *New York Evening Post* (today, the *New York Post*). Bryant was president of the New York Homeopathic Society, and he was the founder of the New York Homeopathic Medical College, today called the New York Medical College. Like many advocates of homeopathy, he was also a major advocate for the abolition of slavery, and in fact, he was one of the leaders of this movement. Bryant was even influential in getting Lincoln to issue his famed Emancipation Proclamation.

Washington Irving (1783–1859) was best known for writing *The Legend of Sleepy Hollow* and *Rip van Winkle* as well as several major biographies, including a four-volume set on America's first President, George Washington. Irving is said to have mentored authors such as Nathaniel Hawthorne, Henry Wadsworth Longfellow, and Edgar Allan Poe, and because Hawthorne and Longfellow were known advocates for homeopathic medicine, it is not surprising to learn that Washington Irving was too.

On February 21, 1854, Irving wrote to a friend: "I have found, in my own case, great relief from homeopathy, to which I had recourse almost accidentally; for I am rather slow at adopting new theories" (Hendrick, 1987, 170). He went on to say that after homeopathic treatment he was more able to continue his literary efforts. Later that same year, he wrote: "You ask me whether the homeopathics still keep me quite well. I really begin to have a great faith in them. The complaint of the head especially, which troubled me last year, and obliged me to throw by my pen, has been completely vanquished by them."

It is not surprising that Irving chose Dr. John C. Peters of New York as his homeopath since he was both a respected clinician and the editor of a leading homeopathic journal of that time, *The North American Journal of Homeopathy*. Irving began consulting with Dr. Peters in 1852 due to recurrent symptoms of dizziness (Wershub, 1965). Dr. Peters prescribed *Cocculus indicus*, made from an herb called Indian cockle (Peters, 1860).[33] Irving continually called on care from Dr. Peters for himself and members of his family. Dr. Peters became a regular visitor at Irving's Sunnyside estate, and they developed a strong friendship.

Dr. Peters determined that one of Irving's problems resulted from his own self-treatment with a conventional patent medicine. Irving treated himself with a remedy for catarrh (mucus) by snuffing it into his nostrils. Although this medicine dried up his nasal discharge temporarily, it soon led to a violent asthma attack.

Dr. Oliver Wendell Holmes, Sr. had written a book extremely critical of homeopathy, though embarrassingly ill-informed on the subject.[34]

Because Dr. Holmes had such respect for Washington Irving, the doctor chose to visit him and suggest treatment for Irving's asthma and cough. He prescribed medicated cigarettes and "Jonas Whitcomb's Cough Remedy" (a nineteenth-century patent medicine), without having examined his patient.[35] Dr. Peters wrote an admirably restrained reply to Holmes, suggesting that his treatment was not based on adequate understanding of this patient.

Dr. Peters gave Irving the patent medicine to show good faith toward Dr. Holmes, despite Holmes's bad-faith actions toward homeopathy. Irving experienced noticeable improvement that first night from this remedy. However, two days later he suffered a severe nervous attack, and Dr. Peters then chose to use only homeopathic medicines for Irving (Hendrick 1987, 174). Temporary improvement followed by the development of different and more serious symptoms are typical results from conventional drugs of the nineteenth century as well as today, and while conventional physicians pride themselves on their ability to reduce or suppress symptoms, homeopaths have sharply criticized such treatments that provide short-term benefits but long-term problems.

At Irving's funeral the famed writer-editor William Cullen Bryant gave the eulogy that was published in the *New York Times* (April 4, 1860). Irving's personal homeopathic medicine kit is on display at his Sunnyside home in Tarrytown, New York, which was bought by fellow homeopathic appreciator, J. D. Rockefeller in 1945 and opened to the public in 1947. Today, Irving's home is a national historical landmark.

Perhaps America's most known and most quoted author is **Mark Twain** (1835–1910) (a pseudonym for Samuel Clemens). Conventional medicine of his day was a relatively frequent target of his barbed wit. In *Harper's Magazine,* he wrote:

> When you reflect that your own father had to take such medicines as the above, and that you would be taking them to-day yourself but for the introduction of homoeopathy, which forced the old-school doctor to stir around and learn something of a rational nature about his business, you may honestly feel grateful that homoeopathy survived the

attempts of the allopathists [conventional physicians] to destroy it, even though you may never employ any physician but an allopathist while you live. (Twain, 1890)

Mark Twain also makes reference to homeopathy in his highly acclaimed novel *A Connecticut Yankee in King Arthur's Court* (1889). This masterpiece tells the story of Hank Morgan, a nineteenth-century firearms and mechanical expert who is transported to sixth-century Britain. Morgan introduces many modern technologies to Arthurian Britain, including the telephone, and eventually, he begins running the country. However, during a family vacation, the Church takes over the government and destroys the many new technologies Morgan has introduced and changes many of the social reforms he enacted. Part of Morgan's new life is that he marries and has a child who eventually is taken ill. Various conventional treatments are ineffective. Morgan then says: "'Quick!' I shouted to Clarence; 'telephone the King's homeopath to come!'"[36] Morgan's archenemy is the magician Merlin, who places a spell on him, causing him to sleep for thirteen centuries. He wakes during the nineteenth century and tells his story.

Mark Twain was particularly critical of doctors who didn't further their medical education after graduation. He considered the New York Postgraduate Medical School to be "one of the two greatest institutions in the country" because of its commitment to continuing education. In a 1909 speech at this school, which awarded him an honorary medical degree, he said: "I am glad to be among my own kind tonight. I was once a sharpshooter, but now I practice a much higher and equally as deadly a profession" (Ober, 1997).

Ultimately, Mark Twain was appreciative of various schools of thoughts in healing. He was a supporter of osteopathic medicine because this form of manipulation alleviated his own daughter's epilepsy and his own chronic bronchitis. And one of his doctors, Cincinnatus Taft, MD, was a homeopathic physician whose obituary said "he exercised a certain eclectic independence, which looked rather to cure than to creed, and was not entirely within the limitations of any one school" (Ober, 1997).

Upton Sinclair (1878–1968) was one of the greatest investigative journalists of his era. He actually wrote more than ninety books in various genres, though he was most famous for his novel *The Jungle* (1906), which dealt with the unhealthy conditions in the U.S. meat packing industry. The book had a powerful impact on American culture and resulted in the passing of one of the most important consumer rights bills of the twentieth century, the Pure Food and Drug Act of 1906.

Sinclair was a vocal advocate of the work of Albert Abrams, MD, a controversial physician who invented the first radionics device. Although conventional physicians contended that Abrams's invention and his use of homeopathic medicines represented the epitome of nonconventionality, Abrams was not your ordinary "quack."

Abrams initially graduated from medical school in Heidelberg, Germany, in 1882, and then graduated from Cooper Medical College (the medical school that later became Stanford Medical School), where he later served as a professor of pathology and Director of Clinical Medicine.[37] In 1894, he was the vice president of the California Medical Association (Scholten, 1999), and even leading skeptics of his work acknowledge that he wrote a dozen reputable textbooks (Gardner, 1957); one of them, on the value of X-ray in cardiac diagnosis, is considered an outstanding contribution to the medical literature of its time (Flaxman, 1953). Although Abrams was initially a bitter opponent and skeptic of homeopathy, his own research on the subject led him to change his opinions (Dean, 2004, 160).

In addition to support from Upton Sinclair, two other advocates of Abrams were Sir James Barr (a past president of the British Medical Association) and Sir Arthur Conan Doyle (author of the Sherlock Holmes detective novels). Sir James Barr duplicated some of Abrams's experiments and described him as one of the greatest medical geniuses of his time (Russell, 1973, 17).[38]

Sinclair was Abrams's strongest advocate in part because Sinclair had interviewed hundreds of health professionals and patients who used or were treated by radionics diagnosis and treatment. Sinclair asserted: "[Abrams] has made the most revolutionary discovery of this or any other age. I venture to stake whatever reputation I ever hope to have that he has discovered the great secret of the diagnosis and cure of all major diseases." Further, Sinclair claimed that Abrams had treated "over fifteen thousand people, and my investigation convinces me he has cured over ninety-five percent."

European Literary Greats

The primary principle of homeopathy, called the law or principle of similars ("treating like with like"), is actually an ancient understanding that great thinkers and healers have acknowledged and utilized since early written history. Chapter 13, Clergy and Spiritual Leaders, highlights the use of the homeopathic principle by Moses. Even the Greeks' Oracle at Delphi was known to have said, "That which makes sick shall heal," and one of the famous stories from Greek mythology is the tale of Telephus, a Trojan hero who was speared and then healed when pieces of the spear were scraped off and placed on the wound. Hippocrates, the father of medicine and an early medical historian, once asserted, "Through the like, disease is produced, and through the application of the like it is cured."

Even Shakespeare wrote about treating "like with like" in his famed play *Romeo and Juliet* (Act I, scene ii), when Benvolio gives comfort and advice to lovesick Romeo, saying:

> Tut, man, one fire burns out another's burning;
> One pain is lessened by another's anguish,
> Turn giddy and be holp by backward turning;
> One desperate grief cures with another's languish.
> Take thou some new infection to the eye,
> And the rank poison of the old will die.

The eminent British poet, John Milton (1608–1674), made direct reference to the concept of the treatment of "similars" in the preface to *Samson Agonistes* (1671): "Things of melancholic hue and quality are used against melancholoy, sour against sour, salt to remove salt humors."

Johann Wolfgang von Goethe (1749–1832) is considered one of the greatest Western literary figures of all time. A German poet, novelist, playwright, courtier, and natural philosopher, Goethe was a contemporary of homeopathy's founder, Samuel Hahnemann, MD (1755–1843), and they both were Freemasons. When Goethe was given an amulet containing a very small gold ornament (September 2, 1820), he wrote: "The jewelers of Frankfort must have heard of the Leipsig Dr. Hahnemann's theory—now, certainly a world-famous physician— ... and taken the best of it from their own purposes ... now I believe more than ever in this wonderful doctor's theory as I have experienced ... and continue to experience so clearly the efficacy of a very small administration." And in another letter he strongly proclaimed himself a "Hahnemannian disciple" (Haehl, 1922, I, 113).

Goethe not only espoused the virtues of homeopathy in his letters to friends and colleagues, but even in his most famous play, *Faust,* in which his lead character, Mephistopheles, asserts the homeopathic credo, making specific reference to the homeopathic principle of similars: "To like things like, whatever one may ail; there's certain help."

Goethe was also a close friend with Karl Wesselhoeft, the owner of a large German publishing company of literary works, and Goethe was a frequent visitor in the Wesselhoeft home. Wesselhoeft's son, William, became Goethe's protégé. As a result of Goethe's influence and due to later correspondence with German doctors who had become homeopaths, the younger Wesselhoeft became a serious student and then practitioner and teacher of homeopathy in America.

One of the other truly great Western literary figures was **Fyodor Dostoevsky** (1821–1888). Dostoevsky suffered from epilepsy which seemed to begin around 1850 while he was imprisoned for his political beliefs. After this time, his father, a conventional physician, treated Dostoevsky for a severe throat affliction, but his conventional treatment didn't provide benefit and even led to a permanent impairment of his voice (Rice, 1983). Dr. Dostoevsky then resorted to prescribing homeopathic medicines for his son, though there isn't evidence that his father was trained in homeopathy and the results were unclear. Later in life, Dostoevsky included in his classic novel, *The Brothers Karamazov* (1880), a dialogue in which one of the brothers tells the other: "Homeopathic doses perhaps are the strongest" (Chapter 9).

Another of the truly great Russian authors was **Anton Chekhov** (1860–1904), playwright and short story writer. Few people know that Chekhov was also a physician. We must be thankful that he wasn't a homeopath because the joys and the benefits from homeopathic practice might have led him to forego his magnificent contributions to literature.

Three of Chekhov's stories make reference to homeopathy. In "Ariadne" (1895), he spoke of a neighbor, a former landowner who was a homeopathic doctor and interested in spiritualism. Chekhov describes him as "a man of great delicacy and mildness, and by no means a fool." In "The Betrothed" (1903), he wrote of a woman betrothed to the son of a priest. Chekhov described the mother of the woman: "She went in for homeopathy and spiritualism, read a great deal, and was fond of talking about her religious doubts."

Chekhov's short story "The Malingerers" (1885) has as its lead character a homeopathic doctor—the widow of a Russian general who has practiced as a homeopathic physician for ten years.[39] She has an extremely busy practice and is especially popular among the poor peasants. The story focuses on one landowner who has sunk into poverty. He expresses extreme gratitude for her prescribing three doses of a homeopathic medicine to him. He falls to his knees to thank her, telling her that his eight years of suffering from rheumatism are over thanks to her medicines. He tells her that he was initially skeptical of these tiny doses, but his skepticism is over. He also tells her how greedy the regular doctors are and how they never really cure people. He asserts: "The doctors did me nothing but harm. They drove the disease inwards. Drive in, that they did, but to drive out was beyond their science." He refers to doctors as "assassins." He cries because he cannot even provide wood to keep his family warm. The doctor shows sympathy for him and gives him wood. The patient then tells her he needs a cow, and the doctor provides that too. As the patient leaves the doctor, three pieces of paper fall out of his pockets, and she discovers that these are the homeopathic medicines she had previously given him, left untouched.

Chekhov closes the story with the homeopathic doctor experiencing doubt for the first time in ten years of practice. The story ends with the words "The deceitfulness of man!"

George Bernard Shaw (1856–1950) was one of Ireland's most respected playwrights. Shaw is the only person ever to have won both a Nobel Prize (Literature in 1925) and an Academy Award (Best Screenplay for *Pygmalion* in 1938). In his play *The Doctor's Dilemma* (1906), Shaw showed the dilemma that doctors inevitably face between their need to care for their patients and their need to practice, often using dangerous drugs and performing unnecessary operations in order to earn a livelihood.

In the play's preface, Shaw wrote:

> The test to which all methods of treatment are finally brought is whether they are lucrative to doctors or not. It would be difficult to cite any proposition less obnoxious to science than that advanced by Hahnemann, to wit, that drugs which in large doses produced certain symptoms, counteract them in very small doses, just as in modern practice it is found that a sufficiently small inoculation with typhoid rallies our powers to resist the disease instead of prostrating us with it. But Hahnemann and his followers were frantically persecuted for a century by generations of apothecary-doctors whose incomes depended on the quantity of drugs they could induce their patients to swallow. These two cases of ordinary vaccination and homeopathy are typical of all the rest.

He continued: "Here we have the explanation of the savage rancor that so amazes people who imagine that the controversy concerning vaccination is a scientific one. It has really nothing to do with science. Under such circumstances vaccination would be defended desperately were it twice as dirty, dangerous and unscientific in method as it really is."

Thankfully, Shaw goes on to assert that times and things are changing, "Nowadays, however, the more cultivated folk are beginning to be so suspicious of drugs, and the incorrigibly superstitious people so profusely supplied with patent medicines that homeopathy has become a way of rehabilitating the trade of prescription compounding, and is consequently coming into professional credit."

In 1932 Shaw wrote an essay, *Doctors' Delusions, Crude Criminology and Sham Education,* which included a story about the homeopathic treatment he received for a hydrocele. This accumulation of fluid around the testicle normally requires surgery, but Shaw experienced a rapid cure without recurrence.

Shaw once challenged Sir Almroth Wright, a noted conventional physician, to look into homeopathy's ability to cure many "incurable" diseases. Wright expressed complete incredulity, while Shaw retorted that Wright had no scientific attitude or simple curiosity. This short conversation was a classic:

> Almroth said, "This thing is absurd and impossible; let me put it this way. Would you, Shaw, trouble to get out of your chair if I called from the next room. 'Do come in here and see what I have done—I have turned a pint of tea leaves into pure gold.'"
>
> Shaw responded back simply saying, "Certainly I would."
> (Coulter, 1994, 409)

A writer that one might predict to have had an interest in homeopathy would be **Sir Arthur Conan Doyle** (1859–1930), author of the Sherlock Holmes detective stories. The Scottish Doyle popularized the field of crime fiction and put Scotland Yard on the map. He was a prolific writer who also wrote science fiction, historical novels, plays, romances, poetry, and nonfiction.

In many ways, being a good homeopath is a lot like being Sherlock Holmes. A good homeopath obtains an enormous amount of detail about the totality of a sick person's symptoms. A good homeopath probes and probes and probes, asking open-ended questions that lead patients to describe what they are experiencing in their own words. A good homeopath is open to hearing things he or she does not expect, and makes the best use of unusual symptoms that the sick person describes. Sherlock Holmes was also known to assert: "That which is out of the common is usually a guide rather than a hindrance." And again: "That which seemingly confuses the case is the very thing that furnishes the clue to its solution." Both of these statements are an integral part of homeopathic casetaking and case analysis. Homeopaths usually conduct a conventional diagnosis, but they then always seek to find the symptoms that are unusual for the diagnosis, and these unique symptoms are vital in selecting the medicine for the patient.

There is an intriguing reference in Doyle's *Lost World* (1912). Many people are familiar with this novel because several movies were made of it (including a pioneering 1925 silent film with stop-motion special effects of the dinosaurs done by the same wizard who later created the special effects for the original *King Kong*). It is one of Doyle's Professor Challenger stories. Challenger was a zoological "Indiana Jones-type" with a reputation for beating up reporters whose interviews were anathema to him. In *Lost World,* the narrator is a reporter who bravely decides to interview the violent professor, and a physician friend of this reporter advises him to take along a new remedy that is reported to be "better than *arnica*" for dealing with the injuries he is sure to suffer from the encounter (Chapter 3). But then, the narrator of the story asserts, "Some people have such extraordinary notions of humor" (as though there could ever be something better than *arnica*).

Arnica is one of homeopathy's most well-known remedies for shock of injury, for sprains and strains, and for certain pre- and post-surgical problems.[40]

Of additional interest is the fact that Doyle originally trained as a medical doctor, but his frustration, bitterness, and even cynicism is well expressed in his great Holmes adventure, "The Adventure of the Resident Patient," a story in *The Memoirs of Sherlock Holmes* (1894). Ultimately, we must all feel quite blessed that Doyle was not so appreciative of homeopathic medicine that he practiced it rather than writing his stories.

Doyle was also strongly interested in and supportive of the work of Emanuel Swedenborg (who is discussed in Chapter 13, Clergy and Spiritual Leaders). Doyle was also a supporter of the controversial work of Albert Abrams, MD, discussed earlier in this chapter.

Alfred, Lord Tennyson (1809–1892) was poet laureate of the United Kingdom and is one of the most popular English poets of all time. Tennyson was one of many highly respected individuals to frequent the spa of Dr. James Gully, who was known to provide cold water treatments and homeopathic medicines. When Tennyson was in his late thirties, he suffered from *petit mal* seizures and a nervous breakdown supposedly due to thwarted romantic hopes, the death of a close friend, and financial anxieties. He first sought care at a spa under the direction of Dr. Edward Johnson, and there is record of him going to two other spas. He was so despondent and ill that friends despaired for his life (Martin, 1980, 278). However, shortly after he went to the spa and homeopathic clinic operated by Dr. Gully, he experienced noticeable benefits. In fact, although Tennyson was not yet fully cured, after Gully's treatment, he no longer wrote to friends that he was suffering from "hypochondria" as he had done so many times previously. Even Tennyson's mother saw the difference and referred to Dr. Gully as "a very clever man" (Martin, 1980, 315). Five years later Tennyson brought his new wife for care from Dr. Gully (Oppenheim, 1991, 136). Tennyson lived a long and fruitful life.

Other patients of Dr. Gully included: **George Eliot** (the pseudonym for British novelist Mary Ann Evans, 1819–1880, who not surprisingly was a friend of another major homeopathic advocate, Henry James), **Edward Bulwer-Lytton** (British novelist, playwright, and politician, 1803–1873), **Florence Nightingale** (leader in the worldwide nursing movement, 1820–1910), **Bishop Samuel Wilberforce** (highly respected clergyman, 1805–1873), **Charles Dickens** (author, 1817–1870), **Thomas Carlyle** (essayist and historian, 1795–1881), and **Charles Darwin** (British naturalist, 1809–1882). (For a detailed and truly amazing story of Darwin's treatment by Dr. Gully, see Chapter 5, Physicians and Scientists.)

Dr. Frederick Hervey Foster Quin, the first British physician to practice homeopathy in England and the first homeopath to British royalty, was also the homeopath to many of the British elite, including literary greats **Charles Dickens** (author of *Oliver Twist, A Christmas Carol, David Copperfield, Great Expectations,* and many others) and **William Makepeace Thackeray** (author of *Vanity Fair,* among many others, 1811–1863).

One of Charles Dickens's short novels, published posthumously, that mentioned homeopathy was *The Mudfog Papers* (1880). The story takes place in the mythic town of Mudfog, and like other Dickens works is full of odd and interesting characters. In this book, Dickens relates the story of a surgeon named Pipkin who tells about a short and interesting communication from Sir William Courtenay, a self-proclaimed messiah whose real name is Thom and who is an ardent believer in homeopathic medicine. He even believes that homeopathic medicines can raise the dead if prescribed immediately upon passing. This gentleman had a premonition that he would drown, and therefore employed a woman to follow him everywhere he went with a pail of water, with the instructions to place one drop of a homeopathic dose of lead and gunpowder under his tongue after death to restore him. Sadly, however, the peasant woman did not understand his instructions, and Dickens concludes, "the unfortunate gentleman had been sacrificed to the ignorance of the peasantry."

The Irish poet **W. B. Yeats** (1865–1939) was a known appreciator of both homeopathic medicine and Swedenborgian thought.

The discussion of European authors with an appreciation for homeopathy would not be complete without mentioning **Dame Ivy Compton-Burnett DBE** (1884–1969), the English novelist whose writings were published as I. Compton-Burnett. Reviewers of her books assert that she is a direct descendant of Joyce, Kafka, and Woolf, and several of her books are New York Review Classics and still in print. She authored twenty books, including *Manservant and Maidservant, More Women Than Men, A Family and a Fortune, A House and Its Head,* and *A God and His Gifts.* She received her DBE in 1967 for her contribution to literature.

Daughter of a famous homeopathic physician, James Compton-Burnett (1840–1901), Ivy was the cousin of Dr. Margery Blackie (1898–1981), who succeeded Ivy's father as the country's leading homeopathic physician, though distinguished herself even further by becoming the physician to Her Majesty Queen Elizabeth II. Before Ivy's mother, Katherine Rees, married her father, she was diagnosed with Bright's disease and was expected to never get well. However, she sought the homeopathic care of Dr. Compton-Burnett who cured her in eight months with homeopathic *Mercurius vivus* (mercury).[41] They were married within the year, and ten months later Ivy was born. Her mother lived another twenty-seven years.

An Eastern Advocate

The appreciation for homeopathy is not limited to literary greats in the Western tradition. **Rabindranath Tagore** (1861–1941) is widely recognized as the greatest writer in modern Indian literature. He was a Bengali poet, novelist, educator, and an early advocate of independence for India. Tagore won the Nobel Prize for Literature in 1913. Two years later he was awarded knighthood, but he surrendered it in 1919 to protest against the massacre of Amritsar, where British troops killed hundreds of Indian demonstrators. Tagore's influence over Gandhi and the founders of modern India was known to be significant.

In 1936, he wrote: "I have long been an ardent believer in the science of homeopathy, and I feel happy that it has got now a greater hold in India than even in the land of its origin. It is not merely a collection of a few medicines, but a real science with a rational philosophy as its base" (Bagchi, 2000).

Modern Literary Greats

The list of modern homeopathic advocates among writers does not compare with with that of the past. However, Norman Cousins, Barbara Cartland, Gabriel Garcia Márquez, and J. D. Salinger are not lightweights by any measurement.

Norman Cousins (1912–1990) was an internationally respected journalist. He was editor of *The Saturday Review* (originally called *The Saturday Review of Literature,* a leading literary magazine for many decades, 1924–1986) and advisor to several American presidents. Despite impressive lifelong work on international peace and disarmament, he achieved his greatest fame from writing an article in the *New England Journal of Medicine* (1976) and then a book, *Anatomy of an Illness as Perceived by the Patient* (1979) that chronicled his personal experience in contracting a deadly illness and curing it. In the mid-1960s, he was diagnosed with ankylosing spondylitis, a normally incurable degenerative disease of the connective tissue of the body. What was truly remarkable about his case was that he claimed to cure himself by taking large doses of vitamin C and by experiencing frequent fits of laughter (he watched numerous TV comedy programs, including *Candid Camera* and *I Love Lucy*).

After writing this article and book suggesting that there was a significant healing effect from simple vitamin C and from the power of the mind (and of humor!) to heal, he received more than 3,000 letters from medical doctors who expressed sincere interest and support for his experience. Cousins then wrote another important article about what he learned from these doctors (Cousins, 1978).

In 1980 he suffered a severe heart attack. He was treated conventionally except for one thing: His wife, who was a serious student of homeopathic medicine, gave him several homeopathic doses of *Cactus*, a homeopathic medicine known to cause and cure "prickly" and constricting pains around the heart. Despite having had a massive heart attack (and without taking vitamin C or watching any comedy programs), he was sitting up in bed reading and writing in a couple of hours. He and his doctors insisted that it was Cousins's will to live that resulted in his healing, though his wife simply disagreed. She even told me personally that she prescribed homeopathic medicines to her husband throughout his earlier disease of ankylosing spondylitis, but because he was so skeptical of homeopathy, she secretly placed his remedies in his morning orange juice. One of their daughters has confirmed these actions.

Many conventional physicians remain skeptical about the curative power of vitamin C and laughter in treating ankylosing spondylitis, and perhaps their skepticism is justifiable. The fact that Cousins's wife prescribed homeopathic medicines for him during both illnesses might better explain his remarkable recoveries.

Despite skeptics' insistence that homeopathic medicines are only placebos and that "belief" is the primary therapy for homeopathic patients, the moral to the Norman Cousins story is that belief is *not* necessary for homeopathic medicines to have profound effect and that the placebo explanation is at best incomplete and inadequate for explaining the real power of these medicines.

Dame Barbara Cartland (1901–2000) was the most successful writer of romance novels of all time, specializing in historical love themes. Dame Cartland authored more than 700 romance novels, which were translated into thirty-six languages and sold over a billion copies worldwide, making her one of the best-selling authors in history. Besides romance novels, Ms. Cartland also had a special interest in natural medicine. In the 1960s she founded and was president of the National Association of Health. She advocated for organic foods, homeopathy, and acupuncture. She co-owned a health food store in Marylebone, England, and was a patron to a magazine called *Mind and Matter,* which promoted various natural medicines as well as radionics and the work of George de la Warr. She had a special love and appreciation for homeopathic *Arnica.* She also supported efforts for better conditions and wages for midwives and nurses, and advocated for equal rights for gypsies, who commonly experienced great discrimination.

Jerome David Salinger (1919–), known as **J. D. Salinger**, gained his reputation as a result of his novel *The Catcher in the Rye* (1951). Salinger wrote a couple of other books after this and several short stories, but ultimately, he has become one of the most private and reclusive modern-day authors. Very little was known about him, until Joyce Maynard, a *New York Times* columnist who developed a relationship with him and then lived with him for several years, wrote a book about her time with "Jerry" Salinger (Maynard, 1998). Maynard wrote (and Salinger's daughter Margaret confirmed, in her own book, published in 2000) that Salinger has a special deep love for homeopathy. He spends several hours each day studying homeopathic books, and he regularly prescribes homeopathic medicines to people and animals.

At one point, Maynard describes a visit by her mother, who had an infected toe at the time. After an interview with her, Jerry prescribed a homeopathic medicine, and within minutes, her toe swelled considerably and then burst, after which the pain disappeared instantly (Maynard, 1998, 138). Maynard describes Salinger's interest in high-potency homeopathic medicines and his appreciation for constitutional homeopathy (one of the important and sophisticated practices of classical homeopathy, in which a single remedy is prescribed based on the totality of a person's physical, emotional, mental, and genetic characteristics in order to strengthen a person's entire constitution). Maynard also notes Salinger's method of giving a person a homeopathic medicine in water, which is an advanced method of dispensing remedies to people (or animals).

Ultimately, Maynard moved out of Salinger's home, got married, had children, and then got divorced, but throughout this time, she too has sought treatment from professional homeopaths.

Gabriel García Márquez (1927–) is a Colombian novelist and journalist who won the 1982 Nobel Prize in Literature. He is considered one of the greatest South American writers of the twentieth and twenty-first centuries. Perhaps the most well-known of his many novels is *One Hundred Years of Solitude.* Many of his writings are drawn from his own life. Because his father was trained as a medical doctor and a pharmacist who practiced homeopathy, this medical subject has been a part of several of his novels and short stories.

In *Love in a Time of Cholera,* the godfather of the novel's protagonist is a homeopathic doctor, and ironically, the protagonist is fighting for the affections of a woman who is married to a conventional physician. Also, in an autobiographical short story called "Serenade: How My Father Won My Mother," published in the *New Yorker* (February 19, 2001), Garcia Márquez wrote: "Over the course of the year, Gabriel Eligio gave up his worthy profession of telegraph operator and devoted his talent as an autodidact to a science on the decline: homeopathy."

In his most recent novel, *Living to Tell the Tale* (2003), Garcia Márquez chose to incorporate elements of his own life with some fictional twists. His heroine, a much-loved mother, is a "lioness" who fights a long battle with her family to marry a violin-playing telegraph clerk. Then, struggling in poverty when her husband abandons her and her eleven children, she seeks to make a better life for her family by making a living as a homeopathic pharmacist.

References
Albert Abrams, *JAMA,* April 8, 1922, 78(14):1072.
Bagchi, A. K. *Rabindranath Tagore and His Medical World.* New Delhi: Konark Publishers, 2000.
Bingham, M. T. *Emily Dickinson's Home.* New York: Harper and Brothers, 1955.
Coulter, H. L. *Divided Legacy: The Conflict Between Homoeopathy and the American Medical Association.* Volume III. Berkeley: North Atlantic Books, 1973.
Coulter, H. L. *Divided Legacy: A History of the Schism in Medical Thought.* Volume IV: Twentieth-Century Medicine: The Bacteriological Era. Berkeley: North Atlantic Books, 1994.
Cousins, N. Anatomy of an Illness, *New England Journal of Medicine,* 1976, 295:1458–1463.
Cousins, N. *Anatomy of an Illness As Perceived by the Patient.* New York: Norton, 1979.
Cousins, N. What I Learned from 3,000 Doctors, *Saturday Review,* February 18, 1978, 12–16.
Dean, M. E. *The Trials of Homeopathy.* Essen: KVC, 2004.
Emerson, R. W. *English Traits,* Chapter XIV, 1856. Available at www.rwe.org/works/English_Traits_Chapter_XIV_Literature.htm
Emerson, R. W. *The Complete Works of Ralph Waldo Emerson,* Volume VII, Society and Solitude (1870). Available at www.rwe.org/comm/index.php?option=com_content&task=view&id=37&Itemid=215
Fishbein, M. *The Medical Follies.* New York: Boni and Liveright, 1926.
Flaxman, N. A Cardiology Anomaly: Albert Abrams (1863–1924). *Bulletin of the History of Medicine,* 1953, 27(3):252–268.
Gardner, M. *Fads and Fallacies in the Name of Science.* New York: Dover Publications, 1957.
Haehl, R. *Samuel Hahnemann: His Life and His Work.* London: Homoeopathic Publishing Company, 1922. Reprinted, New Delhi: B. Jain.
Hendrick, G. Washington Irving and Homoeopathy, in Wrobel, A., ed., *Pseudo-Science and Society in Nineteenth Century America.* Lexington: University Press of Kentucky, 1987, 166–179.
Hirschhorn, N. Was It Tuberculosis? Another Glimpse of Emily Dickinson's Health. *New England Quarterly,* March 1999, 72(1):102–118.
James, W. *Banner of Light,* March 12, 1898.
James, W. Letter to Henry William Rankin, February 27, 1903. William Ernest Hocking Papers, Houghton Library, Harvard University.
Marshall, M. *The Peabody Sisters: Three Women Who Ignited American Romanticism.* Boston: Houghton Mifflin, 2005.

Martin, R. B. T. *The Unquiet Heart.* Oxford: Oxford University Press, 1980.
Maynard, J. *At Home in the World.* New York: Picador, 1998.
Ober, K. P. The Pre-Flexnerian Reports: Mark Twain's Criticism of Medicine in the United States, *Annals in Internal Medicine,* 1997, 126:157–163.
Oppenheim, J. *Shattered Nerves : Doctors, Patients, and Depression in Victorian England.* Oxford: Oxford University Press, 1991.
Perrin-Wilson, L. Elizabeth Peabody's Foreign Library, *Concord Magazine,* August-September 1999. www.concordma.com/magazine/augsept99/peabody2.html
Peters, J. C. The Illnesses of Washington Irving, *North American Journal of Homoeopathy,* February 1860, 8:451–473.
Rice, J. L. Dostoevsky's Medical History: Diagnosis and Dialectic, *The Russian Review,* 1983, 42:131–161.
Richardson, R. D. William James: *In the Maelstrom of American Modernism.* Boston: Houghton Mifflin, 2006.
Rothstein, W. *American Physicians in the Nineteenth Century.* Baltimore: Johns Hopkins University Press, 1972.
Russell, E. W. *Report on Radionics.* Suffolk, England: Neville Spearman, 1973.
Salinger, M. A. *Dream Catcher.* New York: Pocket Books, 2000.
Sayings and Doings, *Pacific Coast Journal of Homeopathy,* February 1893, 84.
Scholten, P. *Albert Abrams: The Physician Who Made Millions out of Electricity.* San Francisco, Calif.: San Francisco Medical Society, 1999. Available at www.sfms.org/AM/Template.cfm?Section=Home&SECTION=Article_Archives&TEMPLATE=/CM/HTMLDisplay.cfm&CONTENTID=1878.
Seeley B. M., Denton A. B., Ahn M. S., and Maas C. S. Effect of homeopathic Arnica montana on bruising in face-lifts: results of a randomized, double-blind, placebo-controlled clinical trial. *Archives in Facial Plastic Surgery,* January–February 2006 Jan, 8(1):54–59.
St. John, T. Emily Dickinson Daguerreotype (no date), www.geocities.com/seekingthephoenix/d/emily.htm
Thomas, H. K. Emily Dickinson's "Renunciation" and Anorexia Nervosa, *American Literature,* May 1988, 60(2):205–225.
Treuherz, F. The Origins of Kent's Homeopathy, *Journal of the American Institute of Homeopathy,* 1984, 77(4).
Tutorow, N. *The Governor: The Life and Legacy of Leland Stanford.* Norman, Okla.: Arthur H. Clark, 2004.
Tutorow, N. Personal communication, May 1, 2006.
Twain, M. A Majestic Literary Fossil, *Harper's Magazine,* February 1890, 80(477): 439–444.
Weiser, M., Strosser, W., and Klein, P. Homeopathic vs. Conventional Treatment of Vertigo: A Randomized Double-Blind Controlled Clinical Study, *Archives of Otolaryngology—Head and Neck Surgery,* August 1998, 124:879–885.
Wershub, L. P. Washington Irving, *Chironian,* Summer Issue, 1965.
Wilson, J. L. *Stanford University School of Medicine and its Predecessor Schools: A Historical Perspective,* Chapter 26. 1998. Available at http://elane.stanford.edu/wilson/indextext.html.

CHAPTER 4

Sports Superstars: Scoring with Homeopathy

Due to the extremely competitive nature of sports today, athletes and their coaches explore whatever they can do legally to get that extra edge. Just as important as learning ways to condition and challenge an athlete to perform his or her best, it is equally important to know about specific strategies to stay healthy. It is further essential that they know specific treatments that can help speed the healing of an athletic injury. It is therefore not surprising that select high-level athletes and coaches are using homeopathic medicines as a part of their new sports medicine treatment protocols.

In fact, modern sports medicine has recently morphed into one of the most cutting-edge fields of medical and surgical practice. It has become an amalgam of conventional drug and surgical treatments as well as physical therapy, occupational therapy, chiropractic, osteopathy, exercise physiology, kinesiology, massage therapy, ergonomics, nutritional supplements, and herbal and homeopathic medicines.

David Beckham (1975–) is widely considered the world's best soccer ("football" to people outside of the U.S.) player. He used homeopathic medicines after he broke his foot prior to the World Cup in 2003, and a large number of news reports on homeopathy in Europe inevitably mention Beckham's appreciation for homeopathy. In 1998, he married Spice Girl Victoria Adams, and they have had three children. Victoria has openly expressed interest in and use of homeopathic medicines too.

The uses of homeopathic medicines in soccer are appreciated not only by world-class soccer players but also world-class soccer doctors. **Dr. Jean-Marcel Ferret**, physician to the French soccer team from 1993 to 2004, including the World Cup championship team in 1998, has asserted:

> I am a doctor that uses homeopathy and not a homeopath. I am open to all techniques. I consider that there is only one medicine comprising various techniques. We doctors have to know how to use the entire arsenal. As a sports doctor, I quickly discovered that except for anti-inflammatories and muscle relaxants, I was very limited in the care of athletes. I therefore tried to find something else. I began to use homeopathy, first occasionally, and then more and more.

Dr. Ferret also said:

> At first, the athletes were surprised and some of them even wary. So I explained how and why homeopathy acts. The greatest value in sports? Its speed of action. I can use it directly on the soccer field, within seconds of the trauma, and note the results almost immediately. For example, in trauma with *Arnica*,[42] and without any adverse reactions on the stomach or liver. I also use homeopathy to treat ORL, stress or dermatology problems. (www.boiron.com)

David Beckham is not alone in the soccer world in his appreciation for homeopathic medicine. The **Wimbledon Football Club** (known as Wimbledon F.C.) was the name of a now defunct football club that played in south London. In 1963, Wimbledon F.C. won the Football Association Amateur Cup, and in 1988, they beat champions-elect Liverpool in the FA Cup final, thereby becoming the only football club in the country to have won both the amateur and professional versions of the Cup.

During the time of their 1988 championship, the players of the team were known to use massage oil made of homeopathic ingredients *Arnica*, *Ruta*, and *Hypericum*, to help warm up their muscles. A spokesperson for the club even acknowledged that the team's trainer used homeopathic medicines to treat fractures (after bones were set!) (Kindred Spirits, 1989).

One of the greatest professional tennis players of all time is **Martina Navratilova** (1956–). She won eighteen Grand Slam singles titles and forty Grand Slam doubles titles. She won the Wimbledon tournament a record nine times. On July 15, 2000, she was inducted into the International

Tennis Hall of Fame in Newport, Rhode Island. In her acceptance speech, she thanked everyone who had helped her in her career, and she added a thanks to all the "doctors who held me together, homeopathic people, osteopaths, massage therapists" (Roberts, 2000).

Boris Becker (1967–), also a tennis superstar, has won six Grand Slam tournaments, an Olympic gold medal, is the youngest-ever winner of the men's singles title at Wimbledon, and was inducted into the International Tennis Hall of Fame in 2003. Like many leading athletes, he has sought the care of famed Munich homeopathic doctor Hans-Wilhelm Muller-Wohlfahrt.

Golf superstar **José Maria Olazábal** (1966–), who won the Masters in 1994 and 1999, had to pull out of all major tournaments in 1996 because of a severe case of rheumatoid polyarthritis in his feet. There was a real fear in golf that Olazábal would never play again. Then, Olazábal went to see Dr. Hans-Wilhelm Muller-Wohlfahrt, who turned Olazábal from a virtual cripple into Masters champion.

Nancy Lopez (1957–) is one of the most famous women in the history of golf. She starred on the LPGA tour from 1978 to 1997, winning forty-eight tournaments and three majors. Enshrined in the World Golf Hall of Fame, she is now known as Nancy Lopez-Knight, after her marriage to former Major League baseball player and 1986 World Series Most Valuable Player Ray Knight. For her aching knees, she exercises and takes homeopathic medicines (Becker, 1999).

Will Greenwood (1972–) is not well-known in the U.S., even though he is considered one of the leading rugby players in the world. Playing at center position, he is a World Cup winner. During a 1997 rugby tournament, he suffered from an accident in which he stopped breathing for several minutes after hitting his head on the hard ground. Because of Olazábal's fantastic experiences with homeopathic doctor Muller-Wohlfahrt, Greenwood went to see him and made a stunning recovery (Stafford, 1999).

Kelly Slater (1972–) is the most successful professional surfer in the history of the sport. According to peers, he is a surfing genius. Kelly is seven-time world champion (1992, 1994 through 1998, and 2005). While injuries may be one important factor that limits an athlete's abilities, other health issues come to the fore in other sports. When Kelly was asked what his never-fail hangover cure was, he told the reporter: "There's a homeopathic medicine called *Nux vomica*. It consists of little pellets that you put on your tongue every hour or so. It's a real natural way to cure things" (*Australian Cleo*, 2004).

Not only is it important for athletes to be knowledgeable and experienced in using homeopathic medicines, it is particularly important for coaches to be properly informed. **Arnie Kander** is the strength and conditioning coach for the Detroit Pistons, the National Basketball Association's most-winning basketball team in the twenty-first century. Kander has routinely utilized homeopathic and Eastern medicine methods in conjunction with conventional physical therapy training. When Grant Hill, one of the team's best players, was traded to Orlando, Hill tried to hire Kander away to work with him exclusively.

The *Detroit Free Press* reported that the 2006 Pistons set the NBA record for most consecutive starts by the same starting five, and they gave Kander the credit for this impressive result (Watson, 2007).

Russell Nua received his baseball World Series ring at Boston Red Sox's Fenway Park in 2005, but I'm sure that virtually no one has ever heard of him. This is because he is not a baseball player. He is the massage therapist with the Red Sox. What is also a tad unusual about him getting this ring is that he worked for the Arizona Diamondbacks all year as their massage therapist, and he only began working for the Red Sox at the demand of ace pitcher Curt Schilling. One of the special things that Nua does for the players is apply *Arnica* for its anti-inflammatory properties and its powerful healing of soft tissue injuries (Silverman, 2005).

The most winning baseball team in history is the New York Yankees, and one of the team's best players from 1993 to 2001 was **Paul O'Neill** (1963–). The *New York Daily News* (October 24, 1999) reported that his locker is "filled with homeopathic cures." It is interesting to note that O'Neill's great-grandmother, Mary Clemens, was a first cousin of Samuel Clemens (aka Mark Twain), who also was an advocate of homeopathy (see Chapter 3, Literary Greats).

Jim Bouton (1939–) was another New York Yankee, and as a pitcher, he won twenty-one games in 1963 and eighteen games in 1964. He wrote a famous and controversial book about baseball called *Ball Four*. Bouton once told me that he had an experience with homeopathy that amazed him: "I had a severe case of asthma which made it extremely difficult to breathe. I usually need to be hospitalized. A friend gave me the name of a homeopath who gave me a medicine which worked incredibly rapidly. Within 24 hours, my breathing was completely cleared, and I was on the mound that next day ... as the winning pitcher."

David Moncoutié (1975–) is currently France's leading professional cyclist. In 2004 he won a stage of the Tour de France to Figeac, and in the following year he won his biggest victory in the Tour de France stage from Briançon to Digne-les-Bains on Bastille Day, guaranteeing him a place in the hearts of French cycling fans. He has become a role model for the cycling community (as well as for all sports) by his strong anti-drug-abuse stance. But he isn't against all legal drugs because he is a known advocate of homeopathic medicines.

Gabrielle Reece (1970–) is a professional volleyball player and former fashion model. Reece befriended Sheryl Crow, the Grammy Award-winning singer and songwriter, after Crow received an early diagnosis of breast cancer in 2006. Reece contacted Crow through a mutual friend, actress Rita Wilson. *Vanity Fair* (August 2006) reported that Reece felt compelled to tell Crow about "an immunity-boosting homeopathic product" she should try.

Hermann Maier (1972–) is an Austrian skier who has won four over-all World Cup titles, two Olympic gold medals (both in 1998), three World Championship titles (two in 1999, one in 2005), and fifty-three World Cup races. He ranks among the greatest skiers of all time. However, on August 24, 2001, Maier was returning from a workout on his motorcycle when a car swerved in front of him, and he was seriously, nearly fatally, injured. The *New Yorker* describes Austrians as the "masters of this strange art" of sports science, reconstructive medicine, and homeopathy, and Hermann was an agreeable and active patient (Bilger, 2004). Just a year later, he won two silver medals in the Salt Lake City games in 2002, and then won the World Cup in 2003–2004.

The name **Misty Hyman** (1979–) may not be well known but her face is. An American swimmer, she won the gold medal in the 200m butterfly at the Sydney 2000 Summer Olympics; she was so surprised when she won that she looked at the scoreboard three times just to make certain she had won. However, a 2001 shoulder injury led to surgery, and she has not yet competed on the same spectacular level as before. Still, she bragged to the *Los Angeles Times* that she had replaced her antibiotic regimen with homeopathic medicines that are working (Smith, 2004).

Marie-Hélène Prémont, a Canadian who won the 2004 Olympic silver medal in mountain biking, credits homeopathic medicines with helping in her victory. "Homeopathic medicines are safe and work naturally to relieve aches and pains so I can work hard one day and continue what I need to do the next day," Prémont said. The challenging sport of mountain biking occasionally results in accidents for which Prémont uses *Arnica* cream to reduce pain, swelling, and bruising (www.boiron.com).

Elvis Stojko MSC, MSM (1972–), is a Canadian figure skating world champion. Stojko won silver medals at the 1994 and 1998 Winter Olympics, and he won the World Figure Skating championships in 1994, 1995, and 1997. He has told numerous interviewers that he actively seeks out acupuncture and homeopathic treatments. He has worked with a German team doctor who uses homeopathic medicines, and he acknowledged that numerous other leading skaters also seek out this doctor's care (Rod Black Boat Interview, 1996).

Chris Bonington, formally known as **Sir Christian John Storey Bonington, CBE** (1934–), is a British mountaineer. He participated in nineteen expeditions to the Himalayas, including four to Mount Everest and the first ascent of the south face of Annapurna. He has authored fifteen books and was knighted in 1996. Bonington told a London newspaper that he takes homeopathic medicines for various situations, including a homeopathic remedy to counter the effects of altitude sickness. Tony Pinkus, a pharmacist and owner of Ainsworth Homeopathic Pharmacy in London, supplies Bonington with homeopathic medicines. Pinkus told the press that Bonington "sent us a very cheery postcard from the top of Mount Menlungtse" (Middleton, 1999).

The fact that so many athletes appreciate *Arnica* so much is no big surprise. There simply isn't anything like it. When used immediately after an injury, it often creates such rapid healing that the next day the person hardly remembers the injury. Athletes and coaches see its efficacy regularly. Though it is important that *Arnica* be used as soon after an injury as possible, it will still provide benefits if applied twelve hours later.

Scientific studies have verified *Arnica*'s value. An AMA surgery journal showed the benefit of *Arnica* after the trauma of facial plastic surgery (Seeley, et al., 2006). This double-blind and placebo-controlled study included digital photos of people, with measurements of the differences in discoloration and swelling. People who didn't take *Arnica* had 11–41 percent more bruising than those who took this homeopathic medicine and took 50 percent longer to reduce their level of bruising to the level of bruising with the homeopathic treatment.[43]

Some athletes use *Arnica* in special formulas that include homeopathic medicines that help to heal nerve injuries and bone injuries that are sometimes concurrent with soft tissue injuries. One German company that makes such a product has conducted double-blind studies that have also shown great benefit in the healing of sprains and strains (Zell, et al., 1989; Bohmer, 1992). It is interesting to note that the parent company that owns the homeopathic manufacturer is the same company that creates the Bavarian Motor Works (BMW) cars. Homeopathy, again, is in good company.

Dr. E. Petrie Hoyle (1861–1955), a homeopathic doctor who worked for the French Red Cross and the British Mobile Hospital Services during World War I, reported on the incredible successes that he had using *Arnica* during the war. He also talked and wrote about a homeopathic doctor who was the physician to the football team of the University of California at Berkeley and who gave *Arnica* internally as soon as the players came off the field after exercise. The doctor insisted that they take their *Arnica* in just one dose before they got cold after vigorous exercising, thereby preventing soreness the next day (Hoyle, 1942, 70).

The use of homeopathic medicines for professional athletes, Olympic competitors, and the rest of us who engage in sports and exercise holds immense promise that is only just beginning to be realized.

References
Australian Cleo (magazine), Kelly and Sophie Get Cosy, August 2004, 78.
Becker, D. Lopez Confident Despite Knee Pain, *USA Today,* June 2, 1999.
Bilger, B. Twin Peaks, *The New Yorker,* January 26, 2004.
Rod Black Boat Interview–1996, http://members.aol.com/hoacpics/elvis/rodblack.htm.
Bohmer, D. and Ambrus, P. Treatment of sports injuries with Traumeel ointment—Controlled double-blind study (translated from German). *Biologische,* 1992, 21:260–268. www.boiron.com
Hoyle, E. P. Medical and Surgical Experiences in the First World War and Some Statistics and Medical Measures of Greatest Value to All Army Medical Corps, *The Homoeopathic Recorder,* August 1942, 58(2):57–74.
Kindred Spirits, *Daily Telegraph* (London), August 12, 1989.
Middleton, C. Holiday jabs without the needle: Homoeopathic immunisation pills are becoming increasingly popular. But do they work against killer diseases? *Daily Telegraph,* October 10, 1999.
Roberts, S. An Improbable Journey: Navratilova came from bare beginning to become one of the greatest, *New York Times,* July 16, 2000.
Seeley B. M., Denton, A. B., Ahn, M. S., and Maas, C. S. Effect of homeopathic Arnica montana on bruising in face-lifts: Results of a randomized, double-blind, placebo-controlled clinical trial. *Archives in Facial Plastic Surgery,* Jan-Feb 2006, 8(1):54–59.
Silverman, M. Red Sox in Good Hands. *Boston Herald,* May 2, 2005, 88.
Smith, K. Her Reaction Is Priceless, *Los Angeles Times,* July 5, 2004, D1.
Stafford, I. Why won't rugby pick up the bill for Greenwood? *Mail on Sunday,* September 5, 1999.
Watson, M. There's Something in the Water in Detroit, *Detroit Free Press,* March 28, 2007.
Zell, J., et al., "Behandlung von akuten Sprung-geleksdisotrionen: Doppelblindstudie zum Wirksamkeitsnachweis eines Homoopathischen Salbenpraparats," *Fortschr. Medicine,* 1988, 106:96–100. (This study on the treatment of sprains was reprinted in English: Treatment of Acute Sprains of the Ankle: A Controlled Double-Blind Trial to Test the Effectiveness of a Homeopathic Ointment, *Biological Therapy,* 1989, 7(1):1–6.

Homeopathic Sports Medicine Resources
Hershoff, A. *Homeopathy for Musculoskeletal Healing.* Berkeley: North Atlantic Books, 1996. (Dr. Hershoff is a naturopath and chiropractor who specializes in homeopathic medicine.)
Subotnick, S. *Sports and Exercise Injuries: Conventional, Homeopathic, and Alternative Treatments.* Berkeley: North Atlantic Books, 1991. (Dr. Subotnick is a podiatrist

and chiropractor who specializes in homeopathic medicine. He has also authored a respected podiatric textbook that includes information on homeopathic medicine.)

CHAPTER 5

Physicians and Scientists: Coming Out of the Medicine Closet

Despite the vicious attacks against homeopathy and homeopaths for the past 200 years, many respected orthodox physicians and scientists have expressed appreciation for this frequently maligned medical science. These physicians and scientists have not shouted from the rooftops and some of them were so skeptical of homeopathy that they even discounted the benefits that homeopathic treatments created in their own health. Nonetheless, the experiences they had, the experiments they conducted, their own intellectual rigor, and their statements about this medical science and art provide a strong case for its efficacy.

In previous chapters, we looked at the attacks by the orthodox medical establishment against homeopathy and homeopaths. In addition, orthodox physicians and their representative medical societies created "ethical codes" that influenced state and federal laws and made it difficult for homeopathy and homeopaths to persist—but persist they did.

There have been different reasons for this strong animosity.[44] Ultimately, homeopathy and homeopaths presented a serious philosophical, scientific, and economic threat to orthodox physicians. When you also understand something about who were orthodox physicians in the mid- and late-1800s in American society, you can get a better understanding of the source of this drama.

Only since the mid-1900s did medical schools in America (and throughout the world) attract the best and brightest college students, but this was not always the case. In fact, Charles W. Eliot, the president of Harvard (1869–1926), issued a report in 1879–1880 in which he described the average American doctor of that time: "An American physician or surgeon may be, and often is, a coarse and uncultivated person, devoid of intellectual interests outside of his calling, and quite unable to either speak or write his mother tongue with accuracy" (Wershub, 1967, 89). Another historian wrote: "Even as late as 1884, the Harvard Medical School each year received a number of students who failed to pass the entrance examinations for the College and went to the medical school because the requirements for admission were so much less" (Wershub, 1967, 68).

In efforts to create the best medical education possible in the nineteenth century, several homeopathic medical schools were among the first to adopt a three-year graded curriculum, and one of these schools (Boston University) was the first medical school in the United States to offer a four-year graded curriculum (Rothstein, 1972, 239).

Modern-day skeptics of homeopathy may choose to attack this book (or its author) by deriding the anecdotal reports of personal experiences with homeopathy, but they will probably have the most difficulty reading and accepting the information and reports from some of the most respected medical doctors and scientists that are reported below.

It should be noted that some of the respected physicians and scientists discussed in this chapter did not always stand up for homeopathy in the same fashion that they stood up for so many other things they believed. However, when you consider the significant and severe antagonism strewn upon those who simply said or wrote anything positive about homeopathy, when support for homeopathy was actually considered traitorous to conventional physicians and scientists, and when you consider that even those researchers who sought to test homeopathic medicines in a scientific fashion were often personally and professionally attacked, it becomes understandable that so many good physicians and scientists kept their appreciation for homeopathy quiet.

To begin this chapter, it is appropriate to provide some biographical information on the founder of homeopathy, Samuel Hahnemann, MD.

Samuel Hahnemann, MD

In America's capital city, Washington, DC, the only monument honoring a physician is one to the founder of homeopathic medicine, Samuel Hahnemann, MD (1755–1843). This monument was dedicated in 1900 by President William McKinley.

Although trained as a medical doctor, Hahnemann was a learned chemist and author of the leading German textbook for apothecaries (pharmacists) of the day. He was conversant in at least nine languages and even supported himself in his mid-twenties teaching languages at the famed University of Leipzig.

Learning languages enabled Hahnemann to become familiar with the latest developments in medicine and science. He further expanded his knowledge and his growing prestige by translating twenty-two textbooks, primarily medical and chemistry textbooks (several of which were multivolume works). Over a twenty-nine-year period, Hahnemann translated some 9,460 pages.

Prior to his discovery of homeopathy, Hahnemann's respect as a physician brought German royalty to seek his medical care, and modern medical historians confirm that Hahnemann showed sound balance and good judgment in his advocacy of proper diet, fresh air, and exercise as a method of treatment. His promotion of hygienic measures during epidemics won him praise as a public health advocate, and his kind, rather than cruel and harsh, treatment of the insane granted him a place in the history of psychiatry (Rothstein, 1972, 152).

It is not surprising to know that Hahnemann was a Freemason as early as 1777; he was later granted the title of Obermeister, or Grand Master (Jurj, 2007). In this esoteric fraternal organization and secret society, men shared certain moral and metaphysical ideals.

Hahnemann stopped practicing conventional medicine of his day because he felt that he was doing more harm than good. Instead, he made a living for his family of eleven children as a translator. During the translation of a book by William Cullen, the leading physiologist of that time, Hahnemann noted that Cullen asserted that Peruvian bark was an effective drug for malaria because of its bitter and astringent properties. Hahnemann thought this a peculiar statement because he knew other bitter and astringent medicines that provided no benefit in the treatment of malaria. He then conducted an experiment upon himself, taking this herb twice a day until he developed symptoms of its toxicology, and here he discovered that it created a fever with chills as well as other symptoms that mimicked malaria. Hahnemann proposed that Peruvian bark (which contains quinine) may be effective for treating people with malaria because it has the capacity to cause similar symptoms.

Hahnemann ultimately conducted upon himself experiments with ninety other substances, and his colleagues and friends also engaged in these experiments. He found a consistent pattern from these experiments: that various substances in overdose create their own unique syndrome of symptoms and whatever syndrome a substance causes in toxic dose, it can and will elicit a healing response when given in specially prepared small doses to people who have similar symptoms of pathology.

Hahnemann observed that sick people were hypersensitive to the medicine that causes similar symptoms as they were experiencing. Because of this, Hahnemann began using smaller and smaller doses. Being a chemist, he experimented with various ways to make these doses both safe and effective. Over the next forty years, he experimented with diluting the medicines 1:10, 1:100, or 1:50,000, with vigorous shaking between dilutions, and he consistently found that exceedingly small doses of medicines had powerful therapeutic effects when prescribed according to his principle of similars.

Being an incredibly avid experimenter, Hahnemann did not come easily or quickly to his conclusions about the exceptionally small doses he and his colleagues found effective. In fact, he first wrote about homeopathy in 1796, and for the next thirty years (!) he primarily used doses that are today considered low potencies. Further, in 1829, a homeopathic physician wrote him about his successes in using potencies that were diluted 1:10 more than 200 times, and Hahnemann expressed skepticism for such actions until he himself found that these higher potencies were surprisingly effective (Bradford, 1895, 455–456).

Ultimately, Hahnemann authored three major books on homeopathy, including six editions of his seminal work *Organon of the Medical Art*, continually updating and refining this science and art.

Christoph Wilhelm Hufeland, MD (1762–1836), Germany's most well-known and respected physician of his day, was as famous as Goethe and Schiller in the early nineteenth century. As the editor of the leading medical journal in Germany, *Journal of Practical Medicine,* Hufeland published some of Hahnemann's writings and held him in extremely high regard: "I have discovered in him an amplitude of knowledge, clearness of mind, and a spirit of tolerance, which last is the more worthy of notice in him." Hahnemann was described as "one of our most distinguished, intelligent and original physicians" (Everest, 1842, 186).

Even though Robert Koch first discovered the cholera bacteria in 1883, as early as 1831 Hahnemann ascribed the cause of the cholera epidemics raging at that time to "an enormously increased brood of those excessively minute, invisible, living creatures so inimical to human life, of which the contagious matter of the cholera most probably consists" (Hahnemann, 1831).

Nicholas Von Hoffman, a columnist for the *Washington Post,* wrote: "Although this German physician never visited the U.S., for 70 years or more his ideas tore up and divided American medicine. No other single individual caused the settled and comfortable structures of this profession the trouble Hahnemann did, and even now many of the questions he raised have not been answered" (Von Hoffman, 1971).

Many of homeopathy's most severe critics have actually had kind words for Samuel Hahnemann. Morris Fishbein, executive director of the American Medical Association, wrote: "The influence of Hahnemann was, on the whole, certainly for the good. He emphasized the individualization of the patient in the handling of disease ... and he demonstrated the value of testing the actual virtues of a drug by trial" (Fishbein, 1925, 37).

Despite Hahnemann's significant contributions to medicine, pharmacy, chemistry, psychiatry, and public health, he remained a humble man. "I do not ask during my lifetime any recognition of the beneficent truth, which I, without any thought of myself, offer. What I have done, I did from higher motives for the world. *Non inutilis vixi* (I have not lived in vain)" (Neng, 1930).

On the Hahnemann monument in Washington, DC, are those Latin words. Indeed, Dr. Samuel Hahnemann did not live in vain.

Charles Darwin

Charles Darwin (1809–1882) was a British scientist-naturalist who wrote about how evolution and natural selection play a central role in biology and human development. His book *The Origin of Species* (1859) established evolution as a primary principle of nature. Few people have known that he experienced significant benefits under the care of a homeopathic physician. In fact, a case can be made that without the homeopathic treatment Darwin received ten years before his most famous book was published, he might not ever have published this classic work.

When Darwin was just 16 years old, he spent a summer as an apprentice to his father, a doctor. Later, he attended Edinburgh University to study medicine. However, he was repulsed by the brutality of surgery and the primitive medical treatments of his day.

He initially studied to be a naturalist, but his father insisted that he go to Cambridge University to become a clergyman (when members of the clergy earned a better living than many other professions). After graduating from Cambridge in 1831, he began what became a five-year journey on the HMS *Beagle* surveying the coast of South America. On board the ship, Darwin suffered from seasickness, and in October 1833, he caught a fever in Argentina. In July 1834, while returning from the Andes down to the coast of Chile, he fell so ill that he spent a month in bed. From 1837 on, Darwin was frequently incapacitated with episodes of stomach pains, vomiting, severe boils, heart palpitations, trembling, and other symptoms. These symptoms worsened at times of stress, such as when attending meetings or dealing with controversy over his new theories because, like many scientists who proposed new ideas, he initially was severely attacked for them. The cause of Darwin's illness was unknown during his lifetime, and various treatments had no success.

Today, some physicians have speculated that Darwin caught Chagas disease from insect bites in South America, while others have suggested that he suffered from Ménière's disease, but the orthodox physicians of Darwin's day had no idea what his problem was, and all of their treatments simply made him worse.[45]

In 1847, Darwin's illness worsened. He was again experiencing frequent episodes of vomiting and weakness, but he now was also fainting and seeing spots in front of his eyes. Darwin wrote that he was "unable to do anything one day out of three" (Ruddick, 2001, 192). He was so ill that he wasn't even able to attend his father's funeral in November 1848. In March 1849, an old HMS *Beagle* shipmate told him about a different type of medical treatment provided by **James Gully, MD** (1808–1883), and his cousin told Darwin that two friends had benefited greatly from Gully's care. Darwin decided to go and to take the entire family (his wife Emma and their seven children) (Keynes, 2002). Dr. Gully and his health spa were situated in Malvern (just southwest of Birmingham), around 125 miles from the Darwins' home.

Dr. Gully, a medical graduate of the University of Edinburgh, was an unyielding opponent of the use of drugs of that era. His medical practice did not simply provide hydrotherapy or dietary advice; he also prescribed homeopathic medicines and recommended medical clairvoyant readings. After being at Dr. Gully's spa for just nine days, Darwin lamented that Gully had prescribed homeopathic medicine to him: "I grieve to say that Dr. Gully gives me homeopathic medicines three times a day, which I take obediently without an atom of faith." Darwin continued: "I like Dr. Gully much—he is certainly an able man. I have been struck with how many remarks he has made similar to those of my Father" (Burkhardt, 1996, 106). The fact that Darwin saw Gully as being like his father and "able" was still not enough to convince him that homeopathic medicines were effective.

Although Darwin was willing to follow Dr. Gully's advice, he had reservations about having his family members do so because Darwin had doubts about Gully's use of homeopathy, clairvoyance, and other unorthodox treatments.

And even though Darwin was extremely skeptical, just two days later (March 30, 1849) Darwin acknowledged, "I have already received so much benefit that I really hope my health will be much renovated" (Burkhardt, 1996, 107). After eight days a skin eruption broke out all over Darwin's legs, and he was actually pleased to experience this problem because he had previously observed that his physical and mental health improved noticeably after having skin eruptions.[46] He went a month without vomiting, a very rare experience for him, and even gained some weight. One day he surprised himself by being able to walk seven miles. He wrote to a friend, "I am turning into a mere walking and eating machine" (Quammen, 2006, 112).

After just a month of treatment, Charles had to admit that Gully's treatments were not quackery after all. After sixteen weeks, he felt like a new man, and by June he was able to go home to resume his important work (Grosvenor, 2004). Darwin actually wrote that he was "of almost perfect health" (Burkhardt, 1996, 108).

Despite Darwin's greatly improved health, he never publically attributed any benefits directly to homeopathy. However, one must also realize that even though homeopathy achieved impressive popularity among British royalty, numerous literary greats, and many of the rich and powerful at that time, there was incredible animosity to it from orthodox physicians and scientists. Because Darwin was just beginning to propose his own new ideas about evolution, it would have been professional suicide to broadcast his positive experiences with homeopathy. Having to defend homeopathy would have damaged his credibility among his colleagues who were extremely antagonistic to this emerging medical specialty.

Eighteen months after first going to Dr. Gully, he showed his own skepticism of homeopathy when he wrote in a private letter:

> You speak about Homeopathy, which is a subject which makes me more wrath, even than does Clairvoyance.[47] Clairvoyance so transcends belief, that one's ordinary faculties are put out of the question, but in homeopathy common sense and common observation come into play, and both these must go to the dogs, if the infinitesimal doses

have any effect whatever. How true is a remark I saw the other day by Quetelet [a famous statistician of that time], in respect to evidence of curative processes, viz., that no one knows in disease what is the simple result of nothing being done, as a standard with which to compare homoeopathy, and all other such things. It is a sad flaw, I cannot but think, in my beloved Dr. Gully, that he believes in everything. When Miss — was very ill, he had a clairvoyant girl to report on internal changes, a mesmerist to put her to sleep, an homeopathist, viz. Dr. —, and himself as hydropathist! and the girl recovered. (Letter of September 4, 1850, in Darwin, 1903, 341)

Alongside his skepticism in this letter, he also noted the case of a specific woman who had been cured by Dr. Gully and his team.

Darwin occasionally experienced relapses of some symptoms over the years, so he returned to Dr. Gully for more treatments, staying two to eight weeks. Although Darwin complained during his first visit that he experienced "complete stagnation of the mind," he didn't have similar problems during later visits to Gully's clinic and spa. In fact, he asserted that his mind was alert and that his scientific writing was progressing well (Quammen, 2006, 113).

He lived thirty-three more years, and it is surprising and confusing that the magnificent story of Darwin's successful experiences with homeopathy and hydrotherapy has not become an integral part of the history of science and medicine today. After successful treatment of his persistent nausea and vomiting, frequent fainting spells, spots before his eyes, incapacitating stomach pains, severe boils, and heart palpitations, he was considerably more able to do his seminal scientific work.

Some other people of significant notoriety who benefited from Dr. Gully's care include Charles Dickens (novelist and writer), Alfred, Lord Tennyson (poet), Florence Nightingale (famed nurse), George Eliot (British novelist), Thomas Carlyle (Scottish essayist, satirist, and historian), John Ruskin (art critic and social critic), Edward Bulwer-Lytton (British novelist, playwright, and politician), Thomas Babington Macaulay (first Baron Macaulay, poet and politician), and Bishop Samuel Wilberforce (Desmond and Moore, 1992, 363). Further, three prime ministers sought Dr. Gully's care, including William Gladstone, Benjamin Disraeli, and George Hamilton-Gordon, as well as Queen Victoria herself. Hamilton-Gordon described Dr. Gully as "the most gifted physician of the age" (Ruddick, 2001, 2).

Although there is no evidence that Darwin knew that these other people saw Dr. Gully, Darwin was pleased that his second cousin, William Darwin Fox, the man who introduced Darwin to entomology and to Dr. Gully, had seen the doctor and had benefited from treatment (Burkhardt, 1985, VI, 346). Darwin wrote to Fox on December 7, 1855: "Dr. Gully did me *much* good" (his emphasis).

Some of Darwin's biographers never mention the homeopathic treatment he received. Those biographers who mention his longtime health problems tend to emphasize the hydrotherapy ("water cure") that Dr. Gully's spa provided and that Charles Darwin followed up on this treatment by regularly self-treating himself with cold baths and self-percussion of his body. A recent acclaimed biography of Darwin suggested the benefits he received were from a placebo effect, despite the inability to experience a similar placebo effect from the many other physicians he saw and the various treatments he attempted. This biography asserted that "he persuaded himself that the water-torture was working" (Quammen, 2006, 112). (It is interesting to note that this biographer showed disrespect for hydrotherapy by calling it "water-torture.")

Darwin and many of his biographers have highlighted hydrotherapy because they simply could not believe that homeopathic medicines could provide any benefit. However, one must wonder if hydrotherapy alone could have provided these significant health benefits, and even if it could, the fact is that few English spas of that day provided homeopathic treatment from an expert physician, and it is doubtful that the above mentioned elite who sought care from Dr. Gully could all have benefited primarily or simply from water treatment. The more likely explanation is that homeopathic medicines played a key role in Charles Darwin's (and others') health. What is additionally intriguing about this story of Darwin is that it confirms an ultimately essential observation of truly effective healing methods: that they can and will be effective whether or not the person believes they will work.

Hardened skeptics insist that homeopathic treatment could not have helped Darwin (or anyone) and suggest that hydrotherapy must have been the method of therapeutic benefit. And yet, few orthodox physicians of that day or today would even consider using hydrotherapy for people with complex disease processes.

Despite the wide respect that Dr. Gully received from his many illustrious patients, he was disliked greatly by select orthodox physicians. Sir Charles Hastings, a physician who later helped to found the British Medical Association, was Gully's most vitriolic antagonist. Dr. Hastings was so opposed to hydrotherapy that he frequently wrote articles about its "dangers," while he utilized a wide range of orthodox medical treatments that everyone would soon call simply barbaric (Bradley and Depree, 2003).[48]

Darwin's letters also expressed his thoughts about conventional medicine of his time. He said emphatically that he had "no faith whatever in ordinary Doctoring." And yet, after twelve years of persistent nausea and vomiting, Darwin acknowledged in 1856 that Dr. Gully's treatment in 1849 was successful enough that "never (or almost never) the vomiting returns" (Burkhardt, 1985, VI, 238).

When Dr. Gully retired from his full-time practice in Malvern in the late 1850s,[49] he chose Dr. James Smith Ayerst (1824/5–1884) as his replacement. Not surprisingly, Ayerst was also a homeopathic physician. He served as assistant surgeon in the Royal Navy, was physician to Great Malvern, Worcestershire, ran a hydropathic establishment at Old Well House, Malvern Wells in conjunction with that of Dr. Gully, practiced homeopathy and hygienics, and later, practiced in Torquay, Devon.

Darwin's wife Emma wrote to W. Darwin Fox: "We like Dr. Ayerst, tho' he has not the influence of Dr. Gully. Dr. G. it is hopeless to try to see tho' I must say he has been to see Ch. [Charles] twice & he quite approves of his treatment" (September 29, 1863, in Burkhardt, 1985, XI, 643).

Darwin visited other hydrotherapy spas as well. In 1857 and 1859 he visited Moor Park, run by Edward Wickstead Lane, MD, a physician and hydrotherapist (not a homeopath). And perhaps not by happenstance, Darwin's famed book *On the Origin of Species* was at the printing press, while he was at Ilkley Wells, a spa operated by Edmund Smith, MD, another homeopathic physician (Burkhardt, 1985, XI, 361).

On March 5, 1863, Darwin wrote a letter to J. D. Hooker (a botanist), noting: "A good severe fit of Eczema would do me good, and I have a touch this morning & consequently feel a little alive" (Burkhardt, 1985, XI, 200). On this same day, he wrote his cousin W. Darwin Fox: "I am having an attack of Eczema on my face, which does me as much good as Gout does others" (Burkhardt, 1985, XI, 255).

What is interesting here is that Darwin was either taught or learned from his own experience a common observation in homeopathy: that symptoms on the skin or in the extremities (the symptoms of gout manifest in the big toe) are important externalizations of the disease process that should not be suppressed through conventional drugs. Because homeopaths and other advocates of natural medicine recognize the "wisdom of the body," symptoms, even acute and painful ones, are ways that the body is working to push out and externalize internal pathology.

It is also fascinating to note that Darwin himself conducted several experiments evaluating the effects of small doses on an insect-eating plant (*Drosera rotundifolia,* commonly called sundew) that is commonly used in homeopathic medicine. He found that solutions of certain salts of ammonia stimulated the glands of the plant's tentacles and caused the plant to turn inward. He made this solution more and more dilute, but the plant still was able to detect the presence of the salt. On July 7, 1874, he wrote to a well-known physiologist, Professor F. C. Donders of Utrecht, Netherlands, that he observed that 1/4,000,000 of a grain had a demonstrable effect upon the *Drosera* and "the 1/20,000,000th of a grain of the crystallised salt does the same. Now, I am quite unhappy at the thought of having to publish such a statement." (Darwin, 1903, 498).

Astonished by his observation, Darwin likened it to a dog that perceives the odor of an animal a quarter of a mile distant. He said: "Yet these particles must be infinitely smaller than the one twenty millionth of a grain of phosphate of ammonia" (Darwin, 1875, 173). Darwin said about this spectacular phenomenon:

> The reader will best realize this degree of dilution by remembering that 5,000 ounces would more than fill a thirty-one gallon cask [barrel]; and that to this large body of water one grain of the salt was added; only half a drachm, or thirty minims, of the solution being poured over a leaf. Yet this amount sufficed to cause the inflection of almost every tentacle, and often the blade of the leaf.... My results were for a long time incredible, even to myself, and I anxiously sought for every source of error.... The observations were repeated during several years. Two of my sons, who were as incredulous as myself, compared several lots of leaves simultaneously immersed in the weaker solutions and in water, and declared that there could be no doubt about the difference in their appearance.... In fact every time that we perceive an odor, we have evidence that infinitely smaller particles act on our nerves. (Darwin, 1875, 170)

In Darwin's book on his experiments with *Drosera,* he expressed complete amazement at the hypersensitivity of a plant to extremely small doses of certain chemicals: "Moreover, this extreme sensitiveness, exceeding that of the most delicate part of the human body, as well as the power of transmitting various impulses from one part of the leaf to another, have been acquired without the intervention of any nervous system" (Darwin, 1875, 272).

Yet, Darwin also discovered that *Drosera* is not simply sensitive to every substance. He tested various alkaloids and other substances that act powerfully on humans and animals who have a nervous system but produced no effect on *Drosera*. He concluded that the "power of transmitting an influence to other parts of the leaf, causing movement, or modified secretion, or aggregation, does not depend on the presence of a diffused element, allied to nerve-tissue" (Darwin, 1875, 274).

Darwin confirmed an important homeopathic observation that living systems are hypersensitive to only certain substances. Sadly and strangely, conventional scientists have attacked homeopaths for using extremely small doses of substances without any appreciation for the homeopaths' credo that living systems—whether human, animal, or plant—will be hypersensitive to a limited number of substances (and the homeopathic method of individualizing treatment is a refined method to find this substance or substances).

The archive of letters from Darwin includes one other interesting reference to homeopathy in which its significance is obvious but its meaning not perfectly clear. This was in an August 20, 1862, letter to Asa Gray, a professor of botany (of which the first part, shown below in brackets, was probably written by Francis Darwin, his son and assistant, who collated his father's letters):

> [The greater number of the letters of 1862 deals with the Orchid work, but the wave of conversion to Evolution was still spreading, and reviews and letters bearing on the subject still came in numbers. As an example of the odd letters he received may be mentioned one which arrived in January of this year] from a German homoeopathic doctor, an ardent admirer of the "Origin." Had himself published nearly the same sort of book, but goes much deeper. Explains the origin of plants and animals on the principles of homoeopathy or by the law of spirality. Book fell dead in Germany. Therefore would I translate it and publish it in England. (Darwin, 1903, 175)

What is intriguing about Darwin's statement is that he asserted that this writing by a homeopathic doctor is similar to his own but "goes much deeper." Darwin's noting that this homeopath emphasized "the law of spirality" as an integral part of evolution is fascinating, especially since these insights preceded by nearly a century the seminal work of Watson and Crick discovering the spirality of DNA.

Robert Jütte, PhD, chief historian at the Robert Bosch Institute in

Stuttgart, Germany, where Hahnemann's casebooks reside and which may have the largest homeopathic library in the world, has determined that this German homeopath was probably **Augustus Wilhelm Koch** (1805–1886). Koch was a conventionally trained physician who graduated from the University of Tubingen in Germany in 1831. He began to study and practice homeopathy within a couple of years, and at the invitation of some influential families in Stuttgart, he moved there and developed a successful homeopathic practice. In 1846 he wrote a 613-page book called *Die Homöopathie, physiologisch, pathologisch und therapeutisch begründet: oder das Gesetz des Lebens im gesunden und kranken* (The homeopathic, physiologically, pathologically and therapeutically foundations: or the law of the life in the healthy and ill).

Dr. Jütte notes that in the introduction to this book (p. xv) Koch explains homeopathy scientifically by including it in a more general "Grundgesetz des organischen Lebens," which could be translated as "law of spirality." A whole chapter is devoted to the evolution of crystals, plants, and animals.

A year after Dr. Koch published this book he moved to Philadelphia, though before leaving Europe, he was made an honorary member of the Homeopathic Institute of Paris. While in the U.S., he was an active member of the American Institute of Homeopathy and the Pennsylvania state and Philadelphia county homeopathic medical societies. He even served on the board of trustees of Hahnemann Medical College in Philadelphia (Rogers, 1998, 41). A close friend and colleague of the "father of American homeopathy" Dr. Constantine Hering (1800–1880), Dr. Koch was one of his pallbearers.

Although Koch lived in the U.S. and could speak and write in English, he probably still sought Darwin (or someone else) whose mother tongue was English in order to have the most accurate translation. Sadly, his master work was never published in English.

Despite Darwin's personal experiences and significant successes as a homeopathic patient, he never publically acknowledged the benefits he received. And despite his own experiments on plants using homeopathic doses, he never used the word "homeopathic" in his public writings.

Although these actions may seem surprising, Darwin's decision to avoid reference to homeopathy was an important part of his own survival strategy. The story of Sir John Forbes (below) and others about conventional physicians or scientists here show the dire consequences to those who said anything even slightly positive about this controversial but ultimately powerful medical science and art.

Sir John Forbes, MD

Sir John Forbes (1787–1861) was a leading orthodox physician in England in the mid-1800s. He was personal physician to Queen Victoria (1819–1901), who was one of few British royalty who did not have a homeopathic physician as primary caregiver. Besides serving as the editor of a leading four-volume medical textbook, *The Cyclopaedia of Practical Medicine* (1833–1835), he wrote a critique of homeopathy and its extremely small doses, *Homeopathy, Allopathy and Young Physic* (1846). Although a critic of homeopathy, Forbes wrote some kind and accurate comments about homeopathy's founder, Samuel Hahnemann, MD:

> No careful observer of his actions or candid reader of his writings can hesitate for a moment to admit that he was a very extraordinary man, one whose name will descend to posterity as the exclusive excogitator and founder of an original system of medicine, as ingenious as many that preceded it, and destined, probably, to be the remote, if not the immediate, cause of more important fundamental changes in the practice of the healing art than have resulted from any promulgated since the days of Galen himself. Hahnemann was undoubtedly a man of genius and a scholar, a man of indefatigable industry, of undaunted energy. In the history of medicine his name will appear in the same list with those of the greatest systematists and theorists, surpassed by few in the originality and ingenuity of his views, superior to most in having substantiated and carried

out his doctrines into actual and most extensive practice. By most medical men it was taken for granted that the system is not only visionary in itself, but was the result of a mere fanciful hypothesis, disconnected with facts of any kind, and supported by no processes of ratiocination or logical inference; while its author and his apostles and successors were looked upon either as visionaries or quacks, or both. And yet nothing can be farther from the truth. Whoever examines the homeopathic doctrines as enounced and expounded in the original writings of Hahnemann and of many of his followers, must admit, not only that the system is an ingenious one, but that it professes to be based on a most formidable array of facts and experiments, and that these are woven into a complete code of doctrine with singular dexterity and much apparent fairness. Many among his followers are sincere, honest, and learned men. (Forbes, 1846, 3–4; Clarke, 1905, 43–45)

Despite Forbes's standing in orthodox medicine and with British royalty at the time, and despite his book being mostly critical of homeopathy and its very small doses (which he considered "an outrage to human reason"), his nearly positive remarks about homeopathy were severely attacked, and 1,400 doctors withdrew their subscriptions to the respected journal that Forbes edited (Nichols, 1988, 126). Forbes's words proved fatal to his previously successful medical journal.

Forbes even conducted a study in 1846 which he thought could evaluate the efficacy of homeopathic medicines in the treatment of patients suffering from diarrhea. He prescribed conventional medical treatment to one group and "bread pills" to another group. Because he (mistakenly) assumed that homeopathic medicines were the same as bread pills, he thought he was making an adequate evaluation of homeopathic treatment (Dean, 2006). Sadly, there is a long history of conventional doctors testing the efficacy of homeopathic medicines with similar harebrained ideas (Dean, 2004, 143).

Sir William Osler, MD

Sir William Osler, MD (1849–1919), is commonly called the father of modern medicine. Born in Canada, he obtained his medical degree from McGill University and then completed further study in London, Berlin, and Vienna before returning to Canada in 1874, where he joined the medical faculty at McGill. In 1884 he became a professor at the University of Pennsylvania, and in 1889, he became physician-in-chief of the new Johns Hopkins Hospital and a professor of medicine at the Johns Hopkins School of Medicine in 1893. Osler's book *The Principles and Practice of Medicine* (1892) remained the standard text on clinical medicine for the next forty years. In 1905 he accepted the Regius Professorship of Medicine at Oxford University, which at the time was the most prestigious medical appointment in the English-speaking world.

In Osler's farewell address to the American medical profession, he said:

> It is not as if our homeopathic brothers are asleep: far from it, they are awake—many of them at any rate—to the importance of the scientific study of disease. ... It is distressing to think that so many good men live isolated, in a measure, from the great body of the profession. The original grievous mistake was ours—to quarrel with our brothers over infinitesimals was a most unwise and stupid thing to do. (Osler, 1905)

Time magazine reported that before Osler's death in 1919, he expressed even greater support for homeopathy and its founder, asserting that "No individual has done more good to the medical profession than Samuel Hahnemann" (Homeopathy, 1940).[50]

Emil Adolph von Behring, MD

Emil Adolph von Behring, MD (1854–1917), won the first Nobel Prize in medicine or physiology for his discovery of the diphtheria antitoxin. Later, he discovered the tetanus antitoxin. For many years he served as military captain of the medical corps to the Pharmacological Institute at the University of Bonn, and then was given a position at the Hygiene Institute of

Berlin in 1888 as assistant to Robert Koch (1843–1910), one of the pioneers of bacteriology. He then became professor of hygienics in the Faculty of Medicine at the prestigious University of Marburg. Because of his significant discoveries in immunology, Behring retains a highly regarded place in its early history.

In 1892 Behring actually experimented with serial (homeopathic) dilutions and found paradoxically enhanced immunogenic activity, but he was advised to suppress this experiment due to the aid and comfort it would provide to homeopaths. Only after he won the Nobel Prize did he feel comfortable in making public these experiments (Behring, 1905; Coulter, 1994, 97).

Behring broke from orthodox medical tradition by recognizing the value of the homeopathic law of similars:

> In spite of all scientific speculations and experiments regarding smallpox vaccination, Jenner's discovery remained an erratic blocking medicine, till the biochemically thinking Pasteur, devoid of all medical classroom knowledge, traced the origin of this therapeutic block to a principle which cannot better be characterized than by Hahnemann's word: homeopathic. Indeed, what else causes the epidemiological immunity in sheep, vaccinated against anthrax than the influence previously exerted by a virus, similar in character to that of the fatal anthrax virus? And by what technical term could we more appropriately speak of this influence, exerted by a similar virus than by Hahnemann's word "homeopathy"? I am touching here upon a subject anathematized till very recently by medical penalty: but if I am to present these problems in historical illumination, dogmatic imprecations must not deter me. (Behring, 1905)

Behring actually made a plea for homeopathy to be granted "citizenship of medicine" (*medicinisches Bürgerrecht*) and that it no longer be taboo for physicians to practice it. Behring even said he would go to a homeopath himself: "If I were confronted with a hitherto incurable disease and could see no way to treat it other than homeopathy, I can assure you that I would not be deterred from following this course by dogmatic considerations" (Behring, 1905; Coulter, 1994, 98).

Behring also showed a certain sophisticated understanding of Hahnemann's contribution to medicine and pharmacology: "The concept that the sick person reacts differently to medications than the healthy one, which had to be established empirically by therapeutic trials, also played a role in Hahnemann's thinking" (from a Behring article in 1915, quoted in Coulter, 1994, 96).

The point here is that Behring understood that homeopaths determine the effectiveness of a medicine by conducting experiments in toxicology in which relatively healthy people are given repeated doses of a substance until symptoms of overdose are created. Every simple or complex substance will create its own toxicological syndrome of symptoms, and homeopathic doses of that substance can and will heal people who have that similar symptom complex. The logic here is because symptoms of illness, from whatever cause, are adaptive efforts of the body to fight infection or adapt to some sort of stress, the use of a medicinal agent that mimics the body's defenses will provide immunological benefit to the sick person.

In 1898 Behring asserted that Koch's discovery of the Tuberculin bacilli and his use of it to treat people for tuberculosis falls under the homeopathic principle, as does Pasteur's rabies therapy (Coulter, 1994, 96). Koch and Pasteur could not and certainly would not give homeopathy credit for any insight or contribution to their discovery, or if they did, they and their new medicine would have been harshly attacked.

By the mid-1890s, as a result of Koch's claims, London homeopath Dr. James Compton-Burnett (1840–1901)[51] used homeopathic doses of the tuberculous sputum to treat fifty-four people, calling this medicine *Bacillinum*. Compton-Burnett aptly differentiated his medicine from Koch's:

> The difference between our old friend [homeopathic] Tuberculinum or Bacillinum and that of Koch lies in the way it is obtained; our is the virus of the natural disease

itself, while Koch's is the same virus artificially obtained in an incubator from colonies of bacilli thriving on beef-jelly; ours is the chick hatched under the hen. Koch's is the chick hatched in an incubator. (Compton-Burnett, 1890, xiii–xiv)

Sydney Ringer, MD

Sydney Ringer, MD (1835–1910), was a professor at the University College in London, and an extremely influential conventional physician. He is known today for his invention of Ringer's solution, a salt-and-mineral solution that has a consistency similar to blood and is used clinically for burns and wounds, and in many laboratory experiments. Ringer's classic book *Handbook of Therapeutics* (1870) was the first conventional medical textbook to incorporate a significant number of homeopathic medicines. More than 100 of the 474 medicines listed in this textbook were common homeopathic medicines of the day. While Ringer recommended smaller doses of various medicines than were usually recommended for conventional drugs of that day, he didn't recommend them in the extremely small doses used by homeopaths. Moreover, Ringer oversimplified their clinical application by recommending that these medicines be used for specific diseases, without the individualizing process that is inherent in the homeopathic prescription of remedies. Because of these significant problems, homeopathic physicians were highly critical of the book and its author (Coulter, 1994, 476–478).

Mary Everest Boole

The vast majority of people reading this book probably have no idea who Mary Boole (1832–1916) was. She and her family made major contributions to her time and the future, and they were serious advocates for homeopathy. Her father was Rev. Thomas Everest, a minister, who moved the family to France in order to receive homeopathic treatment from Dr. Samuel Hahnemann.[52] Mary's uncle, Colonel Sir George Everest, was Surveyor General of India, and for his contributions to geography, the tallest mountain in the world is named after him.

Mary's husband was George Boole (1815–1864), a mathematician and philosopher and inventor of Boolean algebra, which is the basis of all modern computer arithmetic. Because of this seminal contribution, Boole is regarded today as one of the founders of the field of computer science, even though computers did not exist in his day.

Mary Boole was one of the few leading women mathematicians during the nineteenth century. She considered herself a mathematical psychologist. Her goal was to try "to understand how people, and especially children, learned mathematics and science, using the reasoning parts of their minds, their physical bodies, and their unconscious processes," and her textbook *Philosophy and Fun of Algebra* (1909) was used in classrooms for many decades (Perl, 1993, 56). Many of Mary Boole's contributions can be seen in the modern classroom today.

The *Oxford Dictionary of National Biography* states for Mary Boole: "Although she took homeopathic theories to extremes, she frequently offered sound advice" (2004).

August Bier, MD

Without Dr. August Bier (1861–1949) and his discoveries, many surgeries during the past century would be impossible, and many more women would die during childbirth. After professorships in Greifswald and Bonn, Bier became head of the surgical department at the University of Berlin. Bier's significant contribution to medicine and surgery was the development of the first spinal anesthetic. In 1908 he modified his initial discovery by pioneering the use of intravenous procaine analgesia. Anesthesiologists today still use the term "Bier block" for intravenous regional anesthesia, where a local anesthetic, usually Lidocaine, is injected into a vein in a limb below a tourniquet applied at pressure high enough to trap the anesthetic.

August Bier conducted his own experiment testing homeopathic treatment of a dermatological condition, one of his medical specialties (in addition to surgery). Bier was knowledgeable of the well-known toxicological effects of sulphur, especially for its tendency to create various skin symptoms, including abscesses, eruptions, and furunculosis (recurrent boils). Bier was advised by a respected German homeopath to test *Sulphur iodatum* D3 (aka 3X) in the treatment of people with chronic furunculosis, and chose to test *Sulphur iodatum* D6 in a consecutive series of thirty-four cases, many of whom had undergone various conventional treatments unsuccessfully. In his experiment Bier found that every patient was cured, including three patients who had benefited from D6 of this remedy but had relapsed but then responded favorably to D3.

Bier also tested this homeopathic medicine in the treatment of twenty-eight patients with acute furunculosis, and he again observed consistently effective treatment. Bier then tested this medicine in the treatment of various types of acne, and although he found good results, they were not as consistently effective as in the treatment of boils.

Bier's conclusions were that homeopathic medicines were "better, simpler, and cheaper" than the best that conventional medicine offered (Dean, 2004).[53]

Bier gave a remarkable lecture, "What Shall Be Our Attitude Towards Homeopathy?" that was published in a booklet as well as in a homeopathic journal (1925). Being a conventional physician and respected surgeon who worked in a leading university hospital, his pro-homeopathy statement created a very positive but short-lived spin for homeopathy. Besides speaking in strong support for homeopathy, he praised homeopathy's founder:

> Hahnemann was a very eminent, and in spite of his one-sided homeopathic viewpoint, a singularly well-versed physician. As a dietitian and hygienist he was far ahead of his times. As such he gave excellent instructions, which are exemplary to this day, regarding prophylaxis and disinfection in infectious diseases, regarding the mode of living, ventilation, nursing, bringing up of children, puerperal and infant care (he advocated breastfeeding), civic and prison hygiene.

Emil Grubbe, MD

Emil Grubbe, MD (1875–1960), was the first person to use radiation to treat a person with cancer (Dearborn, 2005). In January 1896, Grubbe applied radiation treatment to Mrs. Rose Lee, a woman with breast cancer, who was referred to him by Dr. Reuben Ludlam, the chairman of pathology, physiology, and clinical medicine at Hahnemann Medical College of Chicago.

At this time, Dr. Grubbe was a student at the Hahnemann Medical College. Grubbe's hand and neck developed blisters and tumors as a result of overexposure to X-rays during the course of his experiments with this new technology. Because radiation was clearly determined to be the cause of tumors, one of the professors at the homeopathic college suggested its therapeutic use in cancers. This incident is but one more example from history in which an insight from a homeopathic perspective has provided an important breakthrough in medical treatment, even if the high doses of radiation used still needs greater refinement for its safest and most effective application.

Although Grubbe had to have one arm amputated, he lived a long life (85 years), in part due to homeopathic treatment. Grubbe became professor of electro-therapeutics and radiography at Hahnemann around 1904 and continued in this position until 1919. Grubbe ultimately claimed to be the first professor of Roentgenology in the world (Hodges, 1964). True to his interests in conveying his discoveries to all doctors, Dr. Grubbe served as professor at four different medical schools in Chicago, including homeopathic, eclectic, and allopathic medical schools. At Hahnemann Medical College, he may have been the first to organize the modern-day precursor to continuing medical education (CME) programs by offering two-week courses in radiation physics and the uses of radiation in the treatment of disease.

Harold Randall Griffith, MD

Although the name of Dr. Harold Griffith (1894–1985) may not be familiar, he was a giant in the field of anesthesia. In fact, one of Dr. Griffith's biographers succinctly summarized his medical contribution: "It has been said there are only two eras in anesthesia, before Harold Griffith and after" (Canadian Anesthesiologists' Society).

Harold Griffith's father was Alexander Randall Griffith, MD, who graduated from New York Homeopathic Medical College in 1891 and from New York Ophthalmic Hospital's specialty program in 1892. Dr. Alexander Griffith was medical chief of the Montreal Homeopathic Hospital from 1898 until his death in 1936, at which time his son, Harold, succeeded him. Harold's brother James was surgeon-in-chief from 1937 to 1966.

As children, Harold and his older brother Hugh contracted diphtheria, and with both conventional and homeopathic treatment, they were among the few people to survive this deadly disease.

Harold Griffith was trained in medicine at McGill University, but due to his special interest in homeopathy, he obtained a homeopathic medical degree from the Hahnemann Medical College in Philadelphia. He moved back to Montreal to work alongside his father and brother, both of whom were homeopathic physicians at the Homeopathic Hospital of Montreal. He became chief of anesthesia at the hospital, where for forty-three years he served as chief anesthetist and thirty-nine years as medical superintendent[54] (today, this hospital is known as Queen Elizabeth Hospital). Under his direction, the Homeopathic Hospital of Montreal was the first in Canada to have a surgical recovery room (Shephard, 2004).

Griffith made medical history in 1942 when he became the first doctor in the world to use curare to relax the muscles of a patient undergoing an appendectomy. He was the first president of the Canadian Anesthetists' Society upon its founding in 1943, and in 1955 became founding president of the World Federation of Societies of Anesthesiologists. In 1951, he became chairman of the department of anesthesiology at McGill University.

One of Griffith's classmates at the Hahnemann Medical College was Henry Ruth, MD, who stayed and practiced in Philadelphia. Ultimately, this fellow homeopath Dr. Ruth became the founding editor of the leading journal in their field, *Anesthesiology,* which was published by the American Society of Anesthetists.[55]

Griffith maintained a lifelong appreciation for homeopathic medicines to prevent the need for surgery, but he was ready, willing, and certainly able to provide his surgical skills when necessary. He prescribed homeopathic medicines to many patients pre- and post-surgery to help in their recovery. During his years at the homeopathic hospital, the most commonly treated diseases included pneumonia, typhoid fever, tuberculosis, puerperal fever as a complication of childbirth, syphilis, pernicious anemia, and diabetes. Despite the serious nature of these and other illnesses, Griffith maintained that homeopathic medicines were a useful therapy in which 60–70 percent of patients responded favorably (Bodman and Gillies, 1996, 38).

Although Griffith was strongly partial to homeopathic treatment, he insisted that the hospital maintain an "open door" policy of employing both homeopathic and allopathic (conventional) physicians.

Charles Frederick Menninger, MD

Charles Frederick Menninger, MD (1862–1953), was the co-founder (with his son, Karl Menninger, MD) of the famed Menninger Clinic, the internationally respected mental health clinic, initially located in Topeka, Kansas. He was a homeopathic physician and the head of his local homeopathic medical society. He also authored numerous articles published in homeopathic medical journals. In one of these articles, he stated with vigor: "Homeopathy is wholly capable of satisfying the therapeutic demands of this age better than any other system or school of medicine." He further asserted: "It is imperative that we *exhaust* the homeopathic healing art before resorting to any other mode of treatment, if we wish to accomplish the greatest success possible" (Menninger, 1897, 430).

In another article, he declared:

> It is no easy matter to conform to all the mathematic requirements that constitute the homeopathic law of cure. It is an easy matter resort to "general principles." But how varied the result! The one has demonstrated the existence

of the great law of therapeutics—*similar similibus curentur* (Latin: "let likes cure like," the basic principle of homeopathy)—the greatest boon God has given to disease-stricken men, and the other has been as barren of fruit as the desert of Sahara. (Menninger, 1896, 317–318)

Later in this article, he further asserted: "I have found that the element of success in homeopathic prescribing lies in the closest study of the details, the faithful writing out of all the symptoms of the case and noting the effects of the minimum dose of the single remedy" (Menninger, 1896, 320).

Clearly, Menninger was not just a homeopath; he was what would be called a "Hahnemannian homeopath."

Biographies of Menninger, like so many other biographies of homeopaths and their patients, report on his homeopathic training and practice in a biased and ill-informed way. For instance, Walker Winslow's *The Menninger Story* (1956) stated that C. F. Menninger "made his final break with that sect and was accepted into the County Medical Society as a full member" in 1898 (p. 104). It is typical for those who disliked homeopathy to call its practitioners a "sect," as though it were some sort of religious order. Further, it should be noted that Menninger may have joined the local medical society, like many homeopathic doctors tried to do, in order to get and share information about new advances in medicine and old tried-and-true medical practices.

However, he was chairman of the Materia Medica Section of the American Institute of Homeopathy's annual conference in 1902 (TAIH, 1902), and he was a dues-paying member of the American Institute of Homeopathy until at least 1908 (TAIH, 1908). Winslow acknowledged that throughout his life Menninger "did not hesitate to use homeopathic remedies when he thought they were needed" (1956, 105), though like too many other historians who were antagonistic to homeopathy, Winslow ignored homeopathy and provided little detail on Menninger's passion for and use of homeopathic medicines.

Grant L. Selfridge, MD

Grant L. Selfridge, MD (1863–?), was a San Francisco otorhinolaryngologist (ear, nose, and throat specialist) who was trained at Hahnemann Medical College and was one of three medical doctors to found the Western Society of the Study of Hay Fever, Asthma, and Allergic Diseases in 1923. This organization later changed its name to the American Association for the Study of Allergy and still later became the American Academy of Allergy (the name that it still holds today). Selfridge was the first President of the Western Society. He was also the first physician to conduct a botanical and pollen survey in the West and was the first physician in San Francisco to remove a patient's tonsils surgically.

In 1931, he resigned from the Western Society to devote his time to popularizing the use of vitamins. He designed a special vitamin B complex called the "Selfridge formula" that he found effective in treating allergies, alcoholism, and hypertension. He also led a vigorous effort to establish a governmental institute of nutrition, and this effort evolved into the National Institutes of Health (Cohen, 1979).

Royal S. Copeland, MD

Royal Samuel Copeland, MD (1868–1938), graduated from the Homeopathic Medical College at the University of Michigan in Ann Arbor in 1889. He later served there as professor of ophthalmology and otology (eyes and ear health), and was elected mayor of Ann Arbor in 1901. He moved to New York City because he was appointed dean of the New York Homeopathic Medical College, and he served in this position from 1908 to 1923. He was elected President of the American Institute of Homeopathy in 1908. He was appointed president of the New York Board of Health from 1918 to 1923, and served in this position during the infamous flu epidemic of 1918.

Metropolitan Hospital was a very large homeopathic hospital on Ward's Island in New York with more than 1,800 beds, and it had the lowest mortality rate from the 1918 flu of any city hospital in the United States (Winston, 1999, 234). Due to having several other homeopathic hospitals in New York City at the time,[56] all of which also had extremely low death rates in this epidemic, Copeland bragged that they had the fewest deaths by percentage than any other city in the world (Robins, 2005, 154).

Homeopathy's success in treating the notorious flu of 1918 is not surprising. The leading reason that homeopathy gained such popularity during the nineteenth century was its significant and obvious successes in treating the many infectious diseases of that era, including epidemics of scarlet fever, typhoid, yellow fever, and cholera (Bradford, 1900, 112–146; Coulter, 1973). And bringing this historical experience up to date, three large modern studies have tested a popular homeopathic medicine from France in the treatment of the flu, and found this medicine to be clinically effective (Casanova and Gerard, 1992; Ferley, et al., 1989; Papp, et al., 1998). Even the internationally respected Cochran Commission issued a report on this homeopathic medicine asserting that, based on the three studies, the efficacy of this remedy is "promising" (Vickers, 2005).

Of additional interest is the fact that the specific medicine tested is a popular homeopathic medicine called *Oscillococcinum,* made from the liver and heart of a duck. With the present (2006) terror about avian flu, it is impressive to note that homeopaths have known that ducks (and birds) are carriers of various flu viruses since 1928 when this medicine was initially used and have turned this knowledge into the creation of an effective remedy for the flu, with replicated clinical trials to confirm personal and clinical experiences.

After Copeland's successful term as president of the New York Board of Health, he ran for the U.S. Senate as a Democrat in 1923, at the encouragement of his friend and major power broker, William Randolph Hearst. Franklin D. Roosevelt served as honorary campaign manager in his first election (Robins, 2005, 166). He was elected to the Senate three times.

Copeland was the primary author of the famous Federal Food, Drug, and Cosmetics Act of 1938. This important law empowered the U.S. Food and Drug Administration (FDA) to regulate food, drugs, and cosmetics, and is considered by some people to be the most important consumer rights legislation ever passed. This Act also gave official and formal recognition to the *U.S. Homeopathic Pharmacopeia* as a legal compendium of drugs. Just two days after this law was passed, Dr. Copeland died.

Copeland expressed frequent concern about the prejudice against homeopathy and homeopaths, asserting that orthodox doctors "have not looked squarely and without bias" at the facts and results of homeopathy, though he felt that this was not the result of ill will but, rather, inertia. He further asserted that orthodox doctors had "an implanted and nurtured skepticism... because in their early years their colleges mocked and vilified us, and ever since they have fed upon a blinding literature of prejudice and injustice" (Robins, 2005, 54).

William J. Mayo, MD, and Charles H. Mayo

William W. Mayo (1819–1911) and his two sons, William J. Mayo, MD (1861–1939), and Charles H. Mayo (1865–1939), founded the famed Mayo Clinic in Rochester, Minnesota, which became, shortly after its founding in the 1890s, one of the most highly respected medical research and treatment centers in the world.

Although the Mayo Clinic has been a longtime bastion of conventional medicine, its founders often had kind and supportive words for homeopathy and homeopaths.

Virginia Johnson, MD, a 1913 graduate of Chicago's Hering Medical College, remembered an interesting experience she had at a surgery conference at the Mayo Clinic in 1917 (Enstram, 1953). William J. Mayo asked those attending the conference if there was a homeopath in the audience, and Dr. Johnson raised her hand. He said that he had great respect for homeopaths. He said lots of surgery was unnecessary, and he expressed confidence that the public would become aware of the "wonderful results of homeopathic prescribing in the elimination of unnecessary surgery," but probably not in his own generation but in two or three generations into the future. He particularly expressed serious concern about the appalling amount of unnecessary surgery on women of his day.

William J. Mayo also said something positive about homeopathy and homeopaths when he asserted, "There has always been a place in organized medicine for minority voices, and may the day never come when they do not rule" (Hertzog, 1949). This somewhat surprising statement must be understood in its context. At the time, many states' examining boards included conventional, homeopathic, and eclectic physicians, and all of the individuals were graduates of various types of medical schools. Mayo's concern was that if the homeopaths and eclectic doctors were not on the examining boards, then the public would be besieged with an onslaught of other non-doctor healers, including herbalists, naturopaths (of their day), hypnotists, midwives, and other "cultists" (as he and other conventional physicians called them) (Hertzog, 1949, 1193).

In 1922 Dr. Charles Mayo was asked to come to the White House to treat the wife of U.S. President Warren Harding. Mrs. Harding was experiencing an infection in the one remaining kidney she had. Dr. Mayo recommended immediate surgery, but Mrs. Harding chose to take the advice of two homeopathic doctors and quickly recovered. Although Dr. Mayo's statement to the public indicated that Mrs. Harding "spontaneously" recovered, but he and his brother had seen many similar impressive clinical results from homeopathic medicines.

One medical historian noted one of the Mayo brothers had enough respect for homeopathy's founder, Dr. Samuel Hahnemann, that he once asserted: "He was 100 years ahead of his time" (Hertzog, 1940, 334).

Charles Best, MD

Sometimes medical history is made not because of a direct influence by a homeopathic doctor but because of an indirect effect, and such is the case with the story of Dr. Charles Best.

Charles Best, MD (1899–1978), was a member of the team of scientists who isolated a secretion from the pancreas that was later called insulin. When his colleagues Frederick Banting and J. J. R. Macleod were awarded the Nobel Prize for this discovery in 1923, the Nobel committee surprisingly didn't acknowledge the role that Best played in the discovery. Frederick Banting was so upset about this oversight that he gave half of his award money to Best.

Although Charles Best was not an advocate for homeopathy, he owed a small amount of his successes to it. Best lived with his uncle and aunt,

Reverend William T. Hallam and Lillian Hallam, when he was in high school, and he continued to live with them when he went to college and then to medical school at the University of Toronto. Reverend Hallam was a professor of Greek and Hebrew at this university, and the Hallams' physician was Pat Hardy, MD,[57] a respected homeopathic doctor (Best, 2003, 24).

In late 1917 and early 1918, Charles Best had difficulty getting accepted into the army because of a systolic murmur caused either by scarlet fever or measles. Finally, he found a recruiting officer on duty at the Toronto armories—Dr. Pat Hardy, the Hallams' homeopath, who pronounced him perfectly fit to serve in the army. Dr. Best ultimately made some important contacts in the military that led him to work in the laboratory with Banting and Macleod.

C. Everett Koop, MD

C. Everett Koop, MD (1916–), was Surgeon General of the United States from 1982 to 1989, and was for many years the most well-known and respected doctor in America. In his autobiography, Dr. Koop wrote: "I can't remember a time when I didn't want to be a doctor. The doctors I knew as a very young child must have helped to plant the desire in me, when I was as young as age five or six. One homeopathic physician, Dr. Justice Gage Wright, was a great model"[58] (Koop, 1992, 35).

Despite this personal and powerful experience, Dr. Koop has kept some distance from homeopathy, at least publicly. Although he has on occasion spoken at alternative medicine conferences and has told others of his early experiences with homeopathy, he has remained silent about homeopathy's history and its present status.

Brian Josephson, PhD

Brian Josephson, PhD (1940–), is a British physicist who won a Nobel Prize in Physics in 1973 for work he completed when he was only 22 years old. He is currently a professor at the University of Cambridge where he is the head of the mind-matter unification project in the Theory of Condensed Matter research group.

Responding to an article in the *New Scientist* (October 18, 1997), Josephson wrote:

> Regarding your comments on claims made for homeopathy: criticisms centered around the vanishingly small number of solute molecules present in a solution after it has been repeatedly diluted are beside the point, since advocates of homeopathic remedies attribute their effects not to molecules present in the water, but to modifications of the water's structure.
>
> Simple-minded analysis may suggest that water, being a fluid, cannot have a structure of the kind that such a picture would demand. But cases such as that of liquid crystals, which while flowing like an ordinary fluid can maintain an ordered structure over macroscopic distances, show the limitations of such ways of thinking. There have not, to the best of my knowledge, been any refutations of homeopathy that remain valid after this particular point is taken into account.
>
> A related topic is the phenomenon, claimed by Jacques Benveniste's colleague Yolène Thomas and by others to be well established experimentally, known as "memory of water." If valid, this would be of greater significance than homeopathy itself, and it attests to the limited vision of the modern scientific community that, far from hastening to test such claims, the only response has been to dismiss them out of hand. (Josephson, 1997)

Josephson's remarks on the structure of water have been confirmed by more recent research (Roy, et al., 2005). Professors of material sciences, in conjunction with an MD/PhD homeopath, have written a review of basic science research on the important but technical subject of the structure of water. These leading scientists described how the process of making homeopathic medicines changes the water to turn it into a medicine and differentiate it from simple or plain water. The shaking process, an integral part of making homeopathic medicines, is now known to create bubbles and nano-bubbles that change the pressure and structure of the water.

Josephson was interviewed by the *New Scientist* (December 9, 2006), and asked to comment on how he became an advocate of unconventional ideas. He responded:

> I went to a conference where the French immunologist Jacques Benveniste was talking for the first time about his discovery that water has a 'memory' of compounds that were once dissolved in it—which might explain how homeopathy works. His findings provoked irrationally strong reactions from scientists, and I was struck by how badly he was treated.

Josephson went on to describe how many scientists today suffer from "pathological disbelief"; that is, they maintain an unscientific attitude that is embodied by the statement "even if it were true I wouldn't believe it."

These stories from many of the most respected scientists and physicians of the past 200 years present its own strong body of evidence for the efficacy of homeopathic medicine. When you add to these significant personal experiences with the large and growing body of evidence from basic sciences as well as from clinical research, it can and must be asserted that only those with a closed and unscientific mind would assume that homeopathic medicines are only or primarily a placebo response.

References
Behring, A. E. von. *Moderne Phthisiogenetische und Phthisotherapeutische: Probleme in Historischer Beleuchtung.* Margurg: Selbsteverlag des Verfassers, 1905.

Best, H. B. M. *Margaret and Charley: The Personal Story of Dr. Charles Best, the Co-Discoverer of Insulin.* Toronto: Dundurn Press, 2003.

Bier, A. What Shall Be Our Attitude Toward Homeopathy? *Homeopathic Recorder,* December 15, 1925, XL(12):529–567.

Bodman, R., and Gillies, D. *Harold Griffith.* Toronto: Dundurn Press, 1996.

Bradford, T. L. *The Life and Letters of Samuel Hahnemann.* Philadelphia: Boericke and Tafel, 1895.

Bradford, T. L. *The Logic of Figures or Comparative Results of Homoeopathic and Other Treatments.* Philadelphia: Boericke and Tafel, 1900, pp. 112–146.

Bradley, J., and Depree, M. A Shadow of Orthodoxy? An Epistemology of British Hydropathy, 1840–1858, *Medical History,* 2003, 47:173–194.

Burkhardt, F., and Smith, S. (eds.). *The Correspondence of Charles Darwin.* Cambridge: Cambridge University Press, 1985.

Burkhardt, F., ed. *Charles Darwin's Letters: A Selection (1825–1859).* Cambridge: Cambridge University Press, 1996.

Campbell, A. K., and Matthews, S. B. Darwin's Illness Revealed, *Postgraduate Medicine Journal,* 2005, 81:248–251.

Canadian Anesthesiologists' Society. Anesthesia Greats. Harold Randall Griffith. www.cas.ca/about/history/greats/griffith.asp

Casanova, P., and Gerard, R. *Bilan de 3 annees d'etudes randomisees multicentriques oscillococcinum/placebo, oscillococcinum rassegna della letterature internationale.* Milan: Laboratoires Boiron, 1992, pp. 11–16.

Clarke, J. C. *Homoeopathy Explained.* London: Homoeopathic Publishing Company, 1905.

Cohen, S. G. The American Academy of Allergy: An Historical Review, *Journal of Allergy and Clinical Immunology,* November 1979, 64(5):332–346.

Compton-Burnett, J. *Consumption and Its Cure.* London: Homoeopathic Publishing, 1890. (Now available in a compendium of his work called *The Best of Burnett,* New Delhi: B. Jain, no date.)

Coulter, H. L. *Homeopathic Influences in Nineteenth Century Allopathic Therapeutics.* St. Louis: Formur, 1973.

Coulter, H. L., *Divided Legacy: A History of the Schism in Medical Thought.* Berkeley: North Atlantic Books, 1973, volume III, p. 39.

Coulter, H. L. *Divided Legacy: A History of the Schism in Medical Thought.* Volume IV: Twentieth-Century Medicine: The Bacteriological Era. Berkeley: North Atlantic Books, 1994.

Cushing, H. W. *Life of Sir William Osler.* London: Oxford University Press, 1940, p. 171.

Darwin, C. *Insectivorous Plants.* New York: D. Appleton & Co., 1875. http://pages.britishlibrary.net/charles.darwin3/insectivorous/insect_fm.htm

Darwin, F., ed. *The Life and Letters of Charles Darwin.* New York: D. Appleton & Co., 1903. (It is interesting to observe how various biographers of Darwin dealt with his longtime and serious illness and his treatment. Many simply ignored it. One placed the quote from Darwin about his skepticism of homeopathy as though he said it several years after treatment, when, in fact, it was said during his first month of treatment. See Keynes, 2002, 169.)

Dean, M. E. *The Trials of Homeopathy.* Essen, Germany: KVC, 2004.

Dean, M. E. An Innocent Deception: Placebo Controls in the St. Petersburg Homeopathy Trial, 1829–1830, *Journal of the Royal Society of Medicine,* July 2006, 99:375–376.

Dearborn, F. *Encyclopedia of 20th-Century Technology* (2 vols.). New York: Routledge, 2005.

Desmond, A., and Moore, J. *Darwin*. New York: Warner, 1992.

Enstram, C. H. Non-surgically yours, *Homeopathic Recorder,* December 1953, 69(6). (This piece was read before the Bureau of Surgery, Gynecology and Obstetrics, IHA (International Hahnemannian Association), in July 1953.)

Everest, Rev. T. R. *A Popular View of Homeopathy.* New York: William Radde, 1842.

Ferley, J. P., Zmirou, D., D'Admehar, D., et. al. A Controlled Evaluation of a Homoeopathic Preparation in the Treatment of Influenza-like Syndrome, *British Journal of Clinical Pharmacology,* March 1989, 27:329–335.

Fishbein, M. *Medical Follies.* New York: Boni & Liveright, 1925.

Forbes, Sir J. *Homeopathy, Allopathy and Young Physic.* Boston: Otis Clapp, 1846.

Grosvenor, P. C. Darwin and the Barnacle: The Story of One Tiny Creature and History's Most Spectacular Scientific Breakthrough (review), *Perspectives in Biology and Medicine,* Autumn 2004, 47(4):624–626.

Hahnemann, S. Cause and Prevention of the Asiatic Cholera, from *Archiv. F. hom. Heilk,* XI, 1831. (Also published in Hahnemann, *Lesser Writings.* New York: William Radde, 1852, p. 758.

Hahnemann, S. *Organon of the Medical Art* (edited and annotated by W. B. O'Reilly). Palo Alto: Birdcage, 1996. (This book has been translated many times over the years; this edition is considered the best translation.)

Hertzog, L. S. The Rise of Homeopathy in Ohio, *Ohio State Archaeological and Historical Quarterly,* 1940, 49: 332–346.

Hertzog, L. High Spots of Ohio Homeopathic History 1890–1949, *Ohio State Medical Journal,* December 1949, 45:1189–1195.

Homeopathy, *Time,* May 27, 1940.

Hodges, P. C. *The Life and Times of Emil H. Grubbe.* Chicago: University of Chicago, 1964.

Josephson, B. D., Letter, *New Scientist,* November 1, 1997.

Jurj, G. Quiet At Koethen, *Simillimum,* Winter/Spring 2007, 20:27–42.

Jütte, R. Personal communication, March 29–30, 2006.

Keynes, R. *Darwin: His Daughter and Human Evolution.* New York: Riverhead, 2002.

Koop, C. E. *Koop: The Memoirs of America's Family Doctor.* New York: Harper, 1992.

Menninger, C. F. The Application as Well as the Similar, *Transactions of the American Institute of Homeopathy,* 1896, pp. 317–324.

Menninger, C. F. Some Reflections Relative to the Symptomatology and Materia Medica of Typhoid Fever, *Transactions of the American Institute of Homeopathy,* 1897:427–431.

Neng, H. Homoeopathy in Germany during the Last Ten Years, *Homoeopathic Recorder,* January 1930, 45, 1.

Osler, Sir W. *Unity, Peace and Concord—A Farewell Address to the Medical Profession of the United States.* Oxford University Press, 1905:12–13. (Osler was also once quoted to say: "No one will deny that as many patients recover under homeopathic treatment as recover under any form of treatment." See the Robins listing, below, page 59.)

Oxford Dictionary of National Biography. Oxford: Oxford University Press, 2004.

Papp, R., Schuback, G., Beck, E., et al. Oscillococcinum in Patients with Influenza-like Syndromes: A Placebo Controlled Double-blind Evaluation, *British Homeopathic Journal,* April 1998, 87:69–76.

Perl, T. *Women and Numbers.* San Carlos, Calif.: Wide World Publishing, 1993, pp. 45–56.

Quammen, D. *The Reluctant Mr. Darwin: An Intimate Portrait of Charles Darwin and the Making of His Theory of Evolution.* New York: W. W. Norton, 2006.

Robins, N. *Copeland's Cure.* New York: Knopf, 2005.

Rogers, N. *An Alternative Path: The Making and Remaking of Hahnemann Medical College and Hospital of Philadelphia.* Piscataway: Rutgers University Press, 1998.

Rothstein, W. *American Physicians in the Nineteenth Century.* Baltimore: Johns Hopkins University Press, 1985.

Roy, R., Tiller, W. A., Bell, I., and Hoover, M. R. The Structure of Liquid Water: Novel Insights from Materials Research; Potential Relevance to Homeopathy, *Materials Research Innovations,* December 2005, 9(4):577–608.

Ruddick, J. *Death at the Priory: Sex, Love and Murder in Victorian England.* New York: Atlantic Monthly Press, 2001.

Shephard, D. E. *Preserving the Heritage of Canadian Anesthesiology: A Panorama of People, Ideas, Techniques and Events.* Saint-Laurent, Quebec, Canada: Abbott Laboratories, 2004.

TAIH, *Transactions of the American Institute of Homoeopathy.* Chicago: Publication Committee, 1902.

TAIH, *Transactions of the American Institute of Homoeopathy.* Chicago: Publication Committee, 1908.

Vickers A. J., and Smith, C. Homoeopathic Oscillococcinum for preventing and treating influenza and influenza-like syndromes, *Cochrane Review,* The Cochrane Library, 2005, Issue 4.

Von Hoffman, N. The Father of Homeopathy, *Washington Post,* July 21, 1971.

Wershub, L. P. *One Hundred Years of Medical Progress: A History of the New York Medical College, Flower and Fifth Avenue Hospitals.* Springfield: Charles C. Thomas, 1967.

Winslow, W. *The Menninger Story.* New York: Doubleday, 1956.

Winston, J. *The Faces of Homoeopathy.* Tawa, New Zealand: Great Auk, 1999.

CHAPTER 6

Stage, Film, and Television Celebrities: Starring in Homeopathy

So many early and modern-day film and television stars have used and appreciated homeopathic medicine that it is somewhat surprising that a major movie has not (yet) been made about their experiences. Well, perhaps it's only a matter of time.

Edwin Booth (1833–1893) was a famous American actor who some theatre historians call the greatest American Hamlet and the greatest American actor of the nineteenth century. His father was an actor, as was his brother, the notorious John Wilkes Booth, who shot U.S. President Abraham Lincoln. Ironically, Edwin Booth saved Lincoln's son, Robert, from serious injury or possibly death by pulling him up onto a train platform after Robert had fallen.

In 1889 Edwin Booth was stricken with paralysis while appearing at Rochester's Lyceum Theatre. Luckily, there was a highly respected homeopathic hospital in Rochester from which he was able to obtain treatment. He lived four more years.[59]

Sarah Bernhardt (1844–1923) was a French stage actress and then movie actress who may have been the most famous actress of the nineteenth century. Her stage career started in comic theatre and burlesque, but she later gained a reputation as a serious dramatic actress. After great success in Europe, she was soon popular in the United States as well.

Bernhardt became one of the pioneer silent movie actresses, debuting as Hamlet in *Le Duel d'Hamlet* in 1900; she ultimately starred in eight motion pictures and two biographical films. Sarah Bernhardt was made a member of France's Legion of Honor in 1914, and she is buried in Père Lachaise Cemetery in Paris, the famous cemetery where the founder of homeopathy, Hahnemann, is buried. Sarah Bernhardt also has a star on the Hollywood Walk of Fame, near the famed corner of Hollywood and Vine.

Madame Bernhardt, as she was often called, not only insisted upon homeopathic treatment of herself but for her cast as well (Enstam, 1943, 489). Confirming this fact, **James Ward, MD** (1861–1939),[60] gave a lecture on homeopathy in which he held up the former homeopathic medicine kit of Sarah Bernhardt. It is of note that all of the medicines in the kit were very high-potency homeopathic medicines (1M through CM) (Ward, 1937). These high-potency medicines were only prescribed by the most expert homeopaths, and as such, this suggests that Madame Bernhardt was either extremely knowledgeable of homeopathy or she was in regular contact with a professional homeopath who helped her prescribe for herself and her cast members.

Douglas Fairbanks, Jr., KBE, DSC (1909–2000) was an American actor and highly decorated naval officer of World War II. He is most famous as a leading man in movies, including *The Prisoner of Zenda, Gunga Din,* and *Sinbad the Sailor.* He was the son of Douglas Fairbanks (1883–1939), another leading man known for his swashbuckling role in various silent movies such as *The Mark of Zorro, The Three Musketeers,* and *Robin Hood.*

Douglas Fairbanks, Jr. was a hale and hearty man who lived to age 90. His wife (and mother of their three daughters) took their children to homeopathic doctors when they lived in England. One of their daughters appreciated the experience enough that she became a professional homeopath and has actively promoted homeopathy by organizing conferences in the San Francisco Bay Area with some of the internationally leading teachers of homeopathy.

Marlene Dietrich (1901–1992) was a German-born actress, entertainer, and singer. She received her first role in the first European talking picture, *The Blue Angel.* She later starred in several dozen movies, including several classics such as *Witness for the Prosecution, Touch of Evil,* and *Judgment at Nuremberg.*

In 1999, a musical play was performed on Broadway called *Marlene.* The play includes a scene in it in which the *New York Times* describes Ms.

Dietrich as "the good friend, who has homeopathic medicine sent to Georges Pompidou" (the president of France during the time in which the play is set).

Dietrich's personal physician was **Elizabeth Wright Hubbard, MD** (1896–1967), a respected homeopath in New York City. Dr. Hubbard was the first woman to be elected president of the American Institute of Homeopathy, and she served for many years as editor of the *Homoeopathic Recorder* and subsequently as editor of the *Journal of the American Institute of Homeopathy*.

John Wayne (1907–1979) is the most well-known actor to play cowboys in movies about the American West. Starting in silent movies in the 1920s, John Wayne acted in more than 150 movies, usually epitomizing the rugged, individualistic American man. In a 1942 movie called *The Spoilers,* in which he co-starred with Marlene Dietrich, Wayne's character, Roy Glennister, was known to recommend using *Arnica* for aches and pains from injury.[61] It is, however, unknown if Ms. Dietrich's personal interest in homeopathic medicine led to having Wayne use *Arnica* in this movie for an injury he sustained. Later in 1963, in the movie *McClintock,* after someone is injured, he asserted, "Better get some *Arnica* for that cowboy."

Catherine Zeta-Jones (1969–) is an Academy Award-winning Welsh actress. She became internationally famous after her leading role in *The Mask of Zorro* with Antonio Banderas, where she was seen as one of the most beautiful woman to ever grace the silver screen. Since then, she has starred in numerous major films, including *Entrapment, Traffic, America's Sweethearts, Chicago, Intolerable Cruelty, The Terminal,* and *Ocean's Twelve*. She won an Academy Award for best supporting actress for the movie *Chicago* in 2003.

The popular American magazine, *Entertainment Weekly* (February 21, 2003) interviewed Ms. Zeta-Jones while she was making *Chicago,* and the article noted:

> Say hello to *Arnica,* Catherine Zeta-Jones's best friend from the set of musical Chicago. The pal isn't a she. It's a homeopathic herbal remedy, and the two got to know each other

intimately during the hamstring-hampering shoot. "The pain wasn't there when I was doing it (applying *Arnica*). I had that sticky stuff glued to me for months. Brings out the bruising, darling."

Ms. Zeta-Jones, like other serious dancers and super-athletes, are great appreciators of *Arnica*.

Lesley Ann Warren (1946–) is an American actress who has received an Oscar nomination, an Emmy nomination, and a Golden Globe award for her numerous film and television roles. At 17 years of age she was reputed to be the youngest actress ever accepted into the Actors Studio. She received her first big TV role starring as Cinderella in the Rodgers and Hammerstein classic. Her numerous film appearances include Mel Brook's *Life Stinks,* Alan Rudolph's *Choose Me,* Blake Edwards's *Victor/Victoria,* the famous Miss Scarlet in *Clue,* and Steven Soderbergh's *The Limey.* She has also appeared on numerous television shows, including a recurring role on *Will & Grace* and *Desperate Housewives,* as well as starring in the award-winning miniseries *79 Park Avenue, Evergreen,* and *Joseph.*

Ms. Warren's personal letter to me is printed below; it is testament to the value, power, and breadth of possibilities of homeopathy:

> I can't say enough about the tremendous transformative and healing benefits of homeopathic medicine. I truly feel in awe of its almost miraculous abilities, to address medical, emotional, and psychological issues, rapidly and with powerful results.
>
> I have been using homeopathy for over twenty years, specifically under the care of Dr. Janet Zand, and Dr. Laura Paris. I have successfully dealt with both acute and chronic problems, living a life filled with vitality, energy, and the resilience to participate in stressful work schedules, while juggling a home, marriage, a child, and all the various and sundry life challenges that occur.

Stage, Film, and Television Celebrities

I chose to raise my child using the gift of homeopathy. My eighty-nine-year-old mother is a convert, as well as my husband and truthfully anyone that is around me for any length of time. I also solely work with Dr. John Limehouse and Dr. Priscilla Taylor, both renowned veterinarians, who use homeopathy, as well as Chinese herbs and acupuncture, for all my animals.

We have all been blessed with utilizing homeopathy successfully, to treat so many, and such a wide range of ailments, from the common cold to a variety of viral or bacterial infections. The use of antibiotics or other medicines is rare and unnecessary. During emotional times of shock or loss, the profound and gentle healing of homeopathy is exquisite.

Having been an actress, at times I get the platform, to speak about something I truly believe in. Here is my opportunity. If I could, I would shout it, from the rooftops—homeopathy is a brilliant medicine and it is with deep gratitude that I may pass on this message.

Wow! We heard you, Lesley!

Pamela Anderson (1967–) is a television actress, model, producer, and author. Ms. Anderson was a regular character on the hit television sitcom *Home Improvement* (1991–1993), though she gained her greatest notoriety for her role as C. J. Parker on *Baywatch* (1992–1997). Anderson is a strict vegetarian and an advocate for animal rights. In 1999, she received the first Linda McCartney Memorial Award for animal rights protectors.

In 2002 Ms. Anderson publicly acknowledged that she has hepatitis C. She even predicted that she would die from the disease within a decade—but this was before she tried homeopathy. After going to **Wendy Hewland**, a Los Angeles homeopath whose family founded Ainsworth's Homeopathic Pharmacy in London, which serves the Queen of England, Pamela is now totally optimistic. In 2004, she told a reporter: "It was very, very frightening in the beginning and sapping my strength, (but now) I am very healthy.... My liver was just tested, and I have stayed exactly the same or slightly improved over the last few years. I feel great. I'm convinced my homeopathic remedy is keeping me strong" (Copley, 2004).

Jane Seymour, OBE (1951–), is an English-born American actress who is best known as the star of the popular TV series and movie *Dr. Quinn, Medicine Woman* (1993–2001). She first attained international attention as Solitaire in the James Bond film *Live and Let Die*, and has played roles in numerous movies since then, most recently in the 2005 hit comedy *The Wedding Crashers*. Seymour was named to the OBE (officer of the Order of the British Empire) by Queen Elizabeth II on New Year's Eve, 1999.

Jane Seymour may live in an age of high-tech medicine, but her secret to staying well is actually more similar to pioneer treatments her character Dr. Michaela Quinn might prescribe. Seymour's sister is a homeopath in England, and she and her entire family (she has six children) are appreciative of what homeopathy has to offer. She told one reporter: "While shooting *Doctor Quinn* I would self-medicate using a homeopathic kit my sister gave me and I never missed a day the entire time." (I hope film producers are reading that line because they could save a lot of money by encouraging their actors and actresses to use homeopathic medicines to stay healthy—and stay at work.)

The story of this television show took place in 1867; the leading character, Dr. Michaela Quinn, graduated from a Boston medical school and then established her practice in Colorado Springs. The only medical school in Boston at that time that accepted women was the New England Female Medical College, a homeopathic medical school. This medical school merged with another homeopathic college, Boston University, in 1873. Ironically (and sadly), the writers and producers of this show were not adequately familiar with homeopathy to show her prescribing homeopathic medicines. Instead, on the TV show, she commonly used herbs.

In real life, however, Jane uses both herbal and homeopathic medicines. As her website proclaims, "My current favorite is *Arnica*, a homeopathic remedy for treating bruises and swelling." She has also made public her love of *Oscillococcinum*, the homeopathic medicine for treating the flu. Her husband, James Keach (1947–), a respected actor and producer (he recently produced *Walk the Line,* the award-winning film about Johnny Cash), is equally supportive of homeopathic and natural medicines.

Suzanne Somers (1946–) is an American actress best known for her role as Chrissy Snow on the sitcom *Three's Company,* and for her bit part as the "Blonde in the T-Bird" in *American Graffiti*. She has released two autobiographies, two self-help books, four diet books, and two books about hormone replacement therapy. Ms. Somers announced in 2001 that she had breast cancer and was using alternative medicine to treat it (along with surgery and radiation therapy). She specifically chose not to undergo chemotherapy and instead used a homeopathic and herbal remedy called *Iscador®* (made from mistletoe).

Iscador has been used by homeopaths, anthroposophical doctors, natural medicine doctors, and cancer physicians since 1917. Information about Iscador and the numerous studies that have shown its biological action and clinical efficacy are available at www.iscador.com. In addition to research showing efficacy in the treatment of certain types of cancer (Augustin, et al., 2005), there is also research showing that it is useful in reducing the side effects of conventional cancer treatment (Bock, 2003; Bock, et al., 2004).

Michael York (1942–) is a prolific British actor who has appeared in numerous Shakespearean works in theatre and film, though he may be more known to the general public for his role of Basil Exposition in the *Austin Powers* series of films. Early in his career York joined the National Theatre and worked with Franco Zeffirelli in staging *Much Ado About Nothing*. York made his film debut as Lucentio in Zeffirelli's *The Taming of the Shrew,* and then was cast as Tybalt in Zeffirelli's adaptation of *Romeo and Juliet*. He also starred in an early Merchant-Ivory film, *The Guru*. In *Cabaret* York played Brian Roberts.

When Michael York was recently asked about his interest in natural medicine, he replied:

> My wife and I have been, you know, medically alternative for thirty years, in fact so long ago we were sort of freaks.

Now, of course, everything has become a little more mainstream. I don't think they even call it alternative anymore. It's called integrated. My wife has a passion that the so-called orthodox and the so-called alternative shouldn't be mutually exclusive, and that they should join forces. And you know there are wonderful, huge, noble things being done in each branch. I love homeopathy and acupuncture. I think that everything that keeps the body in an optimum state rather than waiting for it to break down and then seeking help ... you know, seeking help beforehand. (*Strand Magazine,* online)

In another interview, he got more specific:

I've always been into alternative therapies such as homeopathy. The American drug scene scares me—there's always a new medical quick-fix being peddled on the television shopping channels—so my wife, Pat, and I try and keep things as natural as possible. After a misspent youth of swashbuckling roles, I had to have a hip replacement five years ago. The hospital kept trying to give me more morphine, but I found that the homeopathic remedy *Arnica* helped me more during the healing process. (Nikkhah, 2005)

Lindsay Wagner (1949–) is an actress best known for her starring and Emmy-winning role on *The Bionic Woman* and her socially significant television films. This superwoman has authored books on both vegetarianism and acupressure and has significant respect for homeopathy. She serves on the advisory board of the National Center for Homeopathy (www.homeopathic.org), and she has spoken at a couple of the organization's conferences in the past.

She wrote me personally to acclaim her deep appreciation for homeopathy: "Homeopathy has been the primary form of treatment for my sons and myself since 1980. It is an exquisite and powerful form of bringing the body and emotions back to balance and health. I am eternally grateful to those who brought this special modality to my attention."

Phillip McGraw, PhD (1950–), host of the popular American psychology TV-show *Dr. Phil*, initially gained celebrity status from his appearances on Oprah Winfrey's show. Dr. Phil's wife, Robin, is a regular on his show and has co-hosted numerous television events with him.

On a segment that **Robin McGraw** led, "Hormones from Hell," she talked about her personal experiences with menopause and hot flashes:

> You're not the only person experiencing hormonal imbalance and everything that goes with it. It was very important to me to treat the hot flashes because that was very severe and uncomfortable. Early on, I went to a homeopathic practitioner and she sent me to a health food store to buy *Sepia*. It's a homeopathic remedy that you shake and put under your tongue. Within 24 hours of using this, my hot flashes were gone. (*Dr. Phil*, show 213)

Vanessa L. Williams (1963–) is a Grammy-winning American singer and actress who was the first woman of African descent to be crowned Miss America. Two of her albums have achieved "gold" status for their sales, and she won the NAACP Image award in 1989. She has co-starred in numerous films and Broadway musicals and was nominated for a Tony for best performance by a leading actress in a musical (*Into the Woods*). Starting in 2006, she began co-starring on a television show *Ugly Betty*.

Ms. Williams is the mother of four children and is an admitted bookworm. Williams read voraciously about prenatal care, motherhood, and parenting while pregnant. She is a vegetarian, and has used holistic remedies to treat her children's ear infections and diaper rash. After Iparenting Media gave her the Mother of the Month Award in 2005, she said: "The doctor gives his diagnosis and then I'm in there with homeopathy and herbal books." Williams utilizes various treatment options for her kids and herself, often blending Western, homeopathic, herbal, and nutritional methodologies.

Michael Caine (1933–) is a two-time Academy Award-winning British actor. He has also won three Golden Globe awards and the New York Film Critics Award.

In 2002, the *Times* (of London) reported, "In fact, he is in better shape than most men of his age; the quips fly as fast as ever, and he's considerably fitter than he has been in the past. The waistline has trimmed to a reasonable 38in, and with his glasses, tan and the silvery tinge to his hair, he looks like one of those 'Men of Distinction' ads you used to find in *The New Yorker*. 'I just want to stay here as long as possible. I take care of myself. I've given up smoking. I don't drink in the daytime any more. I take a lot of homeopathic remedies and vitamins. I walk four miles every day.' Where? 'Around my garden.' Doesn't it get boring? 'No, you never get bored walking on land you own'" (Perry, 2002).

Julia Sawalha (1968–) is an English actress, best known as Saffron in the TV comedy *Absolutely Fabulous*. Ms. Sawalha was born into an acting family: her father Nadim appeared in the James Bond movie *The Spy Who Loved Me* while her sister Nadia starred in the soap *EastEnders* and is now a talk show host. Julia starred in the 1995 BBC adaptation of Jane Austen's *Pride and Prejudice* as Lydia Bennett. Ms. Sawalha also voiced "Ginger" in the claymation movie *Chicken Run*.

A 1999 newspaper article highlighted two of Ms. Sawalha's special passions: environmental protection and homeopathic medicine. While on a Greenpeace ship, the Rainbow Warrior, as it was sailing to the Outer Hebrides (islands off northern Scotland) to visit a seal sanctuary on Islay, stormy weather set in, but she wasn't worried at all about seasickness because, as she said, "I also brought my homeopathic remedies, which I swear by" (Hagan, 1999).

Coincidentally (or not), Julia Sawalha's character Saffron is a level-headed teenager and then young adult (the series has continued for ten-plus years) who lives with her daffy mother Edina and the mother's equally daffy friend Patsy. As part of her levelheadedness on the show, Saffron uses and loves homeopathic medicines.

Nadia Sawalha (1964–), Julia's sister, is also an English actress and television presenter and is similarly passionate about homeopathy. Nadia is best known for her role as Annie Palmer in the BBC soap opera *EastEnders,* though she has also appeared in *Celebrity Driving School* for Comic Relief and currently presents daytime television.

Nadia Sawalha is one of the millions of people who have suffered from psoriasis, but since discovering homeopathy, she hasn't been to a conventional doctor in fifteen years. She says, "I was getting stress-related psoriasis on my arms and face and, although I'd been using steroid cream, it wasn't getting any better, so I tried homeopathy. It quickly sorted it out" (Celebrity Sick, 2002). Steroid creams are a leading conventional treatment for the red, scaly patches of psoriasis, but because steroids suppress the body's own immune system and tend to thin the skin, they shouldn't be used for very long.

Nadia has given special public appreciation to her homeopath, Rachel Packer, who "has seen me through every stage of my life," and further explains: "I went to her when severe eczema provoked the worst health crisis of my life and I had to stop working. I had regular consultations with her when I was pregnant and even during labor. And now she has helped me to deal with the terrible sadness I felt after the miscarriages." Packer has also helped Nadia have a successful pregnancy and even prescribed homeopathic medicines to speed up her labor, for which Nadia was eternally grateful (Petty, 2006).

In one interview, Nadia happened to also mention one particular homeopathic medicine that has impressed her: "The miracle hangover cure is *Nux Vomica*. It's homeopathic and it works."

Louise Jameson (1951–) is a British actress who is most famous for playing Leela, the leather-clad barbarian warrior companion of the mysterious Doctor in the long-running British science fiction television series *Doctor Who.* Jameson has also appeared on *Emmerdal* (as Sharon Crossthwaite), *The Omega Factor* (as Dr. Anne Reynolds), *Tenko* (as Blanche Simmons), *Bergerac* (as Susan Young), and *EastEnders* (as Rosa di Marco).

Ms. Jameson and her family are all ardent users of homeopathic remedies. Like many parents, she began exploring homeopathy when one of her sons experienced frequent colds, for which homeopathy provided fast and effective relief.

Alan Bates (1934–2003), knighted as Sir Alan Arthur Bates, CBE, was a British actor who won two Tony Awards for best performance by an actor in a leading role. Bates starred in such international hit films as *Georgy Girl, Far from the Madding Crowd, Zorba the Greek, The Go-Between, An Unmarried Woman,* and *Women in Love.*

In 1972, *Time* magazine reported that two of Bates "eccentricities" were his vegetarianism and his appreciation for homeopathic medicine (Colors of Bates, 1972). (One can only wonder when a person's use of the ever-changing conventional drugs will be considered "eccentric.")

Susan Hampshire, Lady Kulukundis, OBE (1937–), is an English actress who is best known for many television roles and occasional films. Ms. Hampshire received Emmy Awards in the 1970s for her roles in *The Forsyte Saga, The First Churchills,* and *Vanity Fair.* She is vice president of the Blackie Foundation, a leading homeopathic research organization named after Dr. Margery Blackie, former physician to Her Majesty Queen Elizabeth II. Ms. Hampshire first consulted a homeopath in the mid-1960s, and she is known to give homeopathic medicines to entire casts with whom she works.

Ashok Kumar (1911–2001) was an Indian actor. Although he isn't well known internationally, he actually is a cinema icon of the twentieth century. He broke apart from the theatrical role-playing prevalent in Indian cinema and started a natural style of acting. In 1988, he received the Dadasaheb Phalke Award—an annual award given to one person by the Indian government for a lifetime contribution to the Indian film industry. He also won two Filmfare awards (the oldest and most prominent film awards given for Hindi films in India, honoring Bollywood's best talents). Besides acting, he was an avid painter and a practitioner of homeopathy.

Indrani Haldar is a contemporary Indian actress popular in Bengali films, and in 1997, she received a national best-actress award in India for her performance in *Dahan.* She is a serious appreciator of homeopathy, asserting: "Homeopathy worked as a miracle for my father. He was an acute diabetic who developed a major kidney problem in the later stages. It is then that we turned to homeopathy and the results were remarkable. I myself use this treatment in most cases" (Ghosh, 2006).

Stage, Film, and Television Celebrities

Chiranjeevi (1955–) is a popular Telugu film actor (Telugu is the second most popular language in India, second to Hindi), known by his millions of fans as *Mega Star*. In January 2006, Chiranjeevi was honored with the Padma Bhushan, the third highest civilian award in India. He has won Southern Filmfare Award (best actor) for seven years. When he was recently asked the secret to his unbounding energy, he said that it was homeopathic medicines (Andhra Café, 2007). Chiranjeevi was introduced to homeopathy by his late father-in-law who was a homeopathic doctor.

Priscilla Presley (1945–), the wife of Elvis Presley, told me personally back in 1989 that she went to a homeopath to help her with the chronic fatigue that she experienced. She was extremely pleased with the results. This positive experience may help explain why her daughter, **Lisa Marie Presley** (1968–), also turned to homeopathic medicines for treatment of postpartum depression (Berry, 2005).

Ben Vereen (1946–) is an actor, dancer, and singer who has appeared in numerous Broadway theatre shows. He won a Tony for his appearance in *Pippin* in 1973, and he may be most well known for his role as "Chicken" George Moore in *Roots* and for his song-and-dance numbers in *All That Jazz*. When one reporter asked him what three things he keeps in his medicine chest, he bragged, "Mainly what I keep in there is homeopathic medicine" (Metz, 2005).

Kim Cattrall (1956–) is best-known as an actress who co-starred in the television series *Sex and the City*, for which she won a Golden Globe and was nominated for an Emmy. In 2003, the *Los Angeles Daily News* reported her appreciation for a well-known homeopathic medicine: "*Arnica!* I love it. I use it all the time because I bruise easily."

Ashley Judd (1968–) knows enough basic information about homeopathy that during the 2006 Sundance Film Festival, she walked up to one of the Festival's exhibitors of homeopathic medicines and specifically requested *Arnica* for her son's recent neck injury (www.lindzi.com). Ashley is also known to travel with homeopathic medicines, including remedies that help her reduce the effects of jetlag or treat the flu (Spencer, 2000).

Naomi Watts (1968–) is an Oscar-nominated British-Australian actress and producer, who is most famous for her starring role in the Lord of the Ring films, as well as her starring role in Peter Jackson's 2005 remake of the 1933 horror epic, *King Kong*. A *Los Angeles Times* article said that the way to get Nicole Kidman to an event is to invite her friend, Naomi Watts, and to get Naomi, you invite her stylist, her trainer, and her homeopath (Davidow, 2005).

Jennifer Aniston (1969–) is a Golden Globe- and Emmy-winning film and television actress who was introduced to homeopathic and natural medicine through her parents, who enrolled her in a Waldorf school (inspired by the work by Rudolf Steiner; see Chapter 13, Clergy and Spiritual Leaders, for more information about Steiner). She has maintained an interest in homeopathic treatment today.

Tobey Maguire (1975–) is an American actor who has starred in the blockbuster superhero movies as Spider-Man as well as numerous other films such as *Cider House Rules, Wonder Boys,* and *Seabiscuit*. Maguire actually almost had to pull out of the starring role in *Spider-Man 2* due to back pain and the irritation to it that the various web-slinging scenes created, but homeopathy came to the rescue. According to a friend: "Tobey was very skeptical of alternative medicine before but now he's virtually a devotee—as is Spider-Man" (www.AbsoluteNow.com, August 7, 2006).

Orlando Bloom (1977–) is an English actor who achieved significant fame playing Legolas in the Lord of the Rings films, and then established himself as a leading man in numerous major movies, including *Pirates of the Caribbean* (the original and the sequel), *Troy, Elizabethtown,* and *Kingdom of Heaven*. His co-star Naomie Harris (1976–) told British *Vogue*: "I caught a cold on the flight to LA and started losing my voice. I couldn't talk between takes and had to mime what I wanted. Orlando kept bringing me homeopathic remedies, which was lovely of him" (August 2006).

References

Andhra Café, February 26, 2007. www.andhracafe.com/index.php?m=show&id =19430

Augustin, M., et al. Long-term Adjuvant Treatment of Primary Intermediate to High-Risk Malignant Melanoma, *Arzneim.-Forsch./Drug Research,* January 1, 2005. (A long-term Iscador treatment in patients with medium-to-high-risk primary malignant melanoma appears to be safe. A tumor enhancement was not observed. In comparison with an untreated parallel control group from the same cohort the results of the mistletoe treatment show a significant survival advantage in the UICC-/AJCC stages II-III.)

Berry, S. Hey, Jude, Why'd You Have to be So Lewd? *Columbus Dispatch,* July 21, 2005, 8B.

Bock, P. R., Misletoe improves tolerability of breast cancer treatment by Nancy Walsh, *Family Practice News.* February 1, 2003. (A multicenter study showed that mistletoe extract, as a concurrent medical treatment, can increase the tolerability of conventional cancer treatment, improve patient quality of life, and lengthening tumor free survival.)

Bock, P. R, et al. Mistletoe Complementary Treatment in Patients with Primary Nonmetastatic Breast Cancer, *Arzneim.-Forsch./Drug Research,* October 1, 2004. (The results of the study confirmed the safety of the complementary therapy for patients with primary, non-metastatic mammary carcinoma with Iscador® and showed considerably fewer adverse drug reactions attributed to concurrent conventional therapy, as well as reduced disease and treatment-associated symptoms, and suggested a prolonged overall survival in the Iscador group as compared with controls.)

Brantley, B. All That Dazzles Is Not Dietrich, However Real She Looks (theatrical review), *New York Times,* April 12, 1999.

Celebrity Sick Note Psoriasis. *Sunday Mirror,* December 1, 2002.

The Colors of Bates, *Time,* Nov. 6, 1972.

Copley News Service, Pamela Anderson, April 11, 2004.

Davidow, A. Dull Guest List? *Los Angeles Times,* April 2, 2005, p. E1.

Enstam, C. H. What Homeopathy Can Do for You, *Homoeopathic Recorder,* April 1943, 58,10:487–492.

Ghosh, T. Indrani's Chill Pills, Times News Network, June 18, 2006.

Hagan, A. Actress Julia's Mission as a Greenpeace Warrior, *The Mirror,* August 3, 1999.

Iparenting Media. Vanessa Williams: Mom of the Month, October 18, 2005. http://iparenting.com/mom/1101.htm

www.lindzi.com/loves/sundance.htm

Los Angeles Daily News, September 28, 2003.

Metz, N. Getting Spiritual in Brooklyn, *Chicago Tribune,* May 29, 2005.

Nikkhah, R. My Regime: A Bounce in the Garden Peps Me Up, *The Daily Telegraph,* November 1, 2005.

Perry, G. Praising Caine, *Times* (of London), November 24, 2002. Available at www.timesonline.co.uk/tol/life_and_style/education/student/article1181065.ece

Petty, M. TV's Nadia: Homeopathy helped me deal with my miscarriage, *Daily Mail,* July 23, 2006.

Spencer, L. Of Mothers, Victims and Psychos, *The Independent* (London), January 27, 2000.

Strand Magazine, www.strandmag.com/york.htm. (For more details, see Michael York's book, *Dispatches from Armageddon,* Lyme, N.H.: Smith and Kraus, 2001.)

Ward, J. W. Taking the history of the case, *Pacific Coast Journal of Homeopathy,* 1937. (From a presentation made March 3, 1937.)

CHAPTER 7

Musicians:
Singing Out for Homeopathy

Pythagoras (582–507 BC), the Greek philosopher who is recognized as the father of numbers and of mathematics, was one of the earliest scientists. By his measurements of the length of musical tones, he made the first known reduction of a quality (sound) into a quantity (length and ratio). He also discovered that every musical tone generates a series of additional inaudible pitches that add to the richness of the tone. He quantified these inaudible pitches, called overtones, with mathematic ratios. Trying to understand nature through mathematics remains a basic method and objective of science today.

Pythagoras is credited with originating the concept of the "music of the spheres," an ancient philosophical concept that regards proportions in the movements of celestial bodies—the sun, moon, and planets—as a form of music. This music may not be normally audible, but ancient scholars acknowledged that each planet and moon created its own motion, sound, and harmony, which the ancients translated into mathematical concepts.

The Pythagoreans were also known to use music to heal the body and elevate the soul. Plato, Pliny, Cicero, and Ptolemy were some of the philosophers of the ancient world who contemplated and wrote about the music of the spheres. This seminal doctrine was made practical and worldly in medieval Europe, where it developed into its most glorious expression in the architecture of great abbeys and cathedrals that were consciously designed to conform to the proportions of musical and geometric harmony (Plant, 2006).

The great astronomer Johannes Kepler (1571–1630) further studied these phenomena and developed laws of planetary motion, describing the relationships of planets and their orbits through numbers and ratios and using them to explain how they influence events on Earth. He was the first to show that our moon influences the tides on Earth. Kepler's writings are replete with musical references. He desired to create a "symphony of the cosmos," stating that "the movements of the heavens are nothing except a certain everlasting polyphony."

At the most sophisticated level, music, science, nature, and healing are interconnected. It is therefore not surprising that some of the most respected musicians of the past 200 years have explored and experimented with inaudible yet powerful nanodoses of homeopathic medicines.

Ludwig van Beethoven (1770–1827) is generally considered the greatest composer in the history of music. He was born in Bonn, Germany but moved to Vienna in his early twenties to study music with Joseph Haydn. Somewhere around 1800 he began suffering from tinnitus (noises in the ear) and hearing loss. The cause of Beethoven's deafness remains unknown, though various experts have attributed it to syphilis (Hayden, 2003), beatings from his father, lead poisoning, typhoid, or the newest theory, otosclerosis (Mai, 2007).

Beethoven also experienced severe gastrointestinal distress, powerful headaches (he even had several teeth pulled in the hopes of relieving some of his pain), an abscessed jaw, recurrent rheumatic pains, and frequent cardiac arrhythmia (which he set to music in a piano sonata, Opus 81a, *Les Adieux*).

Historians are lucky to have a rich cache of letters to and from Beethoven as well as his *Conversation Books*, the writing pads that he used to communicate with others when he could no longer hear audible speech. There are references by Beethoven to homeopathy in this written documentation, and it is well known that his doctor between 1820 and 1826 was **Dr. Anton Braunhofer**, a professor of biology at the University of Vienna. Beethoven's nephew, Karl, described Dr. Braunhofer as using homeopathic medicine "because he too follows fashions in medicine" (Beethoven, 1981, 21; Mai, 2007, 127). Braunhofer also recommended certain dietary changes, including avoidance of wine, coffee, and spices. Braunhofer admonished Beethoven that he "must live according to nature" (Schweisheimer, 1945).

In late April 1825, Beethoven was suffering from inflammation of his bowel, and in May he was spitting blood. Initially, the prescriptions given him didn't work, and Beethoven's nephew complained that he was required to make him specific meals, one rule of which was serving only steak for lunch. Several sources acknowledge that the treatment allowed him to return to work and finish a quartet in July 1825 (String Quartet in A Minor, Op. 132) (Hellenbroich, 1995; Takacs, 2007). By August 1825, Beethoven wrote to his associate and early biographer, Anton Schindler: "My doctor saved me, because I could no longer write music, but now I can write notes which help to relieve me of my troubles" (Mai, 2007, 126).

Ultimately, Beethoven expressed such appreciation to and for Dr. Braunhofer that he composed two canons in his honor (of forty-three canons in total): the Four-Part Canon in C Major (WoO 189, "*Doktor, sperrt das Tor dem Tod*"—"Doctor, bar the gate to death, notes save from distress") and Canon in Two Parts in C Major (WoO 190, "*Ich war hier, Doktor*"—"I was here, Doctor.").[62]

Over his life Beethoven had sought the care of various conventional physicians and was known to refer to them as "medical asses" (Hayden, 2003, 78). Composers such as Beethoven, literary greats such as Goethe, and many others in the creative arts were known to join the political leaders[63] and the wealthy classes of Germans in going to homeopathic doctors and to spas and natural medicine centers in Teplitz, Marienbad, and Driburg (Maretzki and Seidler, 1985, 395–396).

In early February 1826, Ignaz Schuppanzigh (1776–1830), a violinist, friend, and teacher of Beethoven,[64] assured Beethoven that Braunhofer was very skillful, and further, he told him that their mutual close friend and confident Nikolaus Zmeskall, who had suffered from gout, was particularly enthusiastic about homeopathy (Albrecht, 1996, 132).

In late February 1826, Braunhofer treated Beethoven for symptoms of dysentery and gout, at which time he discouraged Beethoven from drinking coffee, because, the doctor said, it would be bad for his stomach and his nerves over the long term, even though the stimulant effect would seem to provide temporary relief (Mai, 2007, 127). Braunhofer prescribed a homeopathic dose of *Cinchona officinalis* (Peruvian bark, from which quinine is a primary ingredient), and Beethoven later expressed gratitude for the benefits he received from the doctor's treatment.

Although Beethoven moved to Baden, some 300 miles away from Vienna where Braunhofer practiced, the composer sought Braunhofer's care when he traveled to Vienna. When Beethoven asked Braunhofer to come to Baden to treat him, Braunhofer declined, saying that it was too far a distance to travel. Several historians note that Beethoven did not follow the doctor's advice to stop drinking wine in 1826 and that this created some tension between the doctor and his patient. Braunhofer's advice to stop drinking was indeed sound, especially in light of the fact that Beethoven died in 1827 of cirrhosis of the liver (Schweisheimer, 1945). Although Beethoven scholars say that he was not a "drinker," he was very fond of table wines, consumed in moderate quantities, and was very reluctant to abstain.

It should also be noted that even though the emperor of Austria had declared the practice of homeopathic medicine to be illegal in 1819 and even though it remained illegal until that emperor died in 1835, homeopathy was still practiced by a small and select group of highly respected physicians and even priests. **Dr. Matthias Marenzeller**, captain of the medical corps in Vienna, was a leading advocate of homeopathy, as was **Father Veith** (1787–1877), pastor at the famed St. Stephens Cathedral in Vienna. Homeopathy was appreciated enough in 1820 that even Prince Schwarzenberg, commander-in-chief of Austria's allied armies against Napoleon, went to Leipzig, Germany, to seek treatment from Dr. Samuel Hahnemann, the founder of homeopathy.[65]

Another interesting connection between Beethoven and homeopathy is the fact that two days after he died, Dr. Franz Hartmann visited his home and obtained a lock of hair from the famed composer.[66] Dr. Hartmann was the close friend of Schubert as well as the homeopath to Robert Schumann and his wife Clara (see below).

Nicolo Paganini (1782–1840), the famous Italian composer who some consider the greatest violinist who ever lived, was a patient of homeopathy's founder, Samuel Hahnemann, MD. Paganini, like many people of his day, suffered considerably under conventional medical treatment. Hahnemann could not help but notice that all of Paganini's teeth had fallen out, his mouth had become ulcerated, and his jawbone was abscessed due to mercury treatment (probably resulting from being diagnosed with syphilis at an early age).

In choosing a remedy, Hahnemann considered Paganini's personal habits and appearance. There are various stories about Paganini's life that show him to be a man of great frugality. He was known to bargain incessantly for a lower price and to purchase used clothing. Once he purchased clothes, he would wear them and patch them continually, insisting that "an old garment is an old friend." This story is meaningful to homeopaths because it helps explain why Hahnemann prescribed homeopathic *Sulphur* for him.[67]

Because of Paganini's good looks and fame, women were very attracted to him. Hahnemann prescribed for him, but shortly afterwards, the doctor stopped treating the violinist-composer after Hahnemann determined that Paganini had gotten too familiar with his young wife, Melanie (Handley, 1990, 114). After Paganini's death, a love letter to Melanie Hahnemann was found among his possessions.

Frédéric Chopin (1810–1849) was a Polish composer who is one of the most famous and influential composers for the piano.

During the 1840s, half of the population of France and England contracted tuberculosis, and two-thirds of its victims died. When Chopin became ill with tuberculosis, he and his lover at the time, the French novelist and feminist **George Sand** (aka Amandine-Aurore-Lucile Dupin, 1804–1876), sought care from **Dr. Jean Jacques Molin** (1797–1849), a homeopathic physician who became Chopin's most trusted doctor. Dr. Molin was twice elected president of the Society of Homeopathic Medicine in France. Chopin claimed that Molin had the "secret of getting me back on my feet again" (Atwood, 1999, 349). During the harsh winter of 1847, Chopin credited Molin with saving his life.

Jane Stirling, a student and benefactor for whom Chopin named two compositions, was a strong advocate for homeopathy, and she was influential in securing homeopathic medical care for Chopin when he traveled. Stirling wanted to take Chopin to Scotland and England for concerts and new students, but Chopin was resistant due to the wet weather that would exacerbate his condition. Against better judgment, Chopin left for Edinburgh, arriving during a heavy fog. At the train station was **Dr. A. Lyszcynski**, a Polish homeopath who Jane had thoughtfully provided to give Chopin homeopathic treatment during his visit. However, due to the weather and the dampness of his lodging, Chopin's health worsened.

Upon his return to Paris, he was saddened to discover that his homeopath, Dr. Molin, had died. He sought homeopathic treatment from two other homeopathic doctors, Dr. Roth and Dr. Leon Simon, but he wasn't satisfied with either of their treatments. Chopin then resorted to orthodox medical treatment which also provided inadequate relief. He died at only 39 years of age. Chopin was buried in Père Lachaise cemetery, the same cemetery where Samuel Hahnemann was laid to rest.

Robert Schumann (1810–1856) was a German composer and pianist who is considered one of the most famous Romantic composers of the first half of the nineteenth century. Some modern-day historians have suggested that he suffered from syphilis, though there is some controversy about this diagnosis. However, even skeptics of this diagnosis acknowledge that his chronic symptoms and his early death at age 46 may have resulted from overconsumption of mercury (a nineteenth-century treatment for syphilis). Schumann sought treatment from one of Hahnemann's colleagues, **Dr. Franz Hartmann**. He was not cured, but this didn't dissuade him from pursuing other homeopathic treatment (Hayden, 2003). Later, he sought the care of another homeopathic doctor, **Wolfgang Muller**, who determined that Schumann was suffering from drug-induced toxicity.

Schumann's wife, **Clara Wieck Schumann** (1819–1896), was also a famous pianist and composer. In fact, she is considered by many to be the premier female musician of the nineteenth century. Clara was a personal friend of Dr. and Mrs. Hahnemann in Paris. She performed at Hahnemann's Sixtieth Jubilee (the sixtieth anniversary of his doctoral degree), in Paris in 1839 (Haehl, 1922, II, 370–371). Her father, Friedrich Wieck (1785–1873), a noted German piano and voice teacher, had been a patient and a friend of Hahnemann's when they lived near each other in Leipzig, Germany.

Richard Wagner (1813–1883) was a leading German composer and conductor who is primarily known for his operas. His most famous compositions include *Tristan and Isolde, Parsifal,* and *Der Ring des Nibelungen,* commonly referred to as The Ring or The Ring Cycle, all of which are regularly performed throughout the world today.

Wagner's use of leitmotif (a recurring musical theme) has had a strong influence on many twentieth-century film scores, notably John Williams's music for *Star Wars.* Even American producer Phil Spector's "wall of sound" was strongly influenced by Wagner's music.

In March 1839, at the tender age of 26 years, Wagner was struck with typhoid fever. In his autobiography, Wagner described what happened after Karl von Holtei, a theatre owner where he was working, insisted that he conduct music in an icy cold theatre at a time when he was already feeling quite ill.

> Typhoid fever was the consequence, and this pulled me down to such an extent that Holtei, who heard of my condition, is said to have remarked at the theatre that I should probably never conduct again, and that, to all intents and purposes, I "was on my last legs." It was to a splendid homeopathic physician, Dr. Prutzer, that I owed my recovery and my life. (Wagner, 1911, 188)

Despite the significance of this experience, it is interesting to note that a review of a dozen biographies of Richard Wagner found that only one book made any reference to this experience (Watson, 1979). When one considers that Wagner's father died of typhoid just six months after the future composer's birth, it is no exaggeration to say that it is likely that Richard Wagner's contribution to music would not have occurred without the homeopathic treatment he received.

Even though the vast majority of people sought conventional medical care, Wagner and many of the most educated and elite members of society sought homeopathic and natural medical treatment. Even though some people chided Wagner for his "quack cures," the natural medical treatment that he used throughout his life allowed him to live to 69 years of age, despite experiencing various health crises. Wagner was known to frequent water-cure spas, and one of his doctors was **Dr. Ernst Schwenninger**,[68] who was the author of a book entitled *The Doctor,* a scathing critique of conventional medicine of the day.

Toward the end of Wagner's life, he composed *Parsifal* (1882), a story in which the protagonist utilizes a central principle of homeopathy to initiate a healing. *Parsifal* is a story about Amfortas, the ruler of the knights who guard the Grail. These knights also protect the sword that was used to wound Jesus while he was on the cross. However, this sword is stolen, and Amfortas is then himself wounded by it. Amfortas suffers for a long time until Parsifal finally retrieves the sword and uses it to heal Amfortas. This application of using something that causes injury to heal injury is a classic metaphor for the homeopathic principle of "like treating like."

Samuel Barber (1910–1981), best known for his hauntingly beautiful Adagio for Strings, was an American composer of classical music. His Piano Sonata (1949) was commissioned by the famed Richard Rodgers and Irving Berlin, and premiered by Vladimir Horowitz. This was the first large-scale American piano work to be premiered by such an internationally renowned pianist. Barber won two Pulitzer Prizes, one for his opera *Vanessa* (1958), and one for a piano concerto, Opus 38 (1963).

Barber's father, **Samuel LeRoy Barber**, graduated from Hahnemann Medical College in Philadelphia in 1901 and practiced homeopathy for forty years. He was a founder of the Homeopathic Hospital of Chester County in 1913. This hospital is now a conventional hospital known as Paoli Hospital.

Sir Yehudi Menuhin (1916–1999) was a Jewish American-born violinist, violist, and conductor who spent most of his adult life in the United Kingdom. He began playing the violin at age 3, and his first public performance, with the San Francisco Symphony, occurred when he was only 7. During World War II, he performed more than 500 concerts for the

Armed Forces, which earned him the French Legion of Honor and Croix de Lorraine, the Belgian Ordre de la Couronne and Ordre Leopold, the Order of Merit from West Germany, and the Order of the Phoenix from Greece. He also received more than fifty additional honors, including the Royal Philharmonic Society's Gold Medal, the Cobbett Medal, the Sonning Prize (from Copenhagen), and an honorary knighthood from Queen Elizabeth II (England's highest honor for a non-British subject).

Due to ailments he experienced from the strain of performing and traveling, he began practicing yoga and meditation and using homeopathic medicines. He became the honorary president of the Hahnemann Society, a leading British homeopathic organization.

In early 1988, I sent him a copy of a book I had written on homeopathy. He responded:

> Homeopathy attracted me because it is so subtle, so discreet and so effective in approach to the whole human being, and I have certainly met some remarkable people who practice it. For me it is a personal preference as I try to steer clear of all doctors, as few have this commitment, and it is because I find that the world deals these days so much in terms of size and mass and volume and is always striving for bigger mass and bigger volume. The mentality that seems to dominate is meeting one mass with a greater one in order to overcome the lesser. This is, of course, nonsense, as any thinking human being knows, for it does not apply to human life. Many people close to me have benefited from homeopathy. (July 5, 1988)

More publically, he asserted with great succinctness: "Homeopathy is one of the rare medical approaches which carries no penalties—only benefits." Sir Yehudi further acknowledged that homeopathy's survival has not been easy as it has had to "withstand the assaults of established medical practice for over 100 years" (Kindred Spirits, 1989).

Dizzy Gillespie (1917–1993) was an American jazz trumpeter, bandleader, singer, and composer. Along with Charlie Parker, Gillespie was a major figure in the development of bebop and modern jazz, and played a major role in defining Afro-Cuban jazz. Ultimately, Gillespie was a trumpet virtuoso and gifted improviser who added layers of harmonic complexity previously not heard in jazz. His unique style and look included a beret, horn-rimmed spectacles, scat singing, a bent horn, and pooched cheeks, matched by a wonderfully lighthearted personality that endeared many people to him and his music.

After being introduced to homeopathic medicine by his protégé, **Jon Faddis,** Dizzy had such remarkable experiences that he once told Faddis: "I've had two revelations in my life. The first was bebop; the second was homeopathy."

Ravi Shankar (1920–) is a Bengali-Indian master musician of the sitar. He played a seminal role in the introduction of classical Indian music to Western culture. Initially, Shankar became famous due to being Beatle George Harrison's sitar teacher.

Ravi Shankar was another appreciator of homeopathy who not only sought homeopathic treatment wherever he lived but also on the road doing concerts. One Boston homeopath who treated him after a concert remarked how open he was with all around him about his strong preference for homeopathic treatment over all other forms of medicine.

Tina Turner (1939–), often called the queen of rock and roll, is an American pop, rock, and soul singer who has won seven Grammies. She has a star on the Hollywood Walk of Fame and was inducted into the Rock and Roll Hall of Fame.

It is hard to imagine, but during the early 1970s this powerful woman was literally brought to her knees by a diagnosis of tuberculosis. She initially sought conventional medical treatment, but continued to suffer, until she sought care from **Chandra Sharma, MD,** a homeopathic doctor in England. Tina considered him her doctor and her friend. He passed away in 1986, and she wrote in her autobiography: "I miss him more than I can say." Tina also noted: "Fortunately, his son, Rajandra, was his protégé and is carrying on his work" (Turner, 1986, 156).

In 1985, *Vogue* magazine reported on Tina's longtime interest in homeopathy and Buddhism: "Tina Turner looks about thirty-six, and her skin is flawless. She does not deprive herself. She sips wine at dinner, does not diet, does not take vitamins. If she's feeling particularly stressed, she consults a homeopathic doctor" (Orth, 1985).

In her autobiography, she wrote: "Life in the fast lane wore me down, changes in my diet and homeopathy saved me. Thanks to my homeopathic physician, for bringing me back to health and always being available for me" (Turner, 1986).

Paul McCartney (1942–), formally known as Sir James Paul McCartney, MBE, is best known as a member of the Beatles, and later, as leader of Wings. He is a British singer, musician, and songwriter who the *Guinness Book of World Records* lists as the most successful composer in popular music history. He has written or co-written more than fifty top-ten hits, and innumerable other music artists and orchestras have recorded his songs.

Paul's second wife, **Linda Eastman** (1941–1998), introduced her husband to vegetarianism in 1975, and she authored several best-selling vegetarian cookbooks. In a 1992 interview, Linda McCartney asserted: "We never go anywhere without our homeopathic remedies. We often make use of them—and that goes for Paul too" (Glew, 1992).

Linda's interest in homeopathy began when a friend broke her arm, and Linda was duly impressed at how fast the injury healed with homeopathic treatment. But it wasn't until she had her own case of tonsillitis that she actually tried homeopathy herself. She was prescribed a round of antibiotics that worked but only temporarily. She then went to a homeopathic doctor. Not only did her symptoms go away rapidly, they never returned. She said, "We couldn't cope without homeopathy."

Sadly, Linda McCartney died in 1998 due to breast cancer.

George Harrison (1943–2001), also best known for being a member of the Beatles, was a British lead guitarist, singer, songwriter, record producer, and film producer. The Beatles songs that Harrison wrote and sang lead on include "If I Needed Someone," "Taxman," "While My Guitar Gently Weeps," "Here Comes the Sun," and "Something." After the dissolution of the Beatles, he created an impressive body of eleven albums, including the much honored *All Things Must Pass*. Harrison was inducted into the Rock and Roll Hall of Fame as a solo artist in 2004.

Harrison also was a film producer, including important films such as Monty Python's *The Life of Brian*, plus *Time Bandits*, *Withnail and I*, and *Mona Lisa*.

Harrison's interest in Indian music and Hinduism sparked international awareness of Eastern music and beliefs. He organized the first large-scale charity concert, for Bangladesh, on August 1, 1971.

A 1992 interview with George Harrison took place in the London office of **Dr. Chandra Sharma**, a practitioner of homeopathy and Ayurvedic medicine. Dr. Sharma was also known to treat members of Pink Floyd, The Police, and numerous other major rock stars (Beatles Ireland, 1992).

George's first wife, **Patti Boyd**, was one of many celebrities who supported a British organization called Frontline Homeopathy that provides treatment to people in underdeveloped countries. Patti introduced George to Maharishi Mahesh Yogi, the founder of Transcendental Meditation, who was not simply a teacher of yoga and meditation but also practiced homeopathy. Later, Patti encourage her second husband, Eric Clapton, to go through drug detoxification with the aid of acupuncture (Greene, 2006, 207).

George's second wife, **Olivia Harrison**, also had a special appreciation for natural medicine and encouraged its use by George (Greene, 2006, 221).

Pete Townshend (1945–) is an influential English rock guitarist and songwriter who is best known as guitarist for The Who. Townshend has authored more than 100 songs, and the rock opera *Tommy*. Townshend suffers from partial deafness and tinnitus due to exposure to loud music during concerts and through the use of headphones. His condition is attributed in part to an infamous 1967 television appearance during which fellow Who musician, Keith Moon, set off a large amount of explosives inside his drums while Townshend was standing in front of them.

In 2000, Pete told a magazine reporter: "I've had some treatment for it. I found a homeopathic practitioner who has really helped reduce it tremendously" (Wilkerson, 2006, Chapter 18, note 6).

Cher (1946–) is a total entertainer. This singer and actress has achieved true diva-hood. She has won a Grammy (1999), an Oscar (1989), three Golden Globe awards (1974, 1984, and 1989), and an Emmy (2003). One of the best-selling singers of all time, she has recorded thirty-four albums, seven with her former husband (Sonny Bono), twenty-seven solo albums, and eight compilations of previous work. Films in which she has starred include *The Witches of Eastwick, Moonstruck, Tea with Mussolini, Mermaids, Silkwood,* and *Mask.* Madame Tussaud's Wax Museum immortalized her in 1992 with a life-size statue as one of the five most beautiful women of history.

In 1987 Cher was struck by a debilitating viral illness that manifested in chronic fatigue and bouts of pneumonia. She was disabled from working for two years: "I tried regular medicine and it just didn't work. Doctors said any illness was all in my head. People thought I was crazy."

Then she decided to do something different: "I turned to a Sikh homeopathic doctor, almost in desperation. He started doing homeopathic stuff with herbs and vitamin therapy. Many doctors didn't believe in all that back then. Within four months, he'd got me up and back on the road again."

In addition to seeking care from this unnamed Sikh doctor, Cher sought treatment from a French homeopathic doctor, **Dr. Marcel Dinnet**. According to famed gossip columnist Liz Smith, Dr. Dinnet is reported to have 10,000 devoted patients in Los Angeles, including Sarah Ferguson (the Duchess of York) and Elizabeth Taylor (Smith, 1988).

Cher pledged her support for the Glasgow Homeopathic Hospital after seeing a TV news report that the government was slashing the city's health budget by 58 million pounds (around $100 million). She intended her donation of $24,000 to encourage others to pledge cash to help keep the hospital open. The hospital treats 500 in-patients a year. The hospital's staff and patients have sharply criticized the budget reduction for both medical and economic reasons. They asserted that closing this important natural medicine hospital could lead to higher health care costs for the

Greater Glasgow Health Board. Cher further asserted: "I'm not quite sure exactly what that will mean but I'd be prepared to do anything I can to help." (Sloan, 2004).

Bob Weir (1947–) is an American singer, songwriter, and guitarist who was a founding member of the Grateful Dead, one of the most popular bands to ever come out of San Francisco. Bob's first experience with homeopathy occurred in 1972 when the Dead were touring England and all came down with a nasty flu. Their tour manager, Sam Cutler, who had previously worked for the Rolling Stones, arranged to obtain homeopathic medicines, which got them up, playing, and "truckin'" in short order.

During a recent lunch with the Weir family, Bob and his wife, **Natascha**, told me that they sought the care of a homeopathic pediatrician, **Ifeoma Ikense, MD**, shortly after they had their first daughter, Monet. Natascha told me that she has called Dr. Ikense dozens of times during various music tours to treat someone in the family and "homeopathy works every time." Bob and Natascha swear by homeopathy, and they both "wonder how other parents do without it." Even Bob's father (a former colonel and B-52 pilot in the U.S. Air Force) and his stepmother, both in their eighties, use homeopathic medicines as an integral part of their lives.

Paul Rodgers (1949–) is a British singer who is most well known for being a member of the bands Free and Bad Company. He collaborated on two albums with Jimmy Page in The Firm, and has created albums and toured with David Gilmour (Pink Floyd), Kenny Jones (The Who), Bryan Adams, Muddy Waters, and Journey. Rodgers has also had a successful career as a solo artist.

In a 2001 interview, he stated:

> I like for the vocals to challenge and stretch me. It keeps it interesting. A voice is not just a voice, it is your whole self. You have got to look after yourself physically, mentally and spiritually to keep the level of what you put out as a singer. Part of my meditation that I do includes a lot of deep breathing. It is very beneficial to breath in a lot of clean air.

> There is also a homeopathic medication that I take. There is a guy I see that gives me *Argentum nitricum* [silver nitrate]. I would not recommend just taking that. You have to see the proper guy. It helps keep my voice nice and clear. (Wright, 2001)

Annie Lennox (1954–) is a Scottish rock musician and vocalist who has won an Oscar, a Grammy, and a BRIT. In the 1980s she was lead singer for a duo called the Eurythmics with British musician David A. Stewart. She wrote and performed the soundtrack cut for Francis Ford Coppola's 1992 movie *Dracula* ("Love Song for a Vampire"). She also made a magnificently memorable appearance with David Bowie and the surviving members of Queen at the Freddie Mercury tribute concert at London's Wembley Stadium. Inevitably, when singers travel, they carry certain must-have tour supplies, and Annie Lennox always includes homeopathic medicines. She admits that she sometimes feels like a witch doctor in her efforts to ward off illnesses (Smith, 2004).

Axl Rose (1962–) is an American hard rock singer and songwriter who is best known as the lead singer of Guns N' Roses. In the late 1980s, Guns N' Roses shot to the top of rock music charts as a result of the massive popularity of the songs "Welcome to the Jungle," "Paradise City," and "Sweet Child O' Mine." In 1992, after performing at the tribute to Freddie Mercury at London's Wembley Stadium, there was a problem with airport security when he asked that his black pouch containing homeopathic medicines not undergo X-ray (Smith, 1992). Rose supposedly flew into a rage because he was concerned that the X-ray would neutralize his homeopathic medicines. (Although X-ray may possibly create some problems for these medicines, there is no conclusive evidence of bad effects.)

According to *Rolling Stone*, Rose has been a powerful, almost evangelical believer in homeopathic medicine for close to a decade. The singer is strongly critical of conventional medicine and conventional physicians and considers the AMA to be populated by greedy doctors. Homeopathic elixirs for his throat were always on hand whenever Rose toured with Guns N' Roses (Rolling Stone, 2000).

Moby (1965–) is an American singer and electronic musician. He took his name from the book *Moby Dick,* whose author, Herman Melville, happens to be his great-great-granduncle. Moby has created numerous albums and scored several movies, including an updated version of the James Bond theme song for the movie *Tomorrow Never Dies.* His breakthrough album, *Play,* was released in 1999, the first album in history to have all of its songs commercially licensed. Despite his great popularity, Moby is known to live a relatively simple life, in a relatively small apartment in New York City, eating a vegan diet. In a 2002 interview, he told salon.com that he is a devout believer in homeopathy and alternative medicine (January 2, 2002).

Nelly Furtado (1978–) is a Grammy Award-winning Canadian singer-songwriter, instrumentalist, and record producer. She came to fame in 2000 with the release of her album *Whoa, Nelly!,* which featured the Grammy Award-winning single "I'm like a Bird."

Nelly, like most working musicians, must travel great distances for gigs. In 2007 she told the *Times* (of London) that she swears by NoJet-Lag, a popular homeopathic medicine that helps reduce the symptoms and discomforts of jet lag (*Times,* 2007).

Jon Faddis (1953–) is an eminent American jazz trumpet player, protégé of Dizzy Gillespie. In December 1991 Faddis was appointed music director of the Carnegie Hall Jazz Band, an eighteen-piece all-star orchestra that typically includes some of the greatest names in jazz. Faddis was the music director of the 1995 Lincoln Center Jazz Orchestra, "The Majesty of Louis Armstrong Tour," and the "Newport Jazz Festival 40th Anniversary Tour." Jon's distinctive trumpet voice is heard on albums by superstar performers as disparate as Duke Ellington, the Rolling Stones, Frank Sinatra, Luther Vandross, Quincy Jones, Billy Joel, and Stanley Clarke. His horn was heard on the theme of *The Cosby Show* and on the soundtrack of Clint Eastwood's films *The Gauntlet* and *Bird.*

When speaking about Jon Faddis, Dizzy Gillespie once said, "He's the best ever—including me!" Faddis's trademark is the very high range in which he plays. He doesn't simply hit those higher notes, he plays and stays in that range.

When teaching master classes on trumpet technique, Jon Faddis first emphasizes the need for jazz players to acquire solid fundamental skills on the instrument, but he is known to quickly move the discussion to his interest in homeopathy, and to "treating the whole trumpet player" (Donaldson, 1999).

Shirley Verrett (1931–), an American mezzo-soprano opera singer, has enjoyed great fame since the late 1960s. She has sung with the New York City Opera, had repeated roles with the Bolshoi Theatre, the Metropolitan Opera, the Royal Opera House, and the Philadelphia Philharmonic Orchestra. In the late 1970s she began to tackle soprano roles, including Tosca, Norma, Lady Macbeth, and Aida. In 1990, Verrett sang Dido in *Les Troyens* at the inauguration of the Opera Bastille in Paris.

Opera News reported that it is extremely rare for an opera singer's voice to actually improve after turning 50 years of age, but the magazine writer insists that it is true with Verrett. She credits her improvement to homeopathic medicine. For thirty years allergies to mold spores clogged her bronchial tubes. Her allergies were so bad that she planned to give up her singing career on numerous occasions, but the real and practical benefits she received from homeopathy helped her regain her health and recapture and even improve upon her magnificent voice (Dyer, 1990).

Carl Davis, CBE (1936–), is a conductor with the London Philharmonic Orchestra, and regularly conducts the Royal Liverpool Philharmonic Orchestra. He has written music for more than 100 television programs and dozens of films, but he is best known for creating musical scores to films that were originally silent. He also assisted in the orchestration of the symphonic works of Paul McCartney.

This modern composer has used homeopathic medicines since the 1960s. He once told a London reporter that he still laughs at the memory of conducting a concert on a platform over the Thames River: "I was cocooned in homeopathic insect repellent while everyone else was besieged by mosquitoes" (Kindred Spirits, 1989).

Appreciation to and for homeopathy among musicians is significant enough that even some recording studios are providing access to homeopathic medicines in the studios themselves. **Grouse Lodge** is a recording studio in County Westmeath, Ireland, that advertises itself as Ireland's only residential studio where musicians can have comfortable lodging as well as access to a health spa with homeopathic and herbal services. Musicians who have recently recorded there include Snow Patrol, Republic of Loose, Bloc Party, Doves, Skinsize Kings, and Muse (Absolution), but this studio became particularly well known in late 2006 when Michael Jackson recorded there.

Wayne Newton (1942–), "Mr. Las Vegas," was reported to shop frequently in a certain Las Vegas pharmacy. When asked what he buys, the pharmacist reported, "Anything homeopathic" (In Style, 2004).

Victoria Beckham (1974–), formerly nicknamed "Posh" of Spice Girl fame, is married to David Beckham, the soccer superstar. Victoria has told the media that she has a special interest in yoga as well as in homeopathic medicine. Homeopathic medicines are also helpful in this celebrity household that presently has three sons.

Many internationally acclaimed classical musicians sought care from **Elizabeth Wright Hubbard, MD** (1896–1967), a respected homeopath in New York City. Some of these musicians included **Darius Milhaud** (1892–1974, a French composer and teacher who was a member of *Les Six*, and who was one of the most prolific composers of the twentieth century); **Georges Auric** (1899–1983, a French composer who scored many films including Jean Cocteau's *Beauty and the Beast, Moulin Rouge,* and *Roman Holiday*); and **Lily Pons** (1898–1976, a French-born American coloratura soprano) (Naifeh and Smith, 1989, 482).

References

Albrecht, T. *Letters to Beethoven and Other Correspondence.* Vol. 3: 1824–1828. Lincoln: University of Nebraska, 1996.

Atwood, W. G. *The Parisian Worlds of Frederic Chopin.* New Haven: Yale University, 1999. (See also www.chopin-society.org.uk/article.htm.)

Beatles Ireland. www.iol.ie/~beatlesireland/harrison/interviews/georgeinterview1.htm

Beethoven, L. van. *Briefwechsel Gesamtausgabe,* Band 6, 1825–1827. Munchen: G. Henle, 1996.

Beethoven, L. van. *Ludwig van Beethovens Konversationshefte,* Band 8, Heft 91–103. Leipzig: VEB Deutscher four Musik, 1981.

Belon, P., Banerjee, P., and Choudhury, S. C. Can Administration of Potentized Homeopathic Remedy, Arsenicum album, Alter Antinuclear Antibody (ANA) Titer in People Living in High-Risk Arsenic Contaminated Areas?: I. A Correlation with Certain Hematological Parameters, *Evidence-Based Complementary and Alternative Medicine,* March 2006, 3(1):99–107.

Collins, S. The man who wants to make Tina Turner live until she's 120, *Sunday Mirror,* November 7, 1999.

Donaldson, J. The International Trumpet Guild, 1999 Conference. www.trumpetguild.org/conferences/conference99/friday/f14a.htm

Dyer, R. Characteristically Verrett, *Opera News,* February 17, 1990, pp. 9–12+.

Glew, J. "We couldn't cope without homeopathy," *Health and Homoeopathy,* Summer 1992, 6–7.

Greene, J. M. *Here Comes the Sun: The Spiritual and Musical Journey of George Harrison.* Hoboken, N. J.: John Wiley and Sons, 2006.

Haehl, R. *Samuel Hahnemann: His Life and Work* (2 vols.). London: Homeopathic Publishing Co., 1922 (reprinted New Delhi: B. Jain).

Handley, R. *A Homeopathic Love Story.* Berkeley: North Atlantic Books, 1990.

Hayden, D. *Pox: Genius, Madness, and the Mysteries of Syphilis.* New York: Basic Books, 2003.

Hellenbroich, A. In Celebration of Ludwig van Beethoven's 225th Birthday, *Fidelio,* Winter 1995.

In Style, November 2004.

Khuda-Bukhsh, A. R., Pathak, S., and Guha, B. Can Homeopathic Arsenic Remedy Combat Arsenic Poisoning in Humans Exposed to Groundwater Arsenic Contamination?: A Preliminary Report on First Human Trial, *Evidence-Based Complementary and Alternative Medicine,* December 2005, 2(4):537–548.

Kindred Spirits, *Daily Telegraph,* August 12, 1989.

Linde, K., Jonas, W. B., Melchart, D., et al. Critical Review and Meta-Analysis of Serial Agitated Dilutions in Experimental Toxicology, *Human and Experimental Toxicology,* 1994, 13:481–492.

Mai, F. *Diagnosing Genius: The Life and Death of Beethoven.* Montreal: McGill-Queen's University, 2007.

Maretzki, T. W., and Seidler, E. Biomedicine and naturopathic healing in West Germany: a historical and ethnomedical view of a stormy relationship. *Culture, Medicine and Psychiatry,* December 1985, 9,4:383–421.

Naifeh, S., and Smith, G. W. *Jackson Pollock: An American Saga.* New York: Charles N. Potter, 1989.

Orth, M. Tina, *Vogue,* May 1985, p. 318.

Plant, D. *Kepler and the Music of the Spheres.* www.skyscript.co.uk/kepler.html

Rolling Stone, What Happened to Axl Rose—The inside story of rock's most famous recluse, May 11 2000.

Schweisheimer, W. Beethoven's Physicians, *Musical Quarter,* 1945, 31:289–298.

Sloan, B. Cher's Ward Rage: Exclusive Star's Fury Over Bid to Close Scots Homeopathic Hospital, *Sunday Mail,* May 16, 2004.

Smith, K. British Pop Greats Go On Tour Together for the First Time, Associated Press, June 1, 2004.

Smith, L. Fergie Told She'll Lose a Fast 50 Pounds, *San Francisco Chronicle,* November 17, 1988.

Smith, L. Axl's Left Holdng Bag, *New York Daily News,* April 24, 1992.
Takacs. 2007. http://ums.org/assets/programbooks/Takacs_Programbook.pdf
Times (of London), Miracle Jet-Lag Cure, February 11, 2007.
Turner, T. *I, Tina.* New York: Avon, 1986.
Ullman, D. *Homeopathic Family Medicine.* Berkeley: Homeopathic Educational Services, 2007. (This is a comprehensive and regularly updated review and description of clinical research in homeopathy. Available as a one-time download or as a subscription from www.homeopathic.com.)
Wagner, R. *My Life, Volume I.* New York: Dodd, Mead and Company, 1911.
Watson, D. *Richard Wagner: A Biography.* New York: McGraw Hill, 1979.
Wilkerson, M. *Amazing Journey: The Life of Pete Townshend.* Lulu Press, 2006. (This specific story was told to Q Magazine's David Cavanaugh in January 2000.)
Wright, J. Interview with Paul Rodgers. *Classic Rock Revisited,* January 12, 2001. Available at www.classicrockrevisited.com/interviews01/PaulEncore.htm

CHAPTER 8

Artists and Fashionistas: Homeopathy in Style

Good art is truly timeless and may even transcend one's culture. Good fashion, in comparison, is fleeting in time and is directly based on a specific culture. Despite the disparity of these two forms of art, various leading artists and fashionistas of the past 200 years have appreciated the art and science of homeopathic medicine—or at least have appreciated the results they got from it.

Vincent Willem van Gogh (1853–1890), a Dutch post-Impressionist painter, is widely considered one of the greatest painters in art history. His brother Theodorus (Theo) (1857–1891) worked as an art dealer, and in 1886, while they lived together in Paris, Theo played an important role in introducing Vincent to various Impressionist painters, including Claude Monet, Pierre-Auguste Renoir, Edgar Degas, and Camille Pissarro.

Vincent was often deeply depressed and suffered from various physical complaints. From May 1889 to May 1890, he was in a mental hospital. After release, he moved to Auvers-sur-Oise near Paris where he could live close to his brother. His friend and fellow artist, Camille Pissarro, enthusiastically recommended that Vincent see **Dr. Paul Gachet** (1828–1909), a homeopathic and eclectic physician who was treating various other artists and was an amateur artist himself (Distel and Stein, 1999).[69]

During the short time in which van Gogh got to know Dr. Gachet, van Gogh developed a strong rapport with the doctor. He wrote, "I have found a friend in Dr. Gachet ... and something of a new brother, since we are so similar both mentally and physically" (Burgess and Phruksachart, 2006).

In June 1890, Vincent painted a portrait of Dr. Gachet. One month later, at the age of only 37, Vincent van Gogh shot himself and died two days later. Hundreds of physicians and art historians have sought to diagnose van Gogh's illness, and dozens of theories presently exist, including schizophrenia, bipolar disorder, syphilis, poisoning from swallowed paints, and temporal lobe epilepsy. All of these diagnoses would have been aggravated by other factors in van Gogh's life, including his fondness for absinthe, malnutrition, tendency to overwork, and insomnia. In the November 2005 issue of *Archives of Pathology and Laboratory Medicine*, Paul L. Wolf, MD, presented a new provocative theory of how disease, drugs, and chemicals might have caused a yellowing of his vision augmented by imbibing absinthe. Made from wormwood, absinthe contains relatively high doses of thujone, a neurotoxin. This theory presents an interesting potential explanation for how van Gogh's disease may have greatly influenced the color in his paintings. Whatever serious health problems van Gogh suffered, his visit to Dr. Gachet was simply too late to save this magnificent artist.

Due to Dr. Gachet's support for so many artists of his day, *The Times* (of London) referred to him as the "unsung godfather and friend of Impressionism and Post-Impressionism" (Macintyre. 1999). Famed artists Claude Monet, Pierre Auguste-Renoir, Paul Cézanne, and Théophile Gautier also sought homeopathic treatment from Dr. Gachet. Many artists sometimes paid medical bills with their own paintings, which Dr. Gachet, being an appreciator and supporter of the arts, accepted gladly (Sparenborg-Nolte and Nolte, 2005). Gachet was also known to treat many actors and musicians (Distel and Stein, 1999, 5).

Although the results of Gachet's treatment for Monet or Gautier are unknown, it is known that he oversaw Renoir's recovery from pneumonia in 1882, and Renoir lived until 1919. Paul Cézanne was so pleased with Gachet's care that he brought his wife and children to the doctor (Negro, 2005).[70]

Dr. Gachet studied under Dr. Jean Jacques Molin, the homeopathic physician to Chopin (Wayne E. Oates Institute, online).[71]

In 1990 (100 years later), van Gogh's painting of Dr. Gachet sold to a

Japanese industrialist for $82.5 million, the highest price for a painting at the time (since then, Picasso's *Garçon à la Pipe* sold for $104.1 million).

Camille Pissarro (1830–1903) is known as the father of Impressionism. He painted rural French life, particularly landscapes and workers in the fields, as well as scenes from Montmartre (a hill and community in Paris). He taught painting to Paul Cézanne and Paul Gauguin, among many others. Although he is generally not considered the best painter of the French Impressionists, he is commonly considered the main conceptualist of Impressionist theory.

Pissarro had a special love for homeopathy that started shortly after his father's death in 1865. His mother, Rachel, became quite ill for several months, and Pissarro sought homeopathic care for her with Dr. Gachet. The results were so fast and so significant that both he and his mother developed a lifelong devotion to homeopathy and Dr. Gachet. Pissarro even became a lay prescriber of homeopathic medicines himself.

Pissarro was appreciative enough of Dr. Gachet that he moved to the lovely town Auvers-sur-Oise just outside of Paris, where the physician had his practice and studio.[72] Van Gogh and several other leading artists of that time followed them to this quaint French town. Gachet himself became an enthusiastic engraver, and although his work wasn't of the same high caliber as his friends, he gained some respect as an artist. Of additional interest is the fact that several of the Impressionists took up etching, working in Gachet's studio and printing their work with the doctor's press (Roe, 2006). Cézanne produced there an etching of Guillaumin, as well as a number of flower pieces arranged in Delft vases for him by the doctor's wife. Gachet was the first person to purchase a Cézanne painting.

It was Pissarro who recommended that van Gogh see the homeopath, even if Gachet's treatment began too late in van Gogh's disease. Pissarro encouraged many people to seek out homeopathic treatment. Pissarro wrote to his friend Octave Mirbeau, a journalist, novelist, and playwright, who was suffering from depression: "What a pity that you have no confidence in homeopathic remedies. Seriously, my dear, I believe that you would be able to fight off these prostrations, this discouragement, this lassitude about all things.... what a pity, I tell you because I have such confidence in it" (Pissarro, 1892).

Pissarro died in 1903 and is buried in Père Lachaise Cemetery in Paris (where Samuel Hahnemann, MD, also rests). Although Pissarro sold few of his paintings during his lifetime, some have recently sold for around $4 million.

Eugène Henri Paul Gauguin (1848–1903) was a leading post-Impressionist painter. Like his friend van Gogh, Gauguin experienced bouts of depression and once attempted suicide. Gauguin paintings are rarely offered for sale, though some have been priced as high as $39.2 million.

Some biographers have determined that Gauguin was infected with syphilis. In 1892 he went to a military hospital in Papeete, Tahiti, where he was diagnosed with syphilis of the heart and prescribed homeopathic doses of digitalis (Hayden, 2003, 166).

In 1872 he moved to the village of Auvers-sur-Oise, where his neighbor Pissarro introduced him to Cézanne and Armand Guillamin. He met Monet, Renoir, and scores of others less known today.

When Gachet was young, he hung out in Paris cafes with various artists and poets who would eventually become world famous, including Jean Désiré Gustave Courbet (leader of the Realist movement in France), Édouard Manet (a French artist who bridged the Impressionism and the Realism movements), and Charles Pierre Baudelaire (one of the most influential poets of the nineteenth century). Gachet was present when Cézanne sneered at Manet's masterful painting, *Olympia,* calling it "mere child's play." Gachet purchased it and later lent it to the 1874 Impressionist exhibition, once again showing his eye for quality art (Robinson, 1999). In his forties, Manet contracted syphilis, and when conventional doctors recommended amputation of his leg due to gangrene, Gachet strongly advised against this surgery. Manet died eleven days later.

Gachet's rule for living was said to be "to cure people, to paint, and to adore art" (Negro, 2005). Obviously, he led a full life.

Jackson Pollock (1912–1956) was a leading American artist who was a major force in the Abstract Expressionism movement. Pollock received significant financial support from heiress Peggy Guggenheim, and married fellow abstract painter Lee Krasner in 1945. Krasner encouraged him to go to her homeopathic doctor due to his very serious bouts of depression and his alcoholism.

Pollock went to Elizabeth Wright Hubbard, MD (1896–1967), a respected homeopath in New York City. Dr. Hubbard graduated in 1921 from the first class to matriculate women from the Columbia College of Physicians and Surgeons. She then left New York to go to Geneva, Switzerland to study homeopathy with **Pierre Schmidt, MD**, who had been taught by **Dr. A. E. Austin** and **Dr. F. E. Gladwin**, two of **Dr. James Tyler Kent**'s most illustrious pupils. She was the first woman to be elected president of the American Institute of Homeopathy, and she served for many years as editor of the *Homeopathic Recorder* and subsequently as editor of the *Journal of the American Institute of Homeopathy*.

Some other people of notoriety who were known to be her patients included: **Marlene Dietrich** (1901–1992, German-American actress, entertainer, and singer known for her many femmes fatale characters), **Darius Milhaud** (1892–1974, French composer and teacher who was a member of *Les Six*), **Georges Auric** (1899–1983, French composer who scored many films including Jean Cocteau's *Beauty and the Beast, Moulin Rouge,* and *Roman Holiday*), **Alexander Calder** (1898–1976, an avant garde American sculptor and artist most famous for inventing the mobile), and **Lily Pons** (1898–1976, French-born American coloratura soprano) (Naifeh and Smith, 1989, 482).

In early 1945, Pollock began Dr. Hubbard's homeopathic treatment just in time. Pollock's patron, Ms. Guggenheim, had scheduled two major art shows for him, including one in New York and another in Chicago, yet he had not produced a single work of art in many months. Shortly after his first homeopathic treatment, Pollock experienced one of his most creative and productive periods in his life (Naifeh and Smith, 1989, 492–493; Gliatto, Burleigh, and Goulding, 1998).

Antoni Gaudi (1852–1926) was a Spanish architect whose style was totally unique. Working mainly in Barcelona, he created startling new architectural forms that paralleled the stylistic development of art nouveau or *modernismo*. Many of his buildings resemble sculptural configurations, and many have a gothic yet futuristic look. Due to chronic rheumatism, Gaudi followed a strict vegetarian diet and was a regular user of homeopathic medicines.

Edgar de Evia (1910–2003) was a prominent American photographer, artist, and author. For many years he was in charge of all photographs for the catalogue of Gimbel's, the once high-style department store. He also photographed virtually every top model in the last half of the twentieth century, and his photographs have graced many ad campaigns of major corporations.

After briefly working for the Associated Press, de Evia became medical research assistant to noted homeopathic physician **Dr. Guy Beckley Stearns**. The doctor gave him his first camera, a Rolleiflex, and taught him to use it. Edgar de Evia co-authored numerous articles and a book with Dr. Stearns entitled *A New Synthesis* (1960).

Hardy Amies, formally known as Sir Edwin Hardy Amies (1909–2003), was an English dressmaker who was awarded a royal warrant by Queen Elizabeth II as her official dressmaker (1955 to 1990). Besides establishing his own fashion house selling haute couture to the rich and famous, he designed costumes for stage and film, most notably for Stanley Kubrick's *2001: A Space Odyssey*. He was knighted in 1989.

Like the queen herself, he was a great appreciator of homeopathic medicine. However, as he got older, he began using less homeopathic medicine. When he was 80, he asserted: "When you get to my age, you want quick results... but homeopathy is most effective in the long term. I don't think that one should be militantly anti-ordinary medicine. The two should go hand-in-hand" (Kindred Spirits, 1989).

Karl (Otto) Lagerfeld (1938–) is widely recognized as one of the most influential fashion designers of the late twentieth and current century. He became famous for his collaboration with high-profile fashion labels, including Chloe, Fendi, and Chanel. In the early 1980s he set up his own label, Lagerfeld, which included perfumes and clothing lines. He has also played a role in dressing leading artists.

Lagerfeld is also famous for a dramatic transformation of his own body, when he lost some 80 pounds (36 kg) in one year. He co-authored *The Karl Lagerfeld Diet* with **Jean-Claude Houdret, MD**, a Parisian homeopathic doctor who teaches medicine at the University of Paris. This book sold several hundred thousand copies in Europe and Asia, and in mid-2005, was released in America. Though the regimen bears the designer's famous name, it's actually the creation of Dr. Houdret. The diet, also called the Spoonlight Program, features a low-carb, low-fat, low-calorie fare that is unmistakably French.

Lagerfeld collaborated with and was treated for many years by another French homeopathic doctor, **Pierre Richand, MD**, who received degrees from the Faculté de Medicine in Paris and the Faculté des Sciences (Petkanas, 1992).

Vidal Sassoon (1928–) was one of the most influential hair stylists of the mid-1960s, and his influence remains today. Sassoon is considered a creator of modernist style, and has been a major player in various commercial hair styling products. He once told a reporter that he attributes his youthful appearance and stamina to homeopathic medicines and natural foods (Ghent, 1983).

Jerry Hall (1956–), the famous model and former wife of Rolling Stone Mick Jagger, was known to receive treatment for her bad back from **Jack Temple** (1918–2004), a "dowsing homeopathic healer." She described Temple as a genius and miracle-worker who was particularly helpful to her when she dealt with the stress of her divorce from Mick Jagger. The benefits she experienced during and after this time were significant enough for her to say that she "regrets not becoming a homeopathic doctor" (Hall, 1999). Jerry has also been one of many celebrities to support a British organization called Frontline Homeopathy, which provides homeopathic treatment to people with AIDS in Africa.

Jade Jagger (1971–), the only child of Mick and Bianca Jagger, was creative director and jewelry designer for Garrard, the high-end British jewelry company known to serve the queen of England. Jade has suffered from eczema throughout much of her life, but homeopathy and acupuncture have been her favorite and most effective treatments. As the mother of two daughters, Jade was concerned that they would also suffer with this condition. She explains: "When I had my first daughter Assisi in 1992 I thought I could prevent her getting it. I fed her only organic vegetarian food and breast milk for the first two years, but despite that, she eventually developed eczema. Fortunately, my homeopath cured her with one remedy" (Raymond, 1997).

Jade is passionate enough about homeopathy that she told me personally that she once considered becoming a homeopath herself and has been an avid reader of homeopathic *materia medica* (Latin for "materials of medicine," detailed information about the various homeopathic medicines and which physical and psychological symptoms each is known to cause and cure). In addition to having her family treated with homeopathic medicines, she has also found that homeopathic medicines act miraculously in treating animals.

Lindka Cierach is one of the UK's leading fashion designers today. Her clients include three generations of the British royal family and international stars and celebrities. She achieved widespread notoriety when she was commissioned in 1986 to design the dress for the wedding of Sarah Ferguson to the Duke of York. On the morning of the royal wedding, she took a homeopathic formula that contained *Kali phos* (potassium phosphate), *Lycopodium* (club moss), *Gelsemium* (yellow jessamine), and *Argentum nit* (silver nitrate) to deal with the stress, and as a result, she said she "sailed through" in royal form (Kindred Spirits, 1989).

It is assumed that models have to do all they can to take care of their skin and looks. Therefore, supermodels know how to take super good care of their appearance. It's not surprising then that supermodel **Cindy Crawford** (1966–) is super into homeopathic and naturalistic products (Finn, 2004).

References

Burgess, C., and Phruksachart, M. Auvers-sur-Oise: Revisiting Vincent van Gogh, *Paris Voice,* May 24, 2006.

Distel, A., and Stein, S. A. *Cézanne to Van Gogh: The Collection of Doctor Gachet.* New York: Metropolitan Museum of Art, 1999.

Finn, K. Crawford Struts into Skin Care, Gale Group, November 12, 2004.

Ghent, J. Sassoon Steps Back, Switches Gears, *Oakland Tribune,* March 10, 1983.

Gliatto, T., Burleigh, N., and Christian Goulding, S. C. Stroke of Genius: Jackson Pollock changed the world of painting with his drips and drabs, *People,* November 23, 1998.

Jerry Hall, *The Times* (London), December 8, 1999.

Hayden, D. *Pox: Genius, Madness, and the Mysteries of Syphilis.* New York: Basic Books, 2003.

Kindred Spirits, *Daily Telegraph,* August 12, 1989.

Macintyre, B. Physician, Paint Thyself, *The Times* (London), January 16, 1999.

Naifeh, S., and Smith, G.W. *Jackson Pollock: An American Saga.* New York: Charles N. Potter, 1989.

Negro, F. E. *Grandi a Piccole Dosi: La Parentesi Omeopatica di Vite Famose.* Milano: Franco Angeli, 2005.

Petkanas, C. Karl Lagerfeld's Weird Weight-Loss Diet, *San Francisco Chronicle,* May 29, 1992.

Pissarro's Letter to Mirbeau. January 10, 1892, in Volkmar, K. F. A Natural Order: Observation and the Four Seasons, *Art Criticism,* 1998, XIII(1):22–40.

Raymond, C. Jade Jagger, *The Mirror* (London), September 17, 1997.

Robinson, W. The Curious Case of Dr. Gachet, *Artnet,* May 17, 1999.

Roe, S. *The Private Lives of the Impressionists.* New York: Harper Collins, 2006.

Sparenborg-Nolte, A., and Nolte, H. Dr. Paul Ferdinand Gachet: Van Gogh's Late Physician, A Disciple of Hahnemann? *Allgemeine Homöopathische Zeitung,* 2005, 250(2):200.

Temple, Jack (obituary). *The Telegraph* (London), February 2, 2004. Available at www.telegraph.co.uk/news/main.jhtml?xml=/news/2004/02/20/db2001.xml&sSheet=/portal/2004/02/20/ixportal.html

Wayne E. Oates Institute Online. www.oates.org/olc/mbr/a0300/meckler/meckler27.html

CHAPTER 9

Politicians and Peacemakers: Voting with Their Lives and Health

At least eleven American presidents have received homeopathic medical treatment or expressed support for it by their political actions. Yet, each was strongly discouraged from committing himself too much to its development, for political reasons. Although the educated and literary elite as well as the wealthy classes of people were using homeopathy in the United States and Europe during the nineteenth century, it still represented a minority school of medical practice. Politicians had to be extremely careful in voicing interest in or support for it, especially because the antagonism toward homeopathy and homeopaths by American and European orthodox physicians and their organizations was so strong.

Numerous heads of state other than those in the United States and Europe also expressed a special interest in homeopathy, including leaders in Asia and South America, but the antagonism against homeopathy in those regions was not nearly as crazed.

Abraham Lincoln

The story of what happened to Abraham Lincoln's Secretary of State, William Seward, is a classical story in medical history that exemplifies conventional medicine's attitude toward and actions against unconventional medical treatments and the physicians who provide them.

William Seward (1801–1872) was one of Lincoln's closest political advisors, and he was also an advocate for homeopathic medicine. On the night Lincoln was assassinated, Seward was stabbed in the multi-person assassination plot against the Union.[73] Thanks to the medical care provided by Joseph K. Barnes, MD, U.S. Surgeon General, Seward survived.

However, because Seward's personal physician was a homeopathic doctor and because the AMA had a policy that it was an ethical violation to consult with a homeopathic doctor or even provide care for a homeopathic patient, Dr. Barnes was denounced by the vice president of the AMA for providing medical care (Haller, 2005, 192).[74]

Abraham Lincoln (1809–1865) himself showed a special interest in homeopathic medicine. In 1854, before Lincoln was elected president, he was retained as a lawyer to prepare a state legislative proposal to charter a homeopathic medical college in Chicago. Because Chicago was the home of the American Medical Association, which had been founded in 1847 in part to stop the growth of homeopathy, Lincoln's job was no simple effort. However, many of Chicago's most prominent citizens and politicians participated on the board of trustees of the proposed Hahnemann Medical College, including Chicago's mayor, two congressmen, an Illinois state representative, a Chicago city councilman, the co-founder of Northwestern University, the founder of Chicago Union Railroad, and several medical doctors who were homeopaths (Spiegel and Kavaler, 2002).[75] Despite significant opposition, Lincoln was successful in obtaining a charter for the homeopathic college.

Today, the Pearson Museum at Southern Illinois University has an exhibit of a nineteenth-century doctor's office and drug store; included in this exhibit is a homeopathic medicine kit from the Diller Drug Store of Springfield, Illinois. The exhibit notes that Abraham Lincoln was a frequent customer of the drug store and a regular user of homeopathic medicines (Karst, 1988, 11).

In addition to choosing Seward to be his secretary of state, several leading advisors were homeopathic advocates. On November 1, 1861, Lincoln appointed Major General George Brinton McClellan (1826–1885) to command the Union army during the Civil War. However, in late December McClellan contracted typhoid fever, which left him unable to go to his office to conduct business (Rafuse, 1997). During the first week of McClellan's illness, two homeopathic doctors arrived from New York to care for the ill general and his father-in-law and chief of staff, Randolph

B. Marcy, who was also ill. McClellan's decision to employ homeopathic doctors is particularly interesting considering the fact that the general came from a family of prominent conventional physicians.[76]

Despite this serious illness, General McClellan remained active, giving regular orders to his subordinates, arranging for troop movement and supply transport, meeting with the president on a weekly basis, issuing court martial orders, and even providing commendations to officers. By January 2, he seemed to be much better and shortly afterwards he had no noticeable physical limitations. McClellan lived another twenty-three years.

Despite the success of this homeopathic treatment on the military leader of the Union army, that very month, January 1862, the Army Medical Board rejected requests by homeopathic doctors to serve in military hospitals, arguing that to grant this request would invite applications from all types of quacks and charlatans claiming medical expertise.

Typhoid fever caused more deaths during the Civil War and the Spanish-American War than the deaths caused by bullets (Wershub, 1967, 175). Despite the fact that homeopathy gained widespread popularity in the United States and Europe due to its successes in treating various infectious disease epidemics of the mid- and late-1800s, including typhoid epidemics (Bradford, 1900; Coulter, 1973), the antagonism against homeopathy and homeopaths led to government regulations stipulating that graduates of homeopathic medical colleges could not receive a commission for military service.

In Connecticut, several "irregular" physicians offered their services to the governor, who accepted them, but the examining board of the Union army rejected them and instead accepted recruits from a hastily graduated class from Yale College.[77]

Although the Union army had strict restrictions against homeopathic physicians, the Confederate army did not. In fact, the physician to the wife of the Confederate army's General Robert E. Lee was a homeopathic doctor, **Alfred Hughes, MD** (Hughes, 1904, 39).[78] At least in one incidence, General Lee himself was known to have taken homeopathic medicines (Mainwaring and Riley, 2005).

Thankfully, the antagonism toward homeopaths was not as severe during World War I; almost 2,000 homeopathic physicians were commissioned as medical officers. Even the American Red Cross authorized a homeopathic hospital unit (Dearborn, 1923).

Lincoln was also known to appoint some homeopathic physicians to political positions. For instance, in 1863 he appointed **Dr. J. G. Hunt**, author of a book on homeopathy and surgery (Hill and Hunt, 1855), to be consul to Nicaragua (King, 1905, I, 177). Lincoln also signed a bill into law that gave the president the authority to make appointments to the Union army's medical department, including homeopaths (Haller, 2005, 187). However, orthodox physicians strongly asserted that they would not work with homeopaths in any way, thus creating new and more difficult problems in military medicine.

Although Lincoln surrounded himself with advocates for homeopathy, that didn't protect the medical science from his famous wit. He once called homeopathy "medicine of a shadow of a pigeon's wing."

On a more serious note, it should also be mentioned that the personal physician to Mary Lincoln (1818–1882) during the later part of her life was a homeopathic physician and surgeon from Chicago, **Dr. Willis Danforth**.[79] Mary Lincoln was known to have experienced serious bouts of depression after her husband was assassinated and two of her children died, one at age 11 (1862) and the other at 18 (1871).

Mary Lincoln became the sole heir of the Lincoln estate and her extravagant spending and unusual behavior later in life concerned her son Robert so much that in 1874, he sought to get her declared insane and sent to a mental asylum. The testimony of her homeopath, Danforth, confirmed her insanity because he noted that Mrs. Lincoln experienced "nervous derangement" and had delusions. She was committed to the asylum, but was free to move about the grounds, and was released three months later. Recent research has uncovered strong evidence to suggest that Mary Lincoln also suffered from syphilis, which may help explain her crazed mental state (Hayden, 2003, 120–132).

William Lloyd Garrison

William Lloyd Garrison (1805–1879) was one of the most prominent anti-slavery activists in the nineteenth century. He is best known as the editor of the radical abolitionist newspaper, *The Liberator,* and as one of the founders of the American Anti-Slavery Society. Garrison was influenced by the ideas of Susan B. Anthony, Elizabeth Cady Stanton, and Lucretia Mott (all of whom were also activists for homeopathy) and other feminists who joined the society, though Garrison's support for the feminists was controversial to many society members, creating a major rift in the organization. In 1839 a rival organization, the American and Foreign Anti-Slavery Society, was formed that did not admit women.

After slavery was abolished, Garrison worked for various social reforms and homeopathy. Speaking at a homeopathic convention, he said:

> Though I am not one of the medical fraternity, I can give substantial evidence of my interest in your school; for homeopathy has been in my family for a quarter of a century as a regular practice. I say I feel drawn to you. I know something about the early struggles of homeopathy, of the universal laughter it created, of the moral courage it required to stand up for it in the midst of a crooked and perverse generation. And a large majority of you have been obliged to give up your old practice, and for the sake of the truth and light vouchsafed to you, you have turned right about and accepted the new doctrine. And so I think you are an extraordinary group of men; and I say this without any desire to flatter.
>
> And if there were nothing else to commend homeopathy, there is the vast amount of suffering it saves in administering medicine to children. The old practice was first to coax, then threaten, and then frighten the little sufferer, to get the potion down. Now nothing is more

acceptable than the (homeopathic) medicine. The children alone would be justified in building to Hahnemann a monument higher than that on Bunker Hill. (Garrison, 1869)

John Tyler

John Tyler (1790–1862) was the tenth president of the United States. Influenced by his secretary of state, **Daniel Webster**, who was an active advocate for homeopathy, President Tyler sought out homeopathic treatment (Meschia, et al., 2001). Tyler had poor health throughout most of his life, and he had little confidence in the medical profession of that era, which led him to seek relief of his ailments by homeopathic means.

Rutherford B. Hayes

President Hayes (1822–1893) was brave enough to appoint a homeopathic doctor, **Tullio S. Verdi, MD**, to a newly created Board of Health (TAIH, 1892, 52). In 1871 President Ulysses S. Grant had appointed Dr. Verdi to the Board of Health of the District of Columbia, and this board chose Dr. Verdi to become its secretary and health officer of the District of Columbia, in which capacity he served two years. In 1875 the Board of Health elected him its president, and in 1876 he was re-elected.

James Garfield

James Garfield (1831–1881) was known to use homeopathic medicines throughout most of his life. The first known time he was prescribed a homeopathic medicine was in 1851, when he was 20. He had a bad cold that was treated by a homeopathic practitioner, **Alpheus Morrill, MD**, a conventionally trained doctor graduate of Dartmouth College who later became a homeopath.

Both Garfield and his wife, Lucretia, were sympathetic to homeopathy. They had both been students at the Western Reserve Eclectic Institute, founded by the Disciples of Christ Church.[80] Later, Garfield returned to this school to teach. Garfield was a classical scholar and taught Greek and Latin, as well as mathematics and geology. When he became the college's president, he significantly expanded the curriculum, which also helped make the college successful. He changed the school's name to Hiram College, the name it still carries today.[81]

Garfield's first cousin and childhood neighbor, **Silas Boynton, MD**, was a homeopathic practitioner. Dr. Boynton initially became the homeopath to Lucretia and her mother, but later Boynton also provided care for Garfield. Boynton was on the faculty of two homeopathic medical schools from 1868 to 1880, serving as professor of physiology, pathology, and microscopic anatomy.

Garfield was a college president, a Civil War general, an attorney, and an Ohio congressman. He had had a longtime appreciation for homeopathy and, even as a congressman, proposed legislation that would prohibit discrimination against homeopathic doctors. The bill passed through committee unanimously but never came to a vote in the U.S. House of Representatives (Deppisch, 1997).

D. W. Bliss, MD, was a conventional physician and a friend of Garfield's. Dr. Bliss was expelled from his local medical society because he had consulted with another conventional physician, C. C. Cox, MD, who had previously been expelled for consulting with a homeopathic doctor in the treatment of Schulyer Colfax, vice president of the U.S. at that time. Then-Congressman Garfield wrote Bliss, congratulating him that the medical profession had "decorated" him with censorship and predicting: "I have no doubt that it will do you good" (Kaufman, 1971, 90). Sadly, however, Bliss's conventional medical practice suffered greatly, as was common when regular doctors en masse shunned an individual practitioner. Eventually, Bliss and Cox were forced to formally apologize in order to be readmitted into the medical society. An editorial in the *New York Times* asserted: "There is no stronger tenet in the orthodox creed than that it is better the patient should die under the old remedies than recover under homeopathic treatment" (Kaufman, 1971, 87).

Just a couple of months after he took office at the tender age of 49, Garfield was shot twice, once in the arm and once in the chest. Despite the efforts of Alexander Graham Bell and his newly invented "induction balance" (better known as the first metal detector), the medical team attending the president was unable to locate or remove the bullet from his chest. During Garfield's final months of life, Dr. Boynton and another homeopath, **Susan Edson, MD** (the first woman doctor to attend an American president), provided care for him (Deppisch, 1997).

Although the official physician of record to President Garfield was Army Colonel Jedediah Hyde Baxter and even though Garfield and his wife also sought homeopathic treatment from Dr. Boynton, Dr. Bliss aggressively seized control of the President's health and even physically prevented Baxter from seeing his patient (Roos, 1961, 330). Garfield went on record in a statement to Dr. Boynton that he did not appoint Bliss to be his physician, but this statement was ignored by Bliss.

Because Bliss was previously kicked out of his local medical society and only just prior to Garfield's shooting had been readmitted into the organization, Bliss sought to establish himself as the sole physician to the president. In order for allopathic and homeopathic doctors to work together, Bliss insisted that whatever time and attention Boynton and Edson provided to President Garfield would be as "nurses" and "watchers," not as physicians. It seems that "homeo-phobia" in the nineteenth century was alive and very active.

Both Doctors Boynton and Edson were critical of the conventional medical treatment that Garfield was getting after being shot; this included high doses of quinine and morphine. Edson, in particular, noted that Garfield's severe intestinal cramping was a known side effect of quinine poisoning. She further noted that Garfield was prescribed Calomel (a mercury derivative), a powerful irritant and purgative commonly prescribed in the nineteenth century but widely known today as a toxic and ineffective drug. After Garfield's death, the bullet was found more than ten inches away from where Dr. Bliss was looking.

Chester A. Arthur

Chester A. Arthur (1829–1886) was Garfield's vice president, and he became president after Garfield died. His photo was one of thirteen famous people known to be advocates for homeopathy on a poster that was widely distributed as a promotion for homeopathy (Haller, 2005, 67). The details of his use of homeopathic medicines are not known.

Benjamin Harrison

Very little is known about the health of President Benjamin Harrison (1833–1901) or of medical care he received. But his wife's physician was **Dr. Franklin A. Gardner**, a homeopathic doctor (Roos, 1961, 341).

Jacob H. Gallinger, MD

Jacob Gallinger (1837–1918) graduated from the Eclectic Medical Institute in Cincinnati in 1859, though he ultimately specialized in homeopathic treatment. He became president of the New Hampshire Homeopathic Medical Society, and received an honorary degree from the New York Homeopathic Medical College in 1868. He served as associate editor of a homeopathic journal, *The New England Medical Gazette.*

He served two terms as U.S. Representative (during 1885–1889), and led the state delegation at the 1888 Republican National Convention, which nominated and then elected Benjamin Harrison. Gallinger was subsequently elected to the U.S. Senate, where he served four consecutive six-year terms, from 1891 until his death in 1918. He also served as chairman of the Republican caucus (1913–1918) and as president pro tempore of the U.S. Senate in 1912 and 1913.

Ultimately, Dr. Jacob Gallinger was the highest elected homeopathic physician in U.S. history, and he may also be the highest elected physician in U.S. history (president pro tempore of the U.S. Senate is the highest ranking senator in the government, and no president or vice president or speaker of the house has been a physician). Throughout his political career, he was a forthright advocate of the homeopathic school of thought and practice. Dr. Gallinger once asserted:

> Homeopathy was destined to be universally accepted by medical men ... although the progress of homeopathy has been wonderful, "similia" [the homeopathic law of similars]

is sneered at and ridiculed by the so-called "regular" profession of today. ... The time is not far distant when all medical men would demand an absolute law to guide them in their selection for drugs, and then homeopathy, or a belief nearly allied to that held by that school, will be the recognized platform upon which all intelligent physicians will stand. (Woodbury, 1930, 93)

William McKinley

William McKinley (1843–1901) was president during the Spanish-American War in 1898. With an executive order, he changed military medicine by allowing *all* physicians who applied for military medical service to undergo examination, thereby enabling homeopathic physicians to serve during this and future wars.

One of the physicians McKinley himself sought treatment from was **Hamilton Fiske Biggar, MD**, the physician and close friend of J. D. Rockefeller, Sr. (see Chapter 11, Corporate Leaders' and Philanthropists' Support for Homeopathy) (Chernow, 1998, 404).

In 1900 McKinley was the keynote speaker at the unveiling of the monument in Washington, D.C., honoring Samuel Hahnemann, MD, founder of homeopathy. This monument is situated at Scott Circle (Massachusetts and 16th Avenue) and is the only monument in the U.S. capital city to a physician. It acclaims Hahnemann as "Leader of the Great Medical Reformation of the Nineteenth Century."

The attorney general in President McKinley's cabinet, **John William Griggs** (1849–1927), gave the following remarks at the unveiling of the Hahnemann monument:

> It was the merit of Hahnemann that he exposed fallacies, uncovered truth and showed things not as they had been believed to be but as they are. It was not his chief glory that, by his doctrine, he founded the Homeopathic School, but rather that he uncovered errors and disclosed secrets of nature which all the world has recognized as correct. He

accepted no dogmatic assertion of any school of philosophy, nor any edict of religions council, where the secrets of nature or of science were concerned. Like Darwin and Pasteur and Koch, and all the tens and hundreds of thousands of scientific investigators of the present day, he believed that truth was to be recognized and found by experiment and observation. He met with persecution. It is not in Jerusalem alone that the prophets are stoned and so this man, for the truth's sake, endured persecution. (Bittinger, 1900, 78–79)

Supporters for creating the Hahnemann monument included key members of both political parties. Colonel J. M. Guffey, of the Democrats' national committee, and Hon. B. F. Jones, chairman of the Republicans' national committee, both contributed support and money to the erection of this monument.

Financial contributions to help build this monument came from: J. D. Rockefeller (founder of Standard Oil), H. J. Heinz[82] (founder of H. J. Heinz Co., the international food company), Mrs. George Westinghouse (wife of the founder of Westinghouse Company), Robert Pitcairn (steel magnate from Pittsburgh, executive with Pennsylvania Railroad, and close friend of George Westinghouse), W. H. Schoen (vice president of Pressed Steel Car Company, one of America's first car companies, starting in 1899), Henry Oliver (founder of Oliver Iron Mining Co., a wholly owned subsidiary of U.S. Steel), and Charles Frederick Menninger, MD (founder of the Menninger Clinic) (Bittinger, 1900).

To honor William McKinley after his assassination and to recognize McKinley's appreciation for homeopathy, Trenton City Hospital in Trenton, New Jersey, changed its name to William McKinley Memorial Hospital in 1902. Originally found in 1887 by six homeopathic doctors, it was created as a free dispensary of homeopathic treatment to the poor. Today, this hospital is a 589-bed, acute-care, teaching hospital and community-based health care provider called Capital Health Systems. Sadly, however, it no longer provides or teaches homeopathic care (www.capital health.org).

Mark A. Hanna

Serious students of American political history know the name Mark A. Hanna (1837–1904); he was one of the developers of the modern political campaign and has been described as "first of the advance men for twentieth-century Madison Avenue" (Murphy, 1974, 8).

Mark A. Hanna, born Marcus Alonzo Hanna, was an industrialist and Republican politician from Ohio who became wealthy early in life, as a shipper and broker for the coal and iron industries. Hanna was one of the early "kingmakers," helping to elect James Garfield U.S. president in 1880 and McKinley in 1896. Both of these presidents, especially Garfield, advocated for homeopathy, as did Hanna. Hanna was chairman of the board of trustees of the Cleveland Homeopathic Hospital during 1887–1904, and the Hanna family gave significant contributions to the endowment of this hospital, which later became Huron Road Hospital, as it is known today (Murphy, 1974). It is now a part of the Cleveland Clinic Health System, though it is no longer homeopathic. But during its day, it was an important and modern urban hospital.[83] Sadly, this hospital also experienced more drama than most, due to conflicts with the allopaths in the community as well as internal squabbles.

Hanna, McKinley, and Rockefeller all shared the same homeopathic physician, **Hamilton Biggar, MD**. Hanna was twice elected to the U.S. Senate representing Ohio, and he became one of the most powerful senators. Hanna loved making deals and bargains on a daily basis over a wide range of products and services. He was one of the few industrialists fascinated less by profit than by the outdoor spectacle and indoor bargaining of politics. He was planning to run for the U.S. presidency in 1904, but he contracted typhoid and died suddenly in the prime of his power.

Warren G. Harding

The parents of Warren G. Harding (1865–1923), **Tyron** and **Phoebe Harding**, studied and practiced homeopathic medicine (Dean, 2004). But because they lived and worked in the small rural town of Caledonia, Ohio, where homeopathy was less popular, their practices were not very successful (homeopathy was much more popular in urban areas because more educated people tended to use it). Phoebe also was a midwife. Tyron treated his son with homeopathic medicines throughout much of Warren's childhood.

Dr. Charles Sawyer (1860–1924), a respected Ohio homeopath, entered the Hardings' lives in 1897 when Phoebe Harding was accused of malpractice as a result of the death of a child. She had prescribed a drug to this child that, unknown to her, contained an opiate that was not listed on the bottle's contents. Sawyer's help absolved her of all responsibility in the affair.

Dr. Sawyer was also a surgeon for the Erie and Hocking Valley railroad companies, the chairman of the American Surgical and Gynecological Association, and president of the American Institute of Homeopathy.

The Sawyers and the younger Hardings became friends, and, starting in 1904, they even traveled together. In 1905, Warren's wife, Florence, had a kidney removed, and later in 1913 she finally sought homeopathic care from Dr. Sawyer. Ultimately, her medical experiences with Dr. Sawyer and homeopathy became so positive that she became dependent upon him and was convinced that only he could keep her alive, which later proved to be true (Deppisch, 1997).

Just a few months before Harding was elected president, he gave the commencement address at Hahnemann Medical College in Philadelphia (Rogers, 1998, 97).

The Hardings insisted that Sawyer become the White House physician, and he even became a member of the twice-weekly White House poker group. In 1922, Florence developed a critical urinary tract illness in her remaining kidney. Two famous conventional physicians, Charles Mayo[84] and John Finney, were called to the White House and wanted to operate immediately. Sawyer disagreed, and Joel T. Boone (see below), who also provided homeopathic advice and care to the Hardings, concurred with Sawyer. Mrs. Harding ultimately recovered without surgery, and yet, the conventional physicians asserted that homeopathic medicines had had no effect and that Mrs. Harding's condition simply healed "spontaneously" (Heller, 2000, 42).

President Harding also received medical care from another distinguished homeopathic physician, **Dr. Joel T. Boone** (1889–1974). He received an MD degree at Hahnemann Medical College in Philadelphia, in 1913, and completed graduate study at the U.S. Navy medical school in Washington, D.C., two years later. He earned the Medal of Honor in World War I, and according to some historians, he won more decorations while serving with the Marines than any other medical officer, ultimately retiring as a vice admiral (Rogers, 1998, 294, note 60). During the Harding administration, Boone was a lieutenant commander in the Navy, medical officer on the presidential yacht the USS *Mayflower*, and assistant to Dr. Sawyer in the care of President Harding. Ultimately, Boone provided care for Presidents Harding, Coolidge, and Hoover (Heller, 2000). The wives of Harding and Coolidge were particularly partial to the homeopathic care provided by Boone, who is known to have saved Mrs. Harding's life several times (Anthony, 1998; Heller, 2000).

President Harding wrote the Foreword to the book *American Homeopathy in the World War* (Dearborn, 1923). This book chronicles the work of the 1,900 homeopathic physicians who were commissioned in the U.S. army and navy to provide homeopathic treatment to troops. New York's homeopathic Flower Hospital was commissioned to create a special hospital unit in association with the American Red Cross.

Harding was an overweight man who was known to exercise rarely (except an occasional round of golf), and who used many forms of tobacco (he smoked two cigars a day, regularly smoked a pipe and an occasional cigarette, and even chewed tobacco). It was his tobacco chewing that endeared him to inventor Thomas Edison, who once told him, "Any man who chews tobacco is all right" (Deppisch, 1997).

Harding's final illness occurred during an extended trip to the West in the summer of 1923. After playing six holes of golf in Vancouver, Canada, he became so tired that he proceeded to the seventeenth hole, and then finished the eighteenth, in order to reduce suspicions of any possible problems. He later called for Dr. Sawyer, complaining of nausea and pain in the upper abdomen. Sawyer found the president had an abnormally high pulse of 120 beats per minute and was breathing forty times per minute. Intensive conventional cardiac therapy, including digitalis, was started, but it was too late, and Harding died (Sawyer, 1923).

Some historians refer to Dr. Sawyer as an incompetent physician, but these accusations only show their lack of knowledge and antagonism toward homeopathic medicine. While it is true that Sawyer did not diagnose Harding's congestive heart failure, physicians of that time typically misdiagnosed this condition (Deppisch, 1997; Heller, 2000). It was not until the 1940s that physicians learned the characteristic symptoms of coronary thrombosis that lead to a heart attack.

Calvin Coolidge

Harding's vice president was Calvin Coolidge (1872–1933). He and his family continued with the homeopathic care provided by Joel T. Boone, MD, but due to criticisms from orthodox medical associations, he felt compelled to have Dr. James F. Coupal, a conventional physician, serve as the official White House physician. During Coolidge's term as president, Boone served as medical officer for the Coolidge family on board the USS *Mayflower,* the presidential yacht, and as second-in-command to Dr. Coupal. Coolidge preferred Boone to Coupal and saw the homeopath much more frequently, as did Mrs. Coolidge, who declared Boone her personal physician.

In a book about Boone written by his son-in-law, Coolidge was described as seeking the advice of both Coupal and Boone, and even though they recommended different therapies, always siding with Boone, saying, "You know best" (Heller, 2000, 113).

Boone's personal memoirs assert that throughout his military career he never experienced direct or indirect prejudice against him because of his training at a homeopathic medical school, though this unique and better treatment may have resulted in part at least from the fact that he was awarded a Medal of Honor from World War I, and he achieved rapid ascension through the military after the war, ultimately becoming vice admiral of the U.S. Navy.

Writing in his memoirs in 1926, Boone further asserted: "I observed that homeopathy had accomplished much in the medical world and would always do so, even though it may not receive full credit for what it had accomplished, but, I further observed, the accomplishing of a mission in life is what counts, not the credit given for its accomplishment" (Boone, 536).

Boone was ever the gentleman and good soldier, but sadly, his and others' work for homeopathy have too often been ignored or suppressed. Even his biography, written by his own son-in-law, never mentions Dr. Boone's use of homeopathic medicine (Heller, 2000). After my own personal discussion with the author, I discovered that this omission was not out of malice toward homeopathy at all; it was simply that he didn't know the degree to which Boone used it. His son-in-law overlooked the above statement from Boone's memoirs.

Herbert A. Hoover

While Herbert Hoover (1874–1964) was president, Joel T. Boone was official physician to the White House. Previously, Boone's naval rank was lieutenant commander, and Hoover elevated him to captain. After serving for seven years as assistant to the physician to the White House, Boone was now the president's number one doctor. Boone was also the first presidential physician to establish a medical office in the White House. Hoover and Boone's relationship was so strong that they were known to have an early morning meeting every day.

Hoover was known to be a frequent cigar and pipe smoker who never exercised. While there is no evidence that Boone tried to change Hoover's smoking habit, Boone did get Hoover to engage in physical exercise by inventing a medicine ball game that became known as "Hoover ball," a game he played with his attorney general, a Supreme Court justice, and cabinet secretaries (Editors, 1929).

Boone asserted that in his long medical and military career, he had never failed to mention the fact that he was a graduate of a homeopathic medical college, even though this was during a time in which people had little knowledge of what it even meant to be a homeopath (Editors, 1929).

José Francisco de San Martín

José Francisco de San Martín (1778–1850), known simply as San Martín, led the liberation movements of Argentina, Chile, and Peru from the Spaniards. In 1810, before battling the Spaniards, he was released from French Napoleonic prison in Spain and traveled to London, where he entered the Lautaro Masonic Lodge that had advocated independence for all of the Americas (North and South) (Martina, 2005). In London, he became acquainted with the innovative homeopathic principles espoused by Hahnemann and cherished them. As he later led his army through the Andes, in wars of liberation, he traveled with a kit of homeopathic medicines.

Benjamin Disraeli

Benjamin Disraeli (1804–1881) served in the British government for three decades; he was twice prime minister. His personal homeopath was a respected Irish physician, **Joseph Kidd, MD** (1824–1918), who was taught homeopathy by **Paul Francois Curie, MD**, the French surgeon and physician who was grandfather of the famed Pierre Curie.

Paul Curie was brought from Paris to London in 1835 by his patron, William Leaf, a rich London silk merchant. But Curie was not brought there just to treat the rich: Leaf funded the first free dispensary for poor people. Then came the infamous Irish potato famine of 1845–1849, when Kidd was challenged to show that homeopathy can be effective in the most adverse conditions. He moved to the rural areas where the worst starvation was happening, and he kept an active record of all of his patients and their diseases and deaths. He recorded 1.8 percent mortality, while the local hospital's rate was 36 percent (Treuherz, 1995, 42–75).

In 1871 Kidd's reputation for effectiveness improved even further, when he became the homeopath to Benjamin Disraeli, Lord Beaconsfield. Disraeli suffered from asthma, bronchitis, and Bright's disease. On the day of Disraeli's first visit (November 7, 1877), he wrote in his journal:

> I had made up my mind never to create a word as to my progress or the reverse, until I had given my new man a fair

> and real trial: I will tell you that I entertain the highest opinion of Dr. Kidd, and that all the medical men I have known, and I have seen the highest, seem much inferior to him, in quickness of observation, and perception, and reasonableness, and at the same time originality, of his measures. (Treuherz, 1995, 37)

Dr. Kidd normally only saw patients in his home office, but he made a rare exception for Disraeli. In July 1878, Kidd had to go to Berlin to treat Disraeli's asthma and gout so that the prime minister could meet with the German leader, Bismarck.

There is even some mention of which homeopathic medicines Disraeli was given at different times: *Ipecacuanha* (ipecac root, a leading remedy known to cause nausea and vomiting and yet cure it in homeopathic doses), *Arsenicum* (arsenic), and *Kali bichromicum* (potassium bichromate, effective medicine for certain serious respiratory problems).[85]

In 1881, during the final days of Disraeli's life, Queen Victoria asked Disraeli to see Sir Richard Quain, a conventional physician. Normally, the harsh and intolerant attitudes of the orthodox medical organizations of that time did not even allow conventional physicians to treat homeopathic patients, but Disraeli was a rare exception. Even in Disraeli's last days and nights, Kidd, Quain, and a third doctor (Mitchell Bruce) provided him with constant attention without worrying or arguing about homeopathic and orthodox doctors working together.

Dr. Kidd's obituary, published in *The Lancet*, was one of the few times in the nineteenth century that this medical journal ever published something positive about a homeopath:

> He always held fast to the opinion that there is a truth contained in the doctrine of homeopathy which supplies a clue to the treatment of obscure cases.... From an early period he adopted the practice of prescribing only one drug at a time so as to be better able to study the action of individual remedies.... A large part of his success must be attributed to his careful survey of small details. (Kidd, 1918)

Mexican Politicians

Portifio Díaz (1830–1915, formally known as José de la Cruz Porfirio Díaz Mori) was a Mexican war hero and president of Mexico, who ruled as a dictator during what is known as the Porfiriato. He ruled Mexico from 1876 until 1911, except for a four-year period. Porfirio Díaz was healed from osteomyelitis, a disease that conventional physicians could not cure, using homeopathic medicine prescribed by **Dr. Joaquin Segura y Pesado**. Because of these impressive results, President Díaz gave recognition to homeopathy in Mexico in the 1890s, leading to the development of a government-run homeopathic medical school and a homeopathic hospital in Mexico City.

The Mexican government formally evaluated the results of homeopathic treatment in this hospital and found such impressive results that the government's support for homeopathy grew.

A bit later **Francisco I. Madero** (1873–1913), the anti-Porfiriato democrat and revolutionary leader, was famous for using homeopathic pills for his peasant troops. Madero was a vegetarian, a mystic, and a liberal capitalist who was ultimately assassinated by counter-revolutionaries. His brother, **Raúl Madero**, was even more passionate for homeopathy. They both carried their homeopathic kits when they traveled, and one of these kits resides today in a museum at Chapultepec castle in Mexico City. Raúl Madero was also known to have once saved the life of Pancho Villa, one of Mexico's most well-known revolutionaries.

Political and Spiritual Leaders of India

In part because India was governed under British rule until 1948, homeopathy achieved relatively widespread popularity in this country, and it has grown considerably since then. As of 2005, there were 300,000 qualified homeopaths, 180 colleges, 7,500 government clinics, 307 hospitals, and 24 state boards for the registration of qualified practitioners of homeopathy (Manchanda and Kulashreshtha, 2005). In fact, an article in the World Health Organization's magazine, *World Health Forum,* stated: "In the Indian subcontinent the legal position of the practitioners of homeopathy has been elevated to a professional level similar to that of a medical practitioner" (Kishore, 1983).

Mahatma Gandhi (1869–1948, spiritual leader for independence) had strong interest in and support for homeopathy, which stimulated interest in this school of medical thought and practice. In *Reminiscences of Gandhi* (Nayyar, 1946), he is quoted to have said, "It was regard for the memory of the late C. R. Das and Pandit Motilal Nehru[86] which had led me to seek homeopathic aid. They had always wanted me to give it a trial."

On August 30, 1936, after Gandhi, and many of his friends and colleagues, had had positive experiences with homeopathy, Gandhi asserted, in his unique speaking and writing style:

> Homeopathy is the latest and refined method of treating patients economically and nonviolently. Government must encourage and patronize it in our country. Late Dr. Hahnemann was a man of superior intellectual power and means of saving of human life having a unique medical nerve. I bow before his skill and the Herculean and humanitarian labour he did. His memory wakes us again and you are to follow him, but the opponents hate the existence of the principles and practice of homeopathy which in reality cures a larger percentage of cases than any other method of treatment and it is beyond all doubt safer and more economical and the most complete medical science. (Das, 1950; All India Homeopathic Medical Conference, 1968)

Pandit Motilal Nehru (1861–1931) was a friend and colleague of Gandhi and leader of the Indian National Congress. He was also the patriarch of India's most powerful political family in history, a family that included three prime ministers and other important leaders of India. His son (Jawaharlal), his granddaughter (Indira Gandhi), and his great-grandson (Rajiv Gandhi) each became prime minister.

The Nehru and Gandhi families have a tradition of appreciation for and use of homeopathic medicines. Today, several homeopathic medical colleges and hospitals are named after them.

Jawaharlal Nehru, Indira Gandhi, and other leaders of Indian society have supported the work of a nonprofit organization called Matru Sewa Sangh for work in providing health services to the poor. Homeopathic treatment has been an important part of these services since the organization's founding in 1921.

Homeopathic medicine is almost as popular as conventional medicine in India today. One of the recognized systems of medicine in India and widely practiced, homeopathy has received considerable support from many leading political and spiritual leaders in India (see Chapter 13, Clergy and Spiritual Leaders, for more details).

There have been and presently are too many politicians who advocate for homeopathy than can be included here. Among them, **Dr. Sarvepalli Radhakrishnan** (1888–1975, the second president of India) said: "Homeopathy did not merely seek to cure a disease but treated a disease as a sign of disorder of the whole human organism. This was also recognized in the Upanishad—which spoke of human organs as combination of body, mind and spirit."

The tenth president of India, who served until 2002, was **Shri K. R. Narayanan** (1921–2005), who asserted: "Homeopathic treatment is my first choice not only for me but also for my family."

Presently (2006), the prime minister of India is **Dr. Manmohan Singh** (1932–), who recently said: "Discovery of homeopathy by Dr. Samuel Hahnemann of Germany proved to be a great boon for humanity for fighting against disease by strengthening the immunity of the body."[87]

Adolf Hitler

Adolf Hitler (1889–1945) is included in this book not because he actually used homeopathic medicines but because numerous respected historical sources have stated that he was prescribed homeopathic medicines (Wainwright, 2004). It seems that Hitler was not actually prescribed homeopathic medicines, but, rather, that historians have incorrectly confused homeopathic remedies with herbal ones.

Because some leading Nazis used and supported homeopathy, discussion of this is appropriate for this book. Inclusion of these people does not infer a scintilla of support for what they did. Reference to these individuals provides additional evidence that just because someone uses homeopathic medicines (or any "natural" treatments) does not mean that the person knows how to use them effectively, and further, even if the patient is being treated correctly with homeopathic medicines, it does not mean that homeopathy can cure everybody of deep-seated hatred and racial or religious prejudice.

Adolf Hitler was chancellor of Germany in 1933 and then *Führer* (leader) of Germany from 1934 until his death. He was leader of the Nazi Party. Hitler was profoundly skeptical of conventional medicine. He was a self-described vegetarian who was regularly treated during his last nine years of life by **Theodor Morell, MD** (1886–1948), who was known for his use of unconventional medical treatments. Although many biographers refer to Morell as a quack, Hitler had such high regard for Morell's skills that the Führer referred Mussolini and Goering to him. Further, Morell turned down invitations to be personal physician to both the shah of Persia and the king of Romania, despite the fact that Morell was notoriously unkempt and smelly (not exactly the "look" that most heads of state typically choose for their personal attendants).

Morell claimed to have studied with Nobel Prize-winning bacteriologist Ilya Mechnikov and to have taught medicine at prestigious universities. In 1936 he treated Hitler's personal photographer, Heinrich Hoffmann, for gonorrhoea and claimed to have cured him. (Skeptics may wonder if natural medicines could cure infections such as gonorrhea, but Hoffman did live for another twenty years.) Hoffman and his assistant Eva Braun (who later became Hitler's wife) introduced Morell to Adolf Hitler.

Many books and articles refer to Morell as a homeopath and his treatments as homeopathic; however, it is common for journalists and researchers who are not familiar with homeopathy to describe many unconventional treatments as homeopathic when this is not always true.

A careful review of the medicines that Hitler was prescribed only shows two medicines that could be construed as homeopathic: *Nux vomica* and *Belladonna* (Morell, 1945). These two herbs, commonly used in homeopathic medicine, were the only medicines that Hitler took in a relatively consistent way for a long time. He took two to four of these pills, called "Dr. Koester's Anti-Gas Pills," at every meal from 1936 to 1945 to combat his intestinal gas build-up. Hitler was convinced these pills saved his life.

Nux vomica and *Belladonna* are herbs that are known to contain poisonous substances (strychnine in *Nux vomica* and atropine in *Belladonna*), though there was only one-half gram of each in each pill, in extract dose (an extract dose usually means that the medicinal substance did not undergo the homeopathic potentization process of serial dilution with vigorous shaking between dilutions). Although one might wonder if the undiluted doses of these herbal extracts might be toxic, Professor Ernst-Günther Schenck (1904–1998), a conventional physician who wrote reliable memoirs of his experiences with Hitler and other leading Nazis, stated that it was a completely harmless medicine. Other experts have noted that these drugs were in such minute quantities that they would be virtually useless.

When you consider that these herbal medicines have known toxic ingredients in them and that they were not potentized (serially diluted), statements that suggest they were too minute to have any medicinal effect show either an absence of knowledge or simply an antagonism to the potential power of nanodoses (Irving, 2005, 25). In essence, Hitler was prescribed homeopathic ingredients, but not in homeopathic dose, and because Hitler was prescribed these medicines in such frequent dosing over such a long period of time, this excessive prescribing (by homeopathic standards) strongly suggests that Morell was not adequately trained in homeopathy.

There is very convincing evidence today that Hitler suffered from syphilis (Hayden, 2003), and even though the classic test for syphilis, the Wassermann test, showed negative findings, such results are common for people, such as Hitler, who actually seemed to have tertiary (late-stage) syphilis. Some recent evidence strongly suggests that Hitler got infected with syphilis early in life, while in Vienna, from a Jewish prostitute (Hayden, 2003). Further confirming that Morell knew that Hitler had syphilis was the many drugs he prescribed for him over the years, including potassium iodine, which was commonly prescribed during that era for late-stage syphilis in the heart. Additional evidence that Morell wasn't trained in homeopathy is that he didn't prescribe any of the homeopathic medicines that are commonly effective for people with syphilis.

Of additional interest is that Morell was one of the earliest German physicians to prescribe penicillin, as early as 1944, and for Hitler. Some historians today wonder if the outcome of the war had been different, Morell might have been regarded as a far-sighted pioneer in his use of antimicrobials (Wainwright, 2004).

Hitler was not known to have written or spoken anything about homeopathy, though he and fellow leading Nazis were interested in herbal and homeopathic medicines derived from Germany (Kenny, 2002). Heinrich Himmler (1900–1945), head of the Nazi's Secret Service, met a former army nurse, **Margarete Boden**, who owned and operated a clinic specializing in homeopathic medicine. They were married in 1928. According to Albert Speer, **Rudolf Hess** (1894–1987), the deputy Führer, "occupied himself with problems of homeopathic medicine," and Hess was known to seek medical care from homeopathic doctors. In 1936, Hess gave the welcoming address at the International Homeopathic Medical League (the international association of MDs who practice homeopathy, founded in 1925 and still active, www.lmhi.net), which met in Berlin that year (Coulter, 1994, 454).

One important contribution during Hitler's rule was the creation of a profession in Germany called *heilpraktiker* ("healing practitioner"). As an alternative to medical doctors (many of whom were Jews who the Nazis killed or scared away), the heilpraktikers were trained to use natural medicines.

August Bier, MD (1861–1949), was a highly respected surgeon and professor in Germany and is today considered the originator of spinal anaesthesia. Although he was not a homeopath himself, he had great admiration and wrote many positive articles about homeopathy (Bier, 1925). Bier also appreciated Hippocratic understandings of health, that is, he respected the "wisdom of the body." He and many other European doctors used injections of animal blood and other substances in order to elicit a fever and inflammation that they found led to healing of various chronic diseases.

Reference to Bier is important here for several reasons. First, his ideas influenced Morell in the treatment of Hitler, who was commonly injected with various unusual medicines. And second, Bier was also a philosopher who created many slogans that were ultimately used by the Nazis as a part of their propaganda, such as "Out of discord comes the fairest harmony" and "War is the father of all things, of all things king." Although Bier's words became an integral part of Nazi propaganda, there is no evidence that he himself was a Nazi (Kenny, 2002).

Muhammad Ayub Khan

Interest in and support for homeopathy is worldwide. In fact, homeopathy is so popular in Pakistan and India that there are almost as many homeopaths as there are conventional physicians.

Muhammad Ayub Khan (1907–1974) was Pakistan's field marshal (highest ranking person in the miliary) during the mid-1960s and was president during 1958–1969. He became Pakistan's first native commander in chief in 1951, and was the youngest full-rank general in Pakistan's military history. He was also the first Pakistani military general to seize power through a (bloodless) coup.

In a speech, he once proclaimed: "My countrymen! God has given you an excellent opportunity to serve your nation through homeopathic medicine. Make full use of it and complete the task assigned to you with devotion, honesty and sincerity."

Karl Carstens

Karl Carstens (1914–1992) served as the fifth federal president of West Germany, from 1979 to 1984. His wife, **Veronica Carstens, MD**, was both a medical doctor and a homeopath. Due to their shared appreciation for homeopathy, they started the Carstens Foundation (www.carstensstiftung.de/eng/the_foundation.shtml), which has as its primary objective the integration and broader acceptance of homeopathy and complementary medicine in today's medical community. As of 2006, they have provided more than 13 million euros (more than $15 million) in grants.

William Jefferson Clinton

Bill Clinton (1946–) was the forty-second president of the United States, serving from 1993 to 2001. He served five terms as governor of Arkansas. *Business Week* reported that a presidential aide would buy homeopathic medicines at a New York homeopathic pharmacy to treat the president's sinus problem (Toy, 1994). Although the press had previously reported that Clinton suffered from recurrent laryngitis, there seemed to be fewer references to this problem after these reports of homeopathic treatment.

It should also be noted that Clinton had a special interest in healthier eating than most previous American presidents. He was known to invite Dean Ornish, MD, to the White House on several occasions. Ornish was a highly respected physician, nutritionist, and researcher known for his low-fat vegetarian and vegan dietary recommendations.

Clinton's wife, **Hillary Rodham Clinton**, is presently in her first term as the junior U.S. senator from New York. George Stephanopoulos, Clinton's former press secretary, wrote a book, *All Too Human: A Political Education,* in which he noted that Hillary sent him some homeopathic medicines to keep him healthy: "Health care reform's slow death in 1994 was particularly disheartening. We fought hard, but were losing. Hillary tried to keep our spirits up. Seeing that I was fluey from fatigue, she sent me a carton of homeopathic cures one day accompanied by a note: 'We need you healthy for health care!'" (Stephanopoulos, 1999, 297).

It is not surprising that during Clinton's presidency, he established the White House Commission on Complementary and Alternative Medicine.

Thorbjørn Jagland

Thorbjørn Jagland (1950–) was prime minister of Norway during 1996–1997, and then minister of foreign affairs during 2000–2001. He was leader of the Norwegian Labour Party from 1992 to 2002. Jagland currently serves as president (speaker) of the Norwegian parliament.

Jagland has publicly declared his interest in and appreciation for homeopathic medicine on several occasions. His support is just one of many reasons that homeopathy is presently the most popular of all alternative therapies in Norway, and one in two Norwegians believes homeopathy should be incorporated into the country's health service (Royal Ministry of Foreign Affairs, 2002).

Tony Blair

Former British prime minister Tony Blair (1953–) and his family have a special interest in homeopathy. Although he is usually tight-lipped on what he and his wife do for their children's health, he has made public the fact that they use homeopathic *Arnica* for treating bruises (Ananova, 2001). In a November 2006 podcast interview with the editor of the *New Scientist,* Blair argued that scientists should not oppose homeopathy. In a direct reference to House of Lords member Dick Taverne, who had recently questioned the government's relaxation of the regulations on the promotion of homeopathic remedies, Blair endorsed homeopathy as a lifestyle choice (Webb, 2006).

His wife, **Cherie Blair**, has been more outspoken in her interest in homeopathy. England's newspaper, *The Guardian,* which is usually critical of Tony Blair, has written very positive things about his wife, who is a human rights lawyer: "Cherie Blair has one of the sharpest legal brains in the country. She is also a committed Catholic, a devoted mother, and an active campaigner for a number of worthwhile causes" (Brooks, 2002).

Cherie's sister, **Lyndsey Booth**, was also trained as a lawyer, but she quit her legal practice to become a homeopath, and she serves on the board of directors of a leading homeopathic organization. Further, it is public knowledge in England that Cherie's and Lyndsey's mother brought them up on homeopathic medicines.

The British press has noted that Cherie had been under the care of an 80-plus-year-old homeopathic dowsing healer[88] for at least six years until he passed away in 2004. The late Princess Diana, the Duchess of York (Sarah Ferguson), and the model Jerry Hall also sought his care and sage advice (Temple, 2004).

References

All India Homeopathic Medical Conference, Hyderabad, December 24–26, 1968. Calcutta: Hahnemann Publishing.

Ananova.com. January 6, 2001.

Anthony, C. S. *Florence Harding.* New York: William Morrow, 1998.

Bier, A. What Shall be Our Attitude Towards Homoeopathy? *Homeopathic Recorder,* December 1925, 38 pages.

Bittinger, Rev. B. F. *An Historic Sketch of the Monument Erected in Washington City (The History of the Hahnemann Monument).* Washington, D.C.: Putnam, 1900.

Boone, J. T. *Prosperity and Thrift: The Coolidge Era and the Consumer Economy, 1921–1929.* Boone Papers. Chapter on President Coolidge from the Memoirs of His Physician. Available at http://memory.loc.gov/cgi-bin/query/r?ammem/coo bib:@field(NUMBER+@band(amrlm+mb01))

Bradford, T. L. *The Logic of Figures or Comparative Results of Homoeopathic and Other Treatments.* Philadelphia: Boericke and Tafel, 1900.

Brooks, L. The Court of Cherie, *The Guardian,* December 6, 2002.

Capital Health System. www.capitalhealth.org/about/history/history_fuld.html

Chernow, R. *Titan: The Life of John D. Rockefeller, Sr.* New York: Vintage, 1998.

Coulter, H. L. *Divided Legacy: A History of the Schism in Medical Thought.* Volume I: The Patterns Emerge—Hippocrates to Paracelsus. Berkeley: North Atlantic Books, 1973.

Coulter, H. L., *Divided Legacy: A History of the Schism in Medical Thought.* Volume IV: Twentieth-Century Medicine: The Bacteriological Era. Berkeley: North Atlantic Books, 1994.

Das, N. C. What Gandhiji Thought of Homoeopathy, *Homeopathic Herald,* March 1950, Vol XIII, 12.

Dean, J. W. *Warren G. Harding.* New York: Times Books, 2004.

Dearborn, F. M. *American Homoeopathy in the World War.* Washington, D.C.: American Institute of Homeopathy, 1923.

Deppisch, L. M. Homeopathic medicine and presidential health: Homeopathic influences upon two Ohio presidents. *Pharos,* Fall 1997, 60:5–10.

Doctor Zebra, *The Medical History of American Presidents.* www.doctorzebra.com/prez/#zree5 (This website is an invaluable source of information on the medical treatment of U.S. presidents, and I used it greatly to confirm various facts in this chapter.)

Editors, *The Homoeopathic Survey.* July 1929, pp. 8–9.

Frass, M., Dielacher, C., Linkesch, M., Endler, C., Muchitsch, I., Schuster, E., and Kaye, A. Influence of potassium dichromate on tracheal secretions in critically ill patients, *Chest,* March 2005.

Garrison, W. L. *New England Medical Gazette,* 1869, pp. 285–286.

Haller, J. S. *The History of American Homeopathy: The Academic Years, 1820–1935.* New York: Pharmaceutical Products, 2005.

Hayden, D. *Pox: Genius, Madness and the Mysteries of Syphilis.* New York: Basic Books, 2003.

Health Minister for Promotion of Homeopathy, *Himalayan Times,* December 31, 2006.

Heller, M. F. *The Presidents' Doctor: An Insider's View of Three First Families.* New York: Vantage Press, 2000.

Hill, B. L., and Hunt, J. G. *Homoeopathic Practice of Surgery and Operative Surgery.* Cleveland: J. B. Cobb, 1855.

Hughes, T. *A Boy's Experience in the Civil War, 1860–1865.* 1904. http://docsouth.unc.edu/fpn/hughest/hughes.html

Irving, D. *The Secret Diaries of Hitler's Doctor.* England: Focal Point, 2005. (Originally published 1983 by Macmillan. Available at www.fpp.co.uk/books/Morell/index.html.)

Karst, F. Homeopathy in Illinois, *Caduceus* (a museum quarterly for the health sciences), Summer 1988, pp. 1–33.

Kaufman, M. *Homoeopathy in America,* Baltimore: Johns Hopkins University Press, 1971.

Kenny, M. G. A Darker Shade of Green: Medical Botany, Homeopathy, and Cultural Politics in Interwar Germany, *Social History of Medicine,* 2002 15(3):481–504.

Kidd, J. Obituary, *The Lancet,* September 21, 1918.

King, W. H. *History of Homoeopathy* (4 volumes). New York: Lewis, 1905.

Kishore, J. Homoeopathy: The Indian Experience, *World Health Forum,* 1983, 3:107.

Mainwaring, R. D, and Riley, H. D. Jr. The Lexington Physicians of General Robert E. Lee, *Southern Medical Journal,* August 2005, 98(8):800–804.

Manchanda, R. J., and Kulashreshtha, M. Cost Effectiveness and Efficacy of Homeopathy in Primary Health Care Units of Government of Delhi: A study. Paper presented at 60th International Homeopathic Congress organized by LIGA at Berlin, Germany from 4th May 2005 to 7th May 2005. www.delhihomeo.com/paperberlin.html

Martina, G. *Hahnemann and the independence of Argentina.* Available at www.thieme-connect.com/ejournals/abstract/ahz/doi/10.1055/s-2005-868643

Meschia, J., Safirstein, B. E., and Biller, J. Stroke and the American Presidency: U.S. presidents who have had strokes, *Saturday Evening Post,* January 2001. Available at www.findarticles.com/p/articles/mi_m1189/is_1_273/ai_68316081

Morell, T. Medicines and preparations administered by Dr. Morell to Hitler during the years 1941–1945. www.adolfhitler.ws/lib/bio/Medicines.html

Murphy, N. A History of Huron Road Hospital, *Centennial edition of Today Magazine* (bulletin of Huron Road Hospital), 1974.

Nayyar, S. *Reminiscences of Gandhi: Light and Shade.* New Delhi, 1946. Available at www.gandhi-manibhavan.org/eduresources/chap18.htm

Other Days, *Homeopathic Recorder,* 1887, p. 6.

Rafuse, E. S. Typhoid and Tumult: Lincoln's Response to General McClellan's Bout with Typhoid Fever during the Winter of 1861–62, *Journal of the Abraham Lincoln Association,* Summer 1997, 18(2). www.historycooperative.org/journals/jala/18.2/rafuse.html

Rogers, N. *An Alternative Path: The Making and Remaking of Hahnemann Medical College and Hospital of Philadelphia.* Piscataway: Rutgers University Press, 1998.

Roos, C. A. Physicians to the Presidents, and Their Patients: A Biobibliography, *Bulletin of the Medical Library Assoc.*, July 1961, 49(3):291–360. Available at www.pubmedcentral.gov/articlerender.fcgi?artid=200603#reference-sec

Royal Ministry of Foreign Affairs, Press Division, *Norway Daily*, March 18, 2002, No. 54/02.

Russell, E. W. *Report on Radionics: Science of the Future.* Suffolk: Neville Spearman, 1973.

Sawyer, C. E., Wilbur, R. L., Cooper, C. M., Boone, J. T. and Work, H. President Harding's Last Illness, *JAMA*, 1923, 81:603.

Spiegel, A. D., and Kavaler, F. The Role of Abraham Lincoln in Securing a Charter for a Homeopathic Medical College, *Journal of Community Health*, 2002, 27(5): 357–380.

Stephanopoulos, G. *All Too Human: A Political Education.* Boston: Little, Brown and Company, 1999.

TAIH. *Transactions of the American Institute of Homoeopathy.* Philadelphia: Herman and Company, 1892.

Temple, J. (obituary), *The Telegraph.* February 2, 2004. Available at www.telegraph.co.uk/news/main.jhtml?xml=/news/2004/02/20/db2001.xml&sSheet=/portal/2004/02/20/ixportal.html

Toy, S. Take Two Eyes of Newt and Call Me in the Morning, *Business Week*, March 28, 1994, pp. 144–145.

Treuherz, F. *Homeopathy in the Irish Potato Famine.* London: Samuel Press, 1995. Available at http://homeoint.org/books/treuherz/index.htm

Wainwright, M. Hitler's Penicillin, *Perspectives in Biology and Medicine*, Spring 2004, 47(2):189–198.

Webb, J. Tony Blair on Science, *New Scientist*, November 4, 2006, Issue #2576.

Wershub, L. P. *One Hundred Years of Medical Progress: A History of the New York Medical College, Flower and Fifth Avenue Hospitals.* Springfield: Charles C. Thomas, 1967.

Woodbury, B. C. Homeopathy in New Hampshire, *The Homoeopathic Survey*, April 1930, pp. 90–94.

CHAPTER 10

Women's Rights Leaders and Suffragists: Pro-Homeopathy

"Too many wives of conventional physicians are going to homeopathic physicians," complained one doctor at the 1883 meeting of the American Medical Association. "And to make it worse," he added, "they are taking their children to homeopaths too" (Coulter, 1973, III, 116).

Ever since the beginning of homeopathy in the early 1800s, women have been attracted to this system of medicine as patients, as home care prescribers for their family, and as professional homeopaths. It is estimated that two-thirds of homeopathic patients in the nineteenth century were women (Kirschmann, 2004). Historians and physicians today assert that nineteenth-century conventional medicine was barbaric. The use of mercury, arsenic, bloodletting, and leeches was common medical practice, and such treatment usually caused considerably more harm than good. The women of that day, therefore, sought safer medical treatment, and they turned to homeopathy in significant numbers.

Women were also attracted to homeopathy because it not only treated their physical complaints but also inquired into and treated various emotional and mental concerns. While the act of listening to patients provided its own therapeutic benefit, the fact is homeopathy became very popular in the U.S. and Europe in the mid- and late 1800s due to its particularly beneficial results in treating the infectious disease epidemics of that day (cholera, typhoid, yellow fever, scarlet fever, and more). These impressive results helped make it clear to women that this new form of medicine was more effective than orthodox medicine—and it was safer (Bradford, 1900; Coulter, 1973).

The 1840s and 1850s witnessed the establishment and growth of "Ladies Physiological Societies," early women's consciousness-raising meetings at which women taught themselves about their own bodies and how to use various natural healing methods to safely and effectively heal themselves and their families.

Women also became known for spreading homeopathy's popularity in communities. One homeopathic doctor asserted at a meeting of the American Institute of Homeopathy: "Many a woman armed with her little stack of remedies, had converted an entire community to homeopathy" (Winston, 1999, 141).

The positive benefits that these women experienced with homeopathic medicines were not simply in their own health care but in that of their children (Coulter, 1975, 114–118). Determining which homeopathic medicine to use for a sick person was not based on the diagnosis of his or her disease but more on the specific syndrome of symptoms that the person had, thus enabling women and other nonmedically trained people to learn how to treat themselves and others for common acute complaints. More serious and chronic ailments required professional homeopathic care, but the homeopathic system allowed women to provide helpful therapeutic care for their families; it was simply more user-friendly than conventional medicine of the day.

These actions became philosophically and economically threatening to orthodox physicians. Not only was homeopathy identified in the public mind with medical reform, it was also closely associated with women's rights, emancipation of slaves, and Republican politics (at a time when Republicans were "liberal" and when Lincoln and other social reformers and abolitionists were Republicans). Homeopathy's connection with social liberalism was important to women because nineteenth-century social norms were so restrictive to women. Women who even considered working in a professional field were scorned.

Elizabeth Cady Stanton (1815–1902), one of the leaders of the nineteenth-century women's rights movement, was a particularly strong advocate of homeopathy, asserting "I have seen wonders in homeopathy" and "I intend to commence life on homeopathic principles" (Wellman,

2004, 158). Ms. Stanton had such good experiences with homeopathy that she even became a lay practitioner (although unlicensed, she prescribed homeopathic medicines for others; Winston, 2004).

Elizabeth Cady Stanton was married to Henry Stanton (1805–1887), who was a successful patent attorney, a state senator, and co-founder of the Free Soil Party, which was later absorbed by the Republican Party. While he was often away doing political work, Elizabeth cared for and raised their seven children. Even though three of their boys contracted malaria, she treated them with homeopathic medicines successfully for this serious illness and for all other health concerns that occurred (Goldsmith, 1998, 39). In her autobiography, which she dedicated to her close friend and colleague, Susan B. Anthony, Stanton wrote that she commonly prescribed homeopathic medicines to various members in her community: "I was their physician, also—with my box of homeopathic medicines I took charge of the men, women, and children in sickness. Thus the most amicable relations were established" (Stanton, 1897). She further asserted that she primarily prescribed homeopathic medicine in high potencies.

One of the most prominent American feminists of the nineteenth century (but whose name is not well-known today) was **Victoria Claflin Woodhull** (1838–1927). Though born quite poor, Woodhull became wealthy as the first woman to own a Wall Street investment firm,[89] the first woman to own a newspaper, and the first woman to run for the U.S. presidency. In 1872, she ran for president in the newly formed Equal Rights Party; her vice presidential candidate was Frederick Douglass, the black statesman, editor, and orator. She lost to a popular incumbent, Ulysses S. Grant.

Woodhull was also known to advocate for and practice homeopathy, though she was never formally trained in it.

Florence Nightingale (1820–1910), pioneer of the nursing profession, was known to have sought care from Dr. James Gully, a homeopathic physician who owned a highly respected hydrotherapy spa in Malvern, England. Dr. Gully helped save Florence Nightingale from a nervous breakdown after she returned home from traumatic experiences during the Crimean War (Ruddick, 2001, 19). She referred to him as a "genius" (Jenkins, 1972, vii). Although Florence Nightingale became an advocate of water cures, she was never known to advocate or write about homeopathy in her public writings; in her private letters, though, she once wrote to her mother that she hoped her father would try homeopathic treatment for an eye problem he was experiencing (Nightingale, 1852).

Many of the leaders of the women's rights movement in the late nineteenth and early twentieth centuries were also advocates of homeopathy. **Mary Coffin Ware Dennett** (1872–1947) was the founder of the National Birth Control League, the first organization in the United States to advocate for population control. Distinct from the work by Margaret Sanger, who sought to circumvent obscenity laws by giving information and devices to physicians so they could distribute them to their patients, Dennett fought for the full repeal of the anti-obscenity laws by arguing that women had a legal right to birth control services and devices (Kirschmann, 2004, 140).

In 1921 Dennett met with Dr. Hubert Work, former AMA president and then assistant postmaster general. Dr. Work asserted that he was "opposed to the entire subject [birth control]," and said that Dennett seemed to advocate instruction on "how to have illicit intercourse without the danger of pregnancy." The next year, when Dr. Work became postmaster general, he instructed post offices throughout the country to post announcements asserting that the simple sending or receiving of information on birth control was a "criminal act" (Kirschmann, 2004, 141). Ms. Dennett was arrested and convicted in 1929 for writing and distributing the YWCA-endorsed pamphlet, "The Sex Side of Life: An Explanation for Young People," which was judged "obscene" under the Comstock Act. This decision was reversed on appeal (Chen, 1997).

Dennett was just as passionate about homeopathy as she was about birth control rights. Born into a family of ardent supporters of homeopathy, her mother and sister were advocates, and her uncle, **Carleton Spencer, MD**, was a leading homeopathic physician and educator in New York City. Dennett even became an employee of the American Foundation for Homeopathy and worked diligently but unsuccessfully to raise money from wealthy homeopathic patients.

The American Institute of Homeopathy voted to admit women into its organization in1869, seven years before the AMA did likewise. Although women were admitted into the AMA in 1876, the bylaws were not changed to formally accept women as members until 1915 (Kirschmann, 2004, 83). By 1915, ten women had already been elected to serve as vice presidents of the American Institute of Homeopathy.

Women who went to homeopathic medical schools did so despite great challenges. Most of these women were considerably older than the male medical students. One survey found that the average age of women attending homeopathic schools was 34 years, and it was not uncommon for them to begin studying medicine in their forties or fifties. Many of these women were mothers, and some faced considerable resistance from within their families.

The First Women Physicians

Although some historians incorrectly credit Elizabeth Blackwell, MD (1821–1910), as being the first woman in America to be awarded a medical degree, she wasn't, and not just because she was British. The first American woman to graduate with a degree from an American medical school was **Lydia Folger Fowler, MD** (1822–1879), who graduated from the Rochester Eclectic Medical College in 1850. Adding a little more Americana history to this story, it is intriguing to note that Dr. Fowler was a relative of Benjamin Franklin.

The first woman ever granted a medical degree was **Melanie d'Hervilly** (1800–1878), the second wife of Samuel Hahnemann, MD, founder of homeopathy.[90] At the age of 34, Melanie married Samuel, who was 79 at the time. Although he lived in Germany, she brought him to Paris, where she apprenticed with him, and he once asserted that she was "better acquainted with homeopathy, both theoretically and practically, than any of my followers" (Haehl, 1922, 446–447). Dr. Hahnemann wrote to the Allentown Homeopathic Academy (America's first homeopathic medical school) to ask if they would grant Melanie a degree, and in 1840, she was awarded a diploma.

Other historians assert that Dr. Blackwell created the first women's medical college. This also is not true. The first women's medical college was the Boston Female Medical College, founded in 1848. Four years later, it changed its name to the New England Female Medical College, and then, in 1873, it merged with a larger homeopathic medical school at Boston University to become a coeducational college of medicine.

Mercy B. Jackson, MD (1802–1877), was one of the early graduates (1850) from the New England Female Medical College. Her story is typical of many women of that time. She was married in 1823 to Rev. John Bisbee, pastor of the First Universalist Society in Hartford, Connecticut, but he died in 1829. She had three children with her first husband and eight more with her second, though five of her children did not survive childhood. Mercy became all too familiar with the limitations and the dangers of conventional medicine as she experienced excessive bleedings, leeches, and purgative and cathartic medications.

Mercy Jackson, her second husband, and her family moved to Plymouth, Massachusetts in 1833. When her husband's cousin and Jackson's good friend, Lydia Jackson, married Ralph Waldo Emerson, Jackson was introduced to a vibrant intellectual circle. In 1839, she began studying homeopathy, and in 1841, she began a limited homeopathic practice among her friends. She expressed an interest in studying medicine to her family physician, **Dr. Robert Capen**, a Harvard-trained doctor. They traveled together to Boston to purchase some books and medicines. Capen also became convinced of homeopathy's value, and in 1842, he became a homeopath and continued to practice until he passed away in 1853.

However, Mercy Jackson wanted to obtain a more formal medical education. When feminist Harriet K. Hunt (1805–1875) was refused admission to Harvard, Mercy wrote to her in support of her efforts. They developed a lifelong friendship as both women became increasingly involved in the women's rights movement. As early as 1854 Mercy wrote a letter to the assessors of the Town of Plymouth protesting "taxation without representation."

Ultimately, Mercy Jackson graduated from the New England Female College in 1850, at the age of 48. In April 1868, Dr. Mercy B. Jackson was nominated to be the first woman member of the Massachusetts Homeopathic Medical Society, but she was refused membership by a 33-to-31 vote, even though the executive committee had recommended her.

In 1867 the question of "female medical education" attracted the attention of the American Medical Association and the American Institute of Homeopathy. A resolution to grant women admittance to the AIH was proposed but lost by a vote of 68 to 56. However, in 1869, a similar resolution was proposed and passed, 80 to 45. In 1871, Dr. Mercy B. Jackson became the first woman admitted to AIH. In 1874, the Massachusetts Homeopathic Medical Society passed a resolution allowing women admittance to their state society, and Dr. Mercy B. Jackson was the first woman to be admitted. She later served on the faculty of Boston University School of Medicine, where she was professor of diseases of children.

The homeopathic profession owes Dr. Jackson gratitude for demonstrating the power of *Pulsatilla* to turn breech babies in the womb to allow a safer and more rapid labor (Cleaves, 1873; King, 1905; Pilgram Hall, online).

Radicalized by her belief in the importance of women's equality, Dr. Jackson argued her medical beliefs in articles on women's diseases for homeopathic journals, and she battled for women's rights in articles written for Lucy Stone's feminist publication, *The Women's Journal*. She chastised a prominent advocate of coeducation for "wishing to make women as nearly as possible like men. ... women are now struggling ... to have the same opportunities to use in a woman's way" (Jackson, 1874).

Clemence Sophia Lozier, MD (1813–1888), opened a homeopathic medical school for women because she insisted "that woman was, by every instinct and aptitude of her nature, better fitted for the medical profession than man" (Lozier, 1888). Distinct from the men's medical schools, where there was great antagonism between conventional and homeopathic faculty and students, the students and faculty at women's medical schools tended to cooperate with each other, at least initially.

Lozier's school, the New York Medical College and Hospital for

Women, opened in 1863, and the therapeutics that were primarily taught were the use of homeopathic medicines. Its board of trustees included several illustrious homeopaths (**Timothy Field Allen, MD, William Guernsey, MD, Edmund Carleton, MD, and Carroll Dunham, MD**—who also happened to be Lozier's cousin), two leaders in the women's rights movement (**Elizabeth Cady Stanton** and **Julia Ward Howe**), and **Clara Barton**, founder of the American Red Cross.

With this board of trustees guiding the college, it is perhaps no surprise that this school was the first medical school in the country to offer a course in hygiene and preventive medicine (Kirschmann, 2004, 59). The school was also one of the earliest to extend its training to three years, doing so before 1874, while the conventional medical college, New York University Medical College, waited until 1892. The faculty of the women's college seemed to be so convinced of the importance of an extended educational program that they declared in their college's announcement that "the medical education of women must be more thorough and carried to a higher degree than the education of men" (Sullivan, 1927, Book 12, Chapter 13, Part 6).

In 1897, with significant support from New York's elite, Lozier's school erected a new building that was designed by William B. Tuthill, the architect of Carnegie Hall. Much later, in 1918, it merged with a larger homeopathic medical school called the New York Homeopathic Medical College and Flower Hospital. Still later, in 1936, the institution changed its name to New York Medical College, and shortly afterwards, it stopped the teaching of homeopathy.

The establishment of Lozier's school was followed by the creation of another women's medical school, founded by Elizabeth Blackwell, MD, called The Women's Medical College. In contrast to Lozier's school, Blackwell's college did not admit women who had suffragist views, and Blackwell even criticized Lozier for her involvement in various social reform movements (Kirschman, 2004, 61).

Despite the differences in medical and social viewpoints, the two schools cooperated. For a period of time, Lozier was the dean of the faculty at Blackwell's school, and several homeopaths taught at both schools.

However, as both schools began to prosper and gain more women students, each school began to focus on different modalities (Lozier's was homeopathic and Blackwell's was orthodox medicine), and still later, the two women developed a strong antagonism for each other. **Susan B. Anthony** (1820–1906), who co-founded the National Women's Suffrage Association with Elizabeth Cady Stanton and who is recognized today as one of America's leaders for women's rights, desperately sought to bring these two powerful women together, but their medical, political, and sociological differences kept an "icy gulf" between them.

The early days of women's medical schools were not easy. In the late 1860s, a group of thirty women homeopathic medical students went to Bellevue Hospital for their clinical training. The women faced such hostility from male professors and students that they carried switchblade knives to fend off their persecutors (Harth, 1999). One day, they were greeted by hundreds of male students who blocked their entrance, pelted them with chewed balls of paper, and laughed and shouted at them. Dr. Lozier, as president of the college, organized a large public meeting with Henry Ward Beecher and Horace Greeley (editor of the *New York Tribune*), who denounced the boorish behavior of the male medical students. After considerable media attention supporting the women, the mayor of New York agreed to send a police force to "protect the ladies in their rights," thereby enabling them to obtain a full medical education (Kirshmann, 2004, 59).

Clemence Sophia Lozier was the most influential homeopathic woman doctor in the United States in the nineteenth century. For twenty-five years she served as president and dean of her college, during which time 219 women graduated. Lozier was to homeopathic women's education what Elizabeth Blackwell was to the conventional medical education of women, though history has a strong tendency to be partial to the dominant medical paradigm. Blackwell's name is known to many people today, while Lozier is known to only a few.

In the late nineteenth century homeopathic doctors usually commanded a better income from their medical practice than conventional doctors. In part because homeopaths attracted more rich and educated patients, homeopaths usually charged more for their services and tended to have fuller practices. In 1870, Lozier reported her yearly income from her medical practice to be more than $25,000—a very considerable income at that time. Elizabeth Cady Stanton, who with Lucretia Mott, led the first women's rights convention in 1848, asserted that Lozier was one of the largest financial supporters of the suffrage movement and of Susan B. Anthony's publication. Lozier served as president of the New York Woman Suffrage Society for thirteen years (1873–1886) and was president of the National Woman Suffrage Association in 1877–1878.

Lozier's home in New York became a virtual headquarters for various social reform movements. Meetings and fundraising events were typical there, whether it was to protest a death sentence for a woman accused of infanticide, to support affordable housing for working women, to prevent the distribution of pornography to children, or to protest against the sentence imposed upon Susan B. Anthony for voting. Lozier and other homeopaths were also advocates of temperance (the movement to reduce the consumption of alcohol).[91]

It is also not surprising that Susan B. Anthony was a homeopathic patient. Her homeopathic physician was **Julia Holmes Smith, MD**, another activist in the social reform movement. Further, Dr. Smith established the first kindergarten, in New Haven, Connecticut, was the first woman elected to a deanship of a coeducational medical school (the National Medical College of Chicago in 1898), the first woman to be appointed trustee at the University of Illinois, and the first woman to be placed on a political ticket in Illinois.

One other woman who was intimately connected to the women's rights movement in the late 1800s and early 1900s was **Julia Ward Howe** (1819–1910), who was also known for her writing of the famous song, "The Battle Hymn of the Republic." Like so many other leaders of the women's rights movement of the time, she was a strong advocate of homeopathy.

Another homeopathic physician who also was extremely active in women's rights issues was **Harriet Clisby, MD** (1830–1931), who founded the Women's Educational and Industrial Union (WEIU) of Boston in

1877 (Harth, 1999). The exploitation of women and children during the mid-nineteenth century, the crowded housing and poor sanitation, and the miserable labor conditions led Dr. Clisby to create the WEIU, an organization that is still active today. By the beginning of the twentieth century, the WEIU established itself as one of Boston's primary service providers and advocacy organizations. Many of the city's most prominent women, including Abby Morton Diaz, Louisa May Alcott, and Julia Ward Howe were an integral part of the Union's early history. Dr. Mercy B. Jackson was on the Union's first board of directors.

Initially, Elizabeth Blackwell had encouraged Clisby to receive medical training in England, but instead, Clisby enrolled in the first graduating class of Dr. Clemence Lozier's Medical College and Hospital for Women. Dr. Clisby's interest in homeopathy was predictable because she followed the religious and spiritual teachings of Emanuel Swedenborg.[92] When Dr. Clisby turned 90, she became the oldest woman physician in the U.S., and she extended this record by living to be 101 years old.

Rebecca Lee Crumpler, MD (1833–1895), was the first African American woman to earn a medical degree, and she graduated from the (homeopathic) New England Female Medical College, in March 1864.

The first black woman physician in New York (and third in the nation) was **Susan Smith McKinney, MD** (1847–1918). She attended Dr. Lozier's homeopathic medical school and became an ardent homeopath. She overcame both race and gender biases to develop a successful practice. When she passed away, the black leader, W. E. B. Du Bois, gave her eulogy (Kirschmann, 2004, 48). Today, a nursing and rehabilitation center in New York City and a junior high school in Brooklyn are named after her. Dr. McKinney would be sadly disappointed that the nursing center provides no homeopathic care.

Mary Harris Thompson, MD (1829–1895), was a graduate of the New England Female Medical College (1863). She founded Chicago Hospital for Women and Children in 1865 and later became the first female surgeon in the U.S.[93] Initially, the hospital was sustained through private benefactions, and through Dr. Thompson's efforts, a college was organized in 1870 for the medical education of women exclusively. The hospital building was totally destroyed in the great fire of 1871, but temporary accommodations were obtained. The following year, with the aid of $25,000 appropriated by the Chicago Relief and Aid Society, a permanent building was purchased. In 1885, a new commodious and well-planned building was erected on the same site, at a cost of about $75,000.

After Thompson's death in 1895, the hospital was renamed the Mary Thompson Hospital for Women and Children. It continued to provide otherwise unavailable clinical opportunities for medical women until 1972, when men were integrated into the medical staff. Financial problems contributed to the closing of the hospital in 1988.

Emily Jennings Stowe, MD (1831–1903), was a pioneer in the struggle for women's equality in Canada, where she became the first woman school principal in 1852 and the first woman to practice medicine in Canada. Before going to medical school, she apprenticed with **Dr. John Lancaster**, who was a family friend and a homeopathic doctor. After applying to medical schools in Canada on numerous occasions and being turned down every time, she applied to and was accepted by the New York Medical College for Women. She graduated from this school in 1867 and immediately returned to Canada.

Like so many other women homeopaths, Emily Stowe was a leading female suffragist and is considered by many to be the mother of the movement in Canada. In 1877, she founded the Toronto Women's Literary Club, which changed its name to the Toronto Women's Suffrage Club in 1882. She organized the country's first suffrage organization, the Dominion Women's Enfranchisement Association, in 1893 and became its first president. In 1896 she was instrumental in creating a mock parliament where a congress of women, using all of the arguments men had used against them, refused to give men the vote. She helped found the Women's Medical College in Toronto in 1883 and the Women's College Hospital in 1888. She died in 1903, fourteen years before women got the vote in Canada.

Florence Nightingale Ward, MD (1860–1919), was not just a homeopath; she was also a surgeon. Ultimately, she was the second woman elected to membership in the American College of Surgeons. Dr. Ward was married to a fellow homeopathic physician, **James Ward, MD**, who was a founder of Hahnemann College of the Pacific and head of the San Francisco Health Department during the famous 1906 earthquake in that city. Dr. Florence Ward ran a three-story hospital and clinic in San Francisco.

By 1884, women represented 31 percent of students at homeopathic medical schools and 19 percent of graduates. And by the turn of the twentieth century, 17 percent of homeopaths were women, compared with only 6 percent of conventional doctors (Haller, 2005, 139). It is interesting to note that women who were conventional physicians tended to establish and become members of separate women's medical societies more than women who were homeopaths did. These differences primarily occurred because women homeopaths tended to be more widely accepted into homeopathic organizations than women who were AMA members. Despite this general trend, homeopaths (men or women) tended to be pioneers of varying sorts. Thus, it is predictable that at a 1904 meeting of the American Institute of Homeopathy, the Women's Homeopathic Fraternity was organized as the first national organization of women in the profession of medicine (Breckinridge, 1933, 62).

Homeopathic medical schools also became pioneers in reaching out to various minority communities. In 1928, the New York Homeopathic Medical College[94] became the first medical school in the nation to establish a scholarship program specifically for minority students, through the efforts of Walter Gray Crump, Sr., MD. Dr. Crump was an alumnus and voluntary faculty member who participated vigorously in the academic life of the college. He also taught surgery, served as staff surgeon at other hospitals, was a founder of the New York Medical College for Women, was a trustee of Tuskegee Institute and Howard University, and assumed a leading role in the advancement of minority education and minority affairs (www.nymc.edu).

Although there were significant tensions and even downright antagonism between conventional medical doctors and homeopathic doctors, there tended to be considerably more cooperative relations between women doctors of the different schools of medical thought and practice.

For instance, in Chicago there were numerous hospitals where women physicians practiced together despite their conventional or homeopathic education and practice (Fine, 2005).

Research on women physicians has also shown that they preferred studying and practicing homeopathic medicine than conventional medicine. According to data from the Illinois Board of Health in 1878 and 1883, 70 percent of men became conventional doctors, while 60 percent of women became homeopathic doctors (Fine, 2005).

There are few statistics today on the percentage of practicing homeopaths who are women, but when going to virtually any homeopathic conference, one finds that the majority of participants are women. One study of professional homeopaths (those not trained in medical schools) in England found that in 1988 women comprised 48 percent of the registered members of the Society of Homeopaths, while from 1996 to 1999 they comprised 77 percent of the membership.

Likewise, the vast majority of homeopathic patients are women, and it isn't hard to understand why this is so. The same reasons that attracted women to homeopathy in the nineteenth century continue to play a role today.

It is therefore no surprise that modern women such as **Coretta Scott King** (1927–2006), wife of the late Martin Luther King, Jr., had a special interest in homeopathic medicine. When Ms. King died in January 2006, in an alternative medicine hospital in Mexico, her family let it be known that her special interest in homeopathic medicine led her to this hospital, even though she arrived there in end-stage disease. Although homeopathy cannot save everyone from disease or death, its history of safety and efficacy will no longer be forgotten as a part of history.

References

Bradford, T. L. *The Logic of Figures or Comparative Results of Homoeopathic and Other Treatments.* Philadelphia: Boericke and Tafel, 1900.

Breckinridge, S. P. *Women in the Twentieth Century: A Study of Their Political, Social and Economic Activities.* New York: McGraw-Hill, 1933.

Chen, C. *The Sex Side of Life: Mary Ware Dennett's Pioneering Battle for Birth Control and Sex Education.* New York: New Press, 1997.

Cleaves Biographical Cyclopedia of Homoeopathic Physicians and Surgeons. Philadelphia: Galaxy, 1873.

Coulter, H. L. *Divided Legacy.* Vol. III: The Conflict Between Homeopathy and the AMA. Berkeley: North Atlantic Books, 1973.

Fine, E. Separatism in Medicine? Regular and Sectarian Women Physicians in Nineteenth-Century Chicago. *Symposium for Women Physicians, Women's Politics, Women's Health: Emerging Narratives.* March 10–11, 2005, National Library of Medicine, National Institutes of Health.

Goldsmith, B. *Other Powers: The Age of Suffrage, Spiritualism, and the Scandalous Victoria Woodhull.* New York: Knopf, 1998.

Haehl, R. *Samuel Hahnemann: His Life and Work* (2 vols.). London: Homeopathic Publishing Co., 1922 (reprinted New Delhi: B. Jain, no date).

Haller, J. S. *The History of American Homeopathy: The Academic Years, 1820–1935.* New York: Pharmaceutical Products, 2005.

Harth, E. Founding Mothers of Social Justice: The Women's Educational and Industrial Union of Boston, 1877–1892, *Historical Journal of Massachusetts,* Summer 1999. Available at www.findarticles.com/p/articles/mi_qa3837/is_199907/ai_n8860523

Jackson, M. B. *The Women's Journal,* February 14, 1874. Available at http://pilgrim hall.org/MedsMercyBJackson.htm

Jenkins, E. *Dr. Gully's Story.* New York: Coward, McCann & Geoghegan, 1972.

King, W. H. *History of Homoeopathy* (4 volumes). New York: Lewis, 1905.

Kirschmann, A. T. *A Vital Force: Women in American Homeopathy.* Piscataway: Rutgers University Press, 2004.

Lozier, A. *In Memoriam: Clemence Sophia Lozier, MD.* New York: New York Historical Society, 1888, p. 17.

Mitchell, K. M. Her Preference Was to Heal: Women's Choice of Homeopathic Medicine in Nineteenth-Century United States. Dissertation, History Dept., Yale University, April 17, 1989.

Nighingale, F. Letter to Mrs. Nightingale, April 1852, Wellcome Medical Library, London, MSS 8993:f82.

www.nymc.edu/today/today.asp (See the heading Nation's First Minority Scholarship Program for information about Crump.)

Ruddick, J. *Death at the Priory: Sex, Love, and Murder in Victorian England.* New York: Atlantic Monthly Press, 2001.

Stanton, E. C. *Eighty Years and More: Reminiscences 1815–1897.* Available at www.gutenberg.org/files/11982/11982-8.txt

Sullivan, J. *The History of New York State.* New York: Lewis Historical Publishing Company, 1927. Available at www.usgennet.org/usa/ny/state/his/bk12/ch13/pt6.html

Wellman, J. *The Road to Seneca Falls: Elizabeth Cady Stanton and the First Woman's Rights Convention.* Chicago: University of Illinois Press, 2004.

Winston, J. *The Faces of Homeopathy.* Tawa, New Zealand: Great Awk, 1999.

Winston, J. History of Women in Homeopathy, *The American Homeopath,* 2004, 10:33–36.

Yasgur, J. Lozier's School, *The American Homeopath,* 1998, pp. 42–47.

CHAPTER 11

Corporate Leaders' and Philanthropists' Support for Homeopathy: A Rich Tradition

In the nineteenth and early twentieth centuries, homeopathy in America was championed as the "new medicine." It attracted America's literary elite, many political leaders, and many leading members of the clergy.

Despite this significant interest and support for homeopathy from so many extremely respected people, their advocacy does not explain how homeopathy was able to create twenty-two homeopathic medical colleges and more than 100 homeopathic hospitals in the United States alone. Establishing and operating colleges and hospitals took money, a lot of money—and homeopaths had money, or access to it, because many of America's richest people were advocates of homeopathy during its "heyday." Although the number of homeopaths in the U.S. was never more than 15–20 percent of practicing medical doctors, the most educated and most wealthy people tended to go to homeopaths. One medical journal in 1889 estimated that over 80 percent of all taxes in Cleveland, Ohio were paid by homeopathic patients (*Medical and Surgical Record,* 1889).

This support from the wealthiest people in America was not unique to this country. Virtually every country in Europe had large homeopathic hospitals as a result of patronage from many of Europe's richest people.

A powerful book of photographs with accompanying text was published by the American Institute of Homeopathy in 1916, entitled *The Hospitals and Sanatoriums of the Homeopathic School of Medicine.* Many of the largest homeopathic hospitals in the world at that time were run entirely or predominantly by homeopathic physicians. An online copy of this book is available at http://homeoint.org/books3/hospital/index.htm.

Other evidence of homeopathy's preeminence was the fact that three of the four largest medical school libraries in 1900 in the U.S. were at homeopathic medical schools, and two of the five medical schools with the greatest assessed value of their buildings were homeopathic (Rothstein, 1972, 237).

Many of the largest corporations in the U.S. maintained clinics with homeopathic physicians providing medical services for their employees. These corporations included General Motors, the Studebaker Company, the Continental Motor Company, Montgomery Ward,[95] General Electric, National Cash Register,[96] and the Chalmers Motor Company[97] (Robins, 2005, 148; American Institute of Homeopathy, 1916).

Given the practical nature of these large American corporations, a decision to devote their medical clinics to homeopathic treatment for the wide variety of acute and chronic ailments that employees experienced resulted from careful thinking and planning as well as a history of impressive clinical results.

John D. Rockefeller, Sr.

John D. Rockefeller (1839–1937) probably had more impact on medicine than anyone else in this chapter, and therefore, his story requires more detail than others. And it is a fascinating story.

America's richest man, John D. Rockefeller was one of homeopathy's most prominent advocates, preferring homeopathic treatment over any other type of medical care. Living to a ripe old age of 97 years, he was known later in his life to have his personal homeopath travel with him. Initially, Rockefeller's homeopath was **Myra King Merrick, MD** (1825–1899), the first woman doctor in Ohio, who helped establish the Cleveland Homeopathic Hospital College for Women in 1867. Dr. Merrick's specialty was obstetrics, and she delivered John D. Rockefeller, Jr. At some point in the 1890s, **Hamilton Fiske Biggar, MD** (1839–1926), began providing homeopathic care to the Rockefeller family. Biggar was J. D.'s golfing buddy as well, and they lived across the street from each other at the time.

Rockefeller had a disease that resulted in the loss of all of his body hair. Although various specialists were consulted, Rockefeller decided to receive care only from Dr. Biggar, who significantly restored his health, though not his hair (Murphy, 1974).

Historians have noted that not only did J. D. Rockefeller go to homeopaths but "all of the Standard Oil families" sought homeopathic care (Kirschmann, 2004, 46), primarily with Dr. Merrick. Merrick was respected enough by both homeopaths and allopaths that it was rumored various conventional obstetricians secretly consulted with her on their more difficult cases (Murphy, 1974).

In 1902, J. D. founded the Rockefeller Institute for Medical Research (RIMR), initially with a small grant of only $20,000 and followed with a gift of $1 million. By 1928 he had given $65 million to RIMR (Brown, 1979, 150). Although Rockefeller's name was on the Institute, the person behind the scenes making all of the decisions about where the money should be going was Frederick T. Gates, a Baptist who previously was executive director of the American Baptist Educational Society (J. D. also was a Baptist, and he believed in tithing 10 percent of his income to his church and charities). J. D. told Gates he didn't have time to administer his philanthropic endeavors, and he wanted Gates to do it.

Rockefeller was also known to not meddle in the affairs of his philanthropic organizations or in the affairs of the organizations to which grants were given. He made it clear that he wanted his money to be supporting homeopathic institutions, but throughout the first three decades of the twentieth century, when Rockefeller and his various foundations gave away $550 million (!), virtually no money supported homeopathic education or research. In 1916 Rockefeller scolded his staff, insisting: "I am a homeopathist. I desire that homeopathists should have fair, courteous, and liberal treatment extended to them from all medical institutes to which we contribute." Again, a few years later, in 1919, when he gave $45 million to the General Education Board, he warned his son and his staff: "Homeopathic teaching should not be excluded; it should be provided for, the same as Allopathic" (Brown, 1979, 109–110).

However, Frederick Gates and J. D.'s son, John D. Rockefeller, Jr., had different ideas. They didn't like homeopathy; Gates referred to Hahnemann as "a little less than a lunatic" (Rockefeller Foundation, 1911), even though Hahnemann was an intellectual giant of his times, author of a leading chemistry text, and physician to various members of the German aristocracy. Although Rockefeller gave significant amounts of money to various homeopathic hospitals and colleges before he hired Gates, these contributions stopped shortly after Gates began running RIMR.

When J. D. asked his lawyer, Starr J. Murphy, to follow up on his recommendations to support the homeopathic colleges and hospitals, Abraham Flexner (1866–1959), a leading executive at one of Rockefeller's philanthropic organizations, was asked to respond, and he wrote to Murphy a boldface lie. Flexner told Murphy and Rockefeller: "We have been in friendly conference with the representatives of the several homeopathic schools and are investigating all schools regardless of their affiliations in precisely the same manner and spirit." This statement was made shortly after Flexner had had some meetings with representatives of the New York Homeopathic Medical College and Flower Hospital, and they were directly told that colleges and hospitals that have "homeopathic" in their name would be considered "sectarian" and therefore inappropriate for funding (Coulter, 1973, III, 464–465).

Strangely enough, even when Rockefeller endeavored to establish a medical institute at the University of Chicago in the mid-1890s "that was neither allopath nor homoeopath, but simply scientific in its investigations into medical science" (Benison and Rivers, 1967, 34), he was dissuaded from doing so by his medical advisors (Nevins, 1940, 263). It seems that Rockefeller's advisors deemed any support for homeopathy inappropriate.

When RIMR was founded in 1902, Gates recommended that the institute be independent and not affiliated with a university so that it would appear impartial. Gates knew that Rockefeller would not want his institute to be affiliated with any allopathic medical school, so he (Gates) found this way to disguise and ultimately hide his support for orthodox medical schools from Rockefeller.

The president of the AMA in 1903 was Dr. Frank Billings, who in his presidential address to the AMA that year stated: "Drugs, with the exception of quinine in malaria and mercury in syphilis, are valueless as cures" (Rand, Dewey, and Hanchett, 1903). Ironically and sadly, even though leading physicians of that day recognized the serious dangers of conventional drugs and their questionable efficacy, conventional physicians and their organizations did not convey this message to the general public, and in fact, they consistently and vigorously attacked any alternatives to conventional treatments.

When Rockefeller started his medical research institute, he hoped that other wealthy people would establish comparable (and competing) research institutes—and they did. For one, Andrew Carnegie (1835–1919), founder of Carnegie Steel Company, which later became U.S. Steel, developed an educational institute, the Carnegie Foundation for the Advancement of Teaching. Henry S. Pritchett was hired to be its head. Pritchett met with Arthur Bevan, head of the AMA's Council on Medical Education, to develop a plan to improve medical education. Ultimately, they conceived of doing a survey of American medical schools. The AMA could not sponsor such a study because it would be seen as too biased, and therefore, Pritchett suggested that the Carnegie Foundation do so—a stroke of public relations genius. The AMA could get what it wanted without seeming to be a party to the report.

To conduct a survey of medical colleges and develop guidelines for a model medical school, Pritchett chose to hire Abraham Flexner, the brother of Gates's appointee Dr. Simon Flexner who was the director of RIMR. At the time Abraham Flexner was an unemployed schoolmaster who had no training or relevant knowledge of medicine. Because he would not be seen as either a homeopath or an allopath, he could be seen as an objective reviewer of medical schools. But the obvious question is, Was he really an objective reviewer?

The AMA and the Carnegie Foundation had a predefined agenda even before Abraham Flexner began his survey of medical schools. Both of these organizations were concerned that America had too many doctors. Representatives from both organizations used the same statistic: Germany had one doctor for every 2,000 people, while the U.S. had one doctor for every 568 people (Flexner, 1910, 14).

The AMA had a strong dislike for the various "irregular" methods of medical treatment (homeopathic, osteopathic, chiropractic, eclectic, and naturopathic), and if something could be done to reduce or eliminate them, orthodox physicians would be in greater demand and therefore earn a better living. The AMA and the Carnegie Foundation were also concerned about the existence of three women's medical colleges. Flexner actually believed that women were less able to withstand the mental rigors of medicine and made better patients than doctors (Brown, 1979, 149).

Flexner consulted frequently with the leadership in the AMA and had no similar relationship with homeopathic physicians or organizations. Representatives of the American Institute of Homeopathy sought to have a meeting with Flexner before the survey began, but there is no record of any such meeting taking place, which signaled that the homeopaths were not going to be treated in a similar fashion to the conventional physicians.

Further, six months before the Flexner Report was published, Pritchett wrote a memo to Bevan of the AMA:

> In all this work of the examination of the medical schools we have been hand in glove with you and your committee. ... When our report comes out, it is going to be ammunition in your hands. It is desirable, therefore, to maintain in the meantime a position which does not intimate an immediate connection between our two efforts. (Berliner, 1985, 110)

This statement—a classic "smoking gun"—clearly shows that Bevan wanted the AMA's and the Carnegie Foundation's collaboration and conspiracy to remain a secret.

If the quoted memo from the Carnegie Foundation to the AMA wasn't strong enough evidence of collusion, a later AMA publication actually bragged: "[Nathan Colwell, secretary of the AMA's Council on Medical Education] provided far more guidance in this famous survey than is generally known" (Coulter, 1973, III, 446).

Historians point out that to conduct his survey Flexner had to visit each of the 155 medical colleges and twelve postgraduate schools in the

U.S. and Canada in just sixteen months. To do so, he usually spent less than a day at a school. He even made some visits with AMA representative Colwell.

Bevan was so anxious to get this information from the Carnegie Foundation's report to the medical community and the general public that he asked Flexner and Pritchett to speak at the AMA meeting several months before the report was to be published. However, Pritchett did not want the public to know about the close tie between the AMA and the Carnegie report (Brown, 1979, 152). Some historians simply and directly assert that the AMA "engineered" this report and the changes it recommended (Roberts, 1986).

Predictably enough, the *Journal of the American Medical Association* (*JAMA*) lauded the Flexner Report, but numerous other medical journals described it as "hasty," "full of errors," "a monumental piece of impudence," and "unfair to small and worthy schools" (Hiatt, 1999).

Sir William Osler, one of America's and Europe's most respected physicians of that day, former professor at Johns Hopkins University and former chief of staff of its hospital, asserted that Flexner had "a very feeble grasp of medicine" and that there were so many errors in his report that Osler was unable to say whether "unfairness or ignorance" was "the more prevalent … but in either case, gross injustice is done" (Chesney, 1963, 177–178).

Osler was particularly critical of Flexner's recommendation that medical school education should focus on laboratory science, rather than clinical science. Flexner insisted that medical schools have only full-time teaching and research faculty who specialized in laboratory research rather than utilize physicians who at least had a part-time medical practice. In 1911 Osler wrote a stern letter to Ira Remsen, MD, president of Johns Hopkins, declaring, "I cannot imagine anything more subversive to the highest ideal of the clinical school than to hand over our young men who are to be our best practitioners to a group of teachers who are ex-officio out of touch with the conditions under which these young men will live" (Osler, 1962).

Because Flexner considered the Johns Hopkins Medical School as his "model" for the best that scientific medical education offered at the time, this criticism should have dealt a death blow to the Flexner Report, but the power and the money behind this report was too considerable to stop this advocacy locomotive from mowing down anything in its way.

It is also ironic that the president of Johns Hopkins at that time was Ira Remsen, MD. Remsen received his medical training at the New York Homeopathic Medical College, graduating in 1865 and later teaching chemistry there. This fact and so many others should have muted any criticisms that homeopathic medical education lacked rigor. But, then, facts were not the primary motivating factor behind the work of Flexner, Gates, and the AMA.[98]

Flexner's attitude toward unorthodox medicine was brutal. He called chiropractors "unconscionable quacks" and eclectic doctors "drug mad" (eclectic doctors went to eclectic medical schools that taught conventional, herbal, and homeopathic medicine). Flexner equated homeopathy with "dogma." He wrote in his report: "The ebbing vitality of homeopathic schools is a striking demonstration of the incompatibility of science and dogma."

It must, however, be noted that only a minority of the educated homeopaths were able to maintain a clinical practice using only homeopathic medicines, while the vast majority of homeopathic doctors were eclectic, usually using homeopathic medicines as their primary method of treatment but also using various orthodox and herbal treatments. A strong case, therefore, can and should be made that it was the orthodox physicians who practiced by dogma, for they would not even consider using homeopathic medicines or many of the common and popular herbal remedies of the day.

Flexner was not interested in creating an "objective" report on medical education. In fact, he asserted that "scientific medicine" did not need to be "democratic" or responsive to the public's interest in alternatives to orthodox medicine. He further maintained that dissent implied ignorance or "blind faith" to "dogma" (Flexner, 1910, 156, 161).

Despite these serious and varied concerns, the Flexner Report had a dramatic impact on American medical education. Flexner recommended that all women's medical colleges be closed, and shortly after his report, all but one were indeed closed, as were five of the seven black medical colleges. The twenty-two homeopathic medical schools in 1900 dwindled to just two by 1923. The naturopathic, eclectic, and chiropractic schools experienced a similar fate. All medical schools teaching homeopathy were forced to change their curriculum to follow the guidelines promoted by Flexner. These changes required a biomedical viewpoint which significantly decreased the amount of homeopathic training. The homeopathic medical schools began producing second-rate homeopaths, and by 1950 all schools teaching homeopathy were closed. Ultimately, the Flexner Report led to creating fewer but richer doctors, with greater homogeneity of race, gender, and type of therapeutic practice.

Shortly after the Flexner Report was published, Abraham Flexner was actually employed at the General Education Board, and he worked tirelessly to augment the "reforms" that his report recommended. The grant-giving organization provided $180 million from 1910 to 1930, and Frederick Gates and Abraham and Simon Flexner held the purse strings to this largesse. This money was used to foster and even force acceptance of the Flexner Report (Brown, 1979, 166), and there is no evidence that a single homeopathic college or hospital was granted a dime. This under-the-radar work was instrumental in closing the homeopathic and eclectic medical schools.

Gates and his top managers were all specifically chosen for their anti-homeopathic perspective, and the group of Rockefeller foundations made certain that no funding would go to any school or college that included the word "homeopathic" in its title. Dr. Biggar, Rockefeller's homeopath, was able to get J. D.'s donation of land and funds for building the Cleveland Homeopathic Hospital College, and J. D. even served as vice president for a short period (Chernow, 1998, 404), but Gates made certain that no other funding was ever obtained from RIMR for other homeopathic institutions. Even Rockefeller's personal secretary, Harry Simms, who married a Rockefeller relative, and who later served on the board of trustees (1922) and became chairman (1936–1956) of the Cleveland Homeopathic Hospital College (Murphy, 1974), was unable to secure any additional funding after the college was built.

Then, because the new medical licensing exams only tested for basic medical science in ever-increasing detail (whether or not these details were actually useful to clinical practice), the homeopathic schools were forced to focus their teaching on these subjects to the exclusion of learning the detailed science and art of homeopathic medicine. The AMA's new strategy to reduce and eliminate the homeopathic and eclectic schools was for the AMA's Council on Medical Education to establish guidelines that "graded" schools depending upon various standards that embodied the biomedical research and the orthodox medical model of treatment. Also, since each school was required to have new and expensive medical equipment that was more useful for orthodox medical treatment than for homeopathic care, and since the Rockefeller foundations supported only the orthodox medical schools' access to this newer equipment, the homeopathic colleges and medical students were put at a great disadvantage.

Homeopaths put up an impressive fight. In 1894, sixteen years before the Flexner Report, the Association of American Medical Colleges had officially recognized that homeopathic medical colleges were as efficient in teaching the essentials of medicine as the orthodox medical colleges. This esteemed organization had also passed a bylaw stipulating that homeopathic graduates could be admitted to advanced standing in orthodox medical colleges and would get every credit except those courses devoted exclusively to homeopathic clinical training (Kaufman, 1971, 146). Even *JAMA* acknowledged the high quality of medical education provided by the homeopathic medical schools, publishing an annual survey that embarrassingly revealed that the graduates of homeopathic medical schools had a lower failure rate on the state medical board examinations than graduates of conventional medical schools (between 1900 and 1905, homeopathic graduates had a 9 percent failure rate, and conventional medical graduates had a 16 percent failure rate; in 1909, the difference was 14.3 percent versus 16.2 percent) (Robins, 2005, 76; JAMA, 1909).[99]

When Gates first met Rockefeller, Gates was a devout Baptist, but soon afterwards, he began reading the Bible more critically and once wrote:

> Christ had neither founded nor intended to found the Baptist Church, nor any church; that neither he nor his disciples during his lifetime had baptized; that the communion was not conceived by Christ as a church ordinance, and that the whole Baptist fabric was built upon texts which had no authority. (Brown, 1979, 125)

Gates had converted from Baptism to the religion of "scientific medicine."[100]

Rockefeller was once asked if he ever studied medicine. He responded: "No, not much, but I have studied doctors." Indeed he had, and perhaps that is why he always preferred homeopathic treatment for himself—and perhaps why he even outlived his own homeopath, who only lived to 87 years of age. Rockefeller's next and last homeopath, **Alonzo Eugene Austin, MD**, was, like his predecessors, a devoted Hahnemannian homeopath.

Ultimately, despite Rockefeller's deep appreciation for homeopathy and his insistence that homeopathic institutions and organizations be funded to the same level as those of conventional medicine, homeopathy did not get any reasonable degree of support from the Rockefeller fortune. When you consider how much money was involved, especially in light of the value of early twentieth-century dollars, it is clear that conventional medicine's financial prowess was significantly augmented, while homeopathic medicine's was substantially hurt. Rockefeller gave $25,000 in 1888, but virtually nothing once Gates took over his philanthropic enterprises.

Rockefeller referred to homeopathy as a "progressive and aggressive step" in medicine (Coulter, 1973, III, 463), but sadly, homeopathy could not survive the power and influence of large amounts of money working against it.

Hiram Sibley

Hiram Sibley (1807–1888), founder of Western Union, was a significant supporter of homeopathy, as was his wife. Living in Rochester, New York, they helped to fund the Rochester Homeopathic Hospital in 1889, and Mrs. Sibley took a very active role in the hospital's administration. When a local congressman, Freeman Clarke, passed away, he donated his stately mansion to the homeopathic hospital, which became its administrative offices. Mrs. Sibley also made a significant donation to Philadelphia's Hahnemann Medical College, becoming one of its "life members."

George Eastman

George Eastman (1854–1932), founder of Eastman Kodak Company (the major photographic camera and film company), was also an avid supporter of homeopathy. Eastman grew up on homeopathy because of his mother's interest in this new medicine. In 1890 his mother Maria underwent successful cancer surgery at the Rochester Homeopathic Hospital. Out of gratitude to Dr. John M. Lee (her homeopath and surgeon), Eastman donated $600 to the hospital. After Maria's death in 1907 he donated $60,000 to help build the nurses' home, named Maria Eastman Hall. The three-story residence was used to house student nurses until the nursing school closed in 1978.

Eastman served on the board of managers of Rochester Homeopathic Hospital. In 1926 the hospital changed its name to Genesee Hospital. Even though the hospital was no longer strictly homeopathic, it developed certain other progressive and liberal medical programs. Because the hospital provided abortion and doctor-assisted suicide services, it became the target of pro-life activity over some fifteen years. Ultimately, it closed its doors in 2001.

Charles F. Kettering

Charles ("Boss") Kettering (1876–1958) served as vice president of General Motors, and was widely recognized as the greatest American inventor and engineer since Thomas Edison. He held more than 300 patents.

Some of his inventions included the all-electric starting ignition, ethyl gasoline, and Duco paint (trade name of a lacquer paint used on cars). He also started the Delco Company (which manufactures car batteries and which GM purchased).

Early in his career, Kettering worked for National Cash Register, which maintained a clinic for employees that was staffed by homeopathic doctors. The company's newsletter often provided health tips on such topics as the necessity of physical fitness, the importance of thorough chewing of the food ("Fletcherism"), the usefulness of fasting, the value of hydrotherapy, and the benefits of health sanitariums like the Battle Creek Sanitarium created by Dr. J. H. Kellogg (the man who also created the famous cereal company).

Kettering publicly acknowledged the health benefits he received due to the skills of **Thomas Addison (T. A.) McCann, MD** (1858–1943), his homeopathic physician from Dayton, Ohio (Enstam, 1943, 489).

T. A. McCann, MD, was a respected homeopathic physician who interacted considerably with conventional physicians. In fact, he was one of the few homeopathic doctors to work with the nationwide Federation of State Medical Examining Boards, serving as vice-president in 1914–1915. Dr. McCann is often quoted today as a result of his report on the impressive successes of homeopathic treatment during the flu epidemic of 1918. In 1921 at the 77th annual convention of the American Institute of Homeopathy in Washington, D.C., he reported that 24,000 cases of flu treated in conventional medical hospitals had a mortality rate of 28.2 percent while 26,000 cases of flu treated in homeopathic hospitals had a mortality rate of 1.05 percent (McCann, 1921; Dewey, 1921).[101]

In 1914 Ohio State University (OSU) formally opened a College of Homeopathic Medicine. To help in these efforts, another homeopathic college (the Cleveland-Pulte Medical College) closed down, donated its medical equipment and library, and sent the proceeds of the sale of its property ($30,000) to the new homeopathic college. In the homeopathic school's first year, an impressive thirty-nine students were enrolled. In 1915, Kettering and Edward A. Deeds (plant manager of National Cash Register, who had initially hired Kettering) gave $2,500 for research work and medical equipment. In 1916 Kettering gave $8,000 more, and in 1920, he donated $7,000 worth of radium for the school's X-ray machine.

Because the governor of Ohio at the time was James Cox, a strong advocate for homeopathy, and one of the governor's appointments to the university's board of trustees was Judge Benjamin McCann (the brother of Kettering's homeopath), the homeopathic college had important political support. This strength was further augmented by the employment of W. B. Hinsdale, dean of the University of Michigan Homeopathic School.[102]

However, the AMA could not stand for the development of a college of homeopathic medicine at a public university. N. P. Colwell, secretary of the AMA's Council on Medical Education, went on the offensive. He sharply criticized the president of OSU and arranged for strongly worded attacks against OSU in *JAMA*, and later, he even threatened to downgrade the accreditation status of OSU. Because Colwell's Council on Medical Education had become the national accrediting agency for medical schools, these threats were significant, and made even worse by Colwell's close relationship with the Carnegie Foundation and its president, Henry S. Pritchett. According to the minutes of OSU's board of trustees, Pritchett made scurrilous attacks upon the motives of OSU's president and trustees (Roberts, 1986).

In 1920 Kettering made a $1 million contribution to OSU with a stipulation that it be used to create a homeopathic research laboratory (Mendenhall Papers, 1920; Hertzog, 1949, 1193; Ohio State University, 1922, 440). This action enraged the AMA and the Carnegie Foundation, thrusting them into further proactive efforts to stop this homeopathic college. When Governor Cox left office in 1920 to run as the Democratic candidate for president of the United States, the homeopaths lost some of their political influence.

In 1922, the board of trustees voted to close down the homeopathic college. OSU was forced to return Kettering's donation as well as other donations that were specifically made to and for the homeopathic college, but OSU actually kept the largest and most valuable possession of the homeopathic community, the Homeopathic Hospital and all of its modern equipment, for its own College of Medicine (Ohio State University, 1923, 441). Kettering never trusted OSU after that. Even though he served on the board of trustees of OSU, he never again gave money to the school.

Dr. John Renner (1890–1989), a homeopathic doctor from Chicago who later retired to southern California, reported that Kettering had also planned to give another $1 million to homeopathy, but the infighting among homeopathic professionals led him instead to work to establish what later became the famed Sloan-Kettering Institute[103] (Suits, 1985, 123). Sadly, the "Boss" is probably turning in his grave, knowing how his institute has turned away from homeopathy and from real healing.

Kettering's philosophy was summarized in the question he asked and answered of an interviewer: "Do you know what an incurable disease is? It's one the doctors don't know anything about. The disease has no objection to being cured at all" (McDowell, 1983). Another reporter asked him about his conquests of the secrets of nature, to which Kettering responded:

> Hah, it's not the conquest of nature, it's the conquest of our own ignorance. And as for secrets, there is only one secret of nature I want to pry into. Why is the human skull as dense as it is? Nowadays we can send a message around the world in one-seventh of a second, but it take years to drive an idea through a quarter-inch of human skull. (Young, 1961, 193–194)

This doggedness and irreverence led Kettering to continually question conventional medical thinking and to have what the *New York Times* called "a long and expensive flirtation with research into homeopathy" (McDowell, 1983).

George Worthington

George Worthington (1813–1871) was a nineteenth-century merchant and banker in Cleveland, Ohio, who founded the George Worthington Company, a wholesale hardware and industrial distribution firm, in 1835 (until 1991, Cleveland's oldest extant business), as well as numerous banking and mining concerns. In 1865, Worthington was among the Cleveland businessmen who founded the Hahnemann Life Insurance Company (named after the founder of homeopathy), which was the first company in the U.S. to offer to insure those whose medical belief and practice were exclusively devoted to homeopathy. Homeopathic patients were offered lower rates than those subjecting themselves to conventional treatment because there was evidence of a lower rate of mortality under homeopathic care. The company was thought to be so well conceived and financed that it was the first western insurance company admitted into the state of New York.

In 1878 the Homeopathic Mutual Life Insurance Company had 7,927 policies for patients whose doctor was a homeopath and had eighty-four deaths (1.06 percent). This same insurance company had 2,258 policies for patients whose doctor was an allopath and sixty-six deaths (2.92 percent), nearly three times higher by percentage (Homeopathic Lives, 1879).

As this life insurance company became popular, many people who were not under homeopathic care sought to obtain their life insurance at reduced rates from this company, creating financial problems for the company. Various homeopathic life insurance companies persisted into the 1890s.

The Rich and Powerful in Four Key American Cities

In order to obtain a deeper sense of the popularity of homeopathic medicine among America's wealthiest families, below are short lists of some of the rich and powerful people in four American cities who advocated for homeopathy (New York City, Boston, Philadelphia, and Chicago).

New York
Some of the advocates and supporters of homeopathy in New York were:

- **Henry G. Stebbins**, president of the New York Stock Exchange (1858–1859) and member of the board of the New York Homeopathic Medical College and Hospital for Women.

Corporate Leaders' and Philanthropists' Support for Homeopathy

- **Cyrus West Field** (1819–1892), businessman and financier who co-founded the Atlantic Telegraph Company, which successfully laid the first telegraph cable across the Atlantic Ocean in 1858.
- **Alexander Turney Stewart**, founder of Manhattan's first department store (1846), called A. T. Stewart. Stewart was one of the three richest men in America and in 1875 developed Long Island's Garden City. He has been called the Merchant Prince and the inventor of the department store.
- **Henry Keep** (1818–1869), president of the New York Central Railroad and president of the Chicago and Northwestern Railway. In 1872, his wife, Emma Keep, donated $100,000 to the New York Homeopathic Ophthalmic Hospital in the memory of her husband.
- **Roswell P. Flower** (1835–1899) was governor of New York (1892–1895). His wife and daughter donated $200,000 to the New York Homeopathic Medical College to help build the Flower Hospital, named after him (Ward, 1900, 100).
- **David Dows** (1814–1890) gave $25,000 to the New York Homeopathic Medical College to help build the Flower Hospital. He was one of the largest grain dealers in the state. His daughter married Carroll Dunham, MD, a leading homeopathic physician, professor, and author.
- **John Englis**, the largest shipbuilder in New York, served on the board of trustees of the Homeopathic Hospital in Brooklyn (Sullivan, 1927).
- **A. Oakey Hall** (1826–1898), mayor of New York City (1869–1872).
- **Horace Webster** (1794–1871), first president of the College of the City of New York (The Gift that Grew, 1965; Wershub, 1967).

Boston

Trustees of the Massachusetts Homeopathic Medical Society included:

- **John Murray Forbes** (1813–1898), president of both the Michigan Central railroad and the Chicago, Burlington and Quincy Railroad in the 1850s. He was one of three brothers sent by their uncle to Canton, China, where he amassed a considerable fortune from the opium trade and China trade during the Opium Wars. His brother was the great-grandfather of 2004 U.S. Democratic presidential candidate John Forbes Kerry.

- **William Pope** (1813–?), chairman of the Marine Midland Trust Company (one of the largest banks in the U.S.) and trustee of both the Massachusetts Homeopathic Hospital and the medical society. Besides being a successful businessman, he served on Boston's first city council and on the school board and was an active abolitionist. Sadly, his grandson, Bayard Foster Pope did not maintain the family's connection to homeopathy; instead, he served on the board of directors of the largest tobacco company in America (Benson & Hedges, which later became Philip Morris). William Pope's son was Boston real estate developer William Carroll Pope.
- **Royal E. Robbins**, president of the Waltham Watch Company, which produced some 40 million high-quality watches, clocks, speedometers, compasses, time fuses, and other precision instruments between 1850 and 1950.

Trustees of the Massachusetts Homeopathic Hospital in the 1880s included:

- **Henry Sturgis Russell** (1838–1905), president of the hospital and the medical society during 1872–1895. He was the son-in-law of John Murray Forbes (see above) and grandson of Jonathan Russell. Jonathan Russell (1771–1832) was U.S. chargé d'affaires in Paris and then in London under President James Madison and a U.S. Congressman from Massachusetts during 1821–1823.
- **R. H. Stearn** was a wealthy merchant whose self-titled department store became one of the largest chains in the Boston area, but eventually failed to compete with comparable chains such as Filene's. His son, Frank W. Stearns, married Emily Williston Clark, eldest daughter of Massachusetts academician and public figure William Smith Clark. F. W. Stearns was a close friend of Calvin Coolidge (another homeopathic patient) from the time Coolidge was a Massachusetts governor.

- **The Hon. Charles R. Codman** was a state senator, school board member, abolitionist, and colonel in the Civil War.
- **Sarah A. Pope** (wife of William Pope; see above) was president of the Ladies' Aid Society of the hospital. William Pope's aunt, **Elizabeth Pope**, was married to Dr. Conrad Wesselhoeft, one of Boston's leading homeopaths.

Philadelphia

In Philadelphia, many "old money" families became homeopathic patients and patrons, including:

- The **Strawbridge** and **Clothier families**, whose members served on advisory boards and were "life patrons" to the Hahnemann Medical College; these families created the large Strawbridge and Clothier (later shortened to Strawbridge's) department stores in the northeastern U.S., which in 2005 were acquired by the Federated Department Stores (Macys).
- The **Widener family**, which founded Widener College, which today is called Widener University.
- **Joseph Wharton** (1826–1909), co-founder of Bethlehem Steel and founder of the Wharton School of Business at the University of Pennsylvania.
- The **Biddle family**, a leading banking family of Philadelphia (Kirschmann, 2004, 45).
- **John Batterson Stetson** (1830–1906), a hat manufacturer, for whom the Stetson hat was named.
- **Anthony Joseph Drexel** (1826–1893), a leading banker, partner at J. P. Morgan, and founder of Drexel University, which now owns the former Hahnemann Medical College of Philadelphia.
- **George C. Thomas**, a leading banker, railroad executive, and large landowner, who donated land worth $60,000 to the Hahnemann Hospital in Philadelphia.

Chicago

In 1871, it was estimated that more than half of the families in the wealthiest part of the city were advocates of homeopathy (Rothstein, 1972, 234). While homeopathy was more popular among the wealthy and the educated classes, conventional medicine was considerably more popular among the poor and uneducated classes. When one AMA member suggested the medical society should induce Chicago's newspapers to work to change this "problem," he was informed that the newspapers were owned and largely edited by advocates of homeopathy.

Many of Chicago's most prominent citizens and politicians participated in the creation of the Hahnemann Medical College in Chicago, including:

- **Orrington Lunt**, a businessman and co-founder of Northwestern University.
- **William H. Brown**, founder of the Chicago Union Railroad. Later, he had a U.S. Navy ship named after him.
- **Joseph B. Doggett**, an Illinois congressman.
- **Thomas Hoyne**, a mayor of Chicago.

Later, other well-known and respected Chicagoans supported the development of three other homeopathic colleges in Chicago, plus several hospitals (Renner, 1974; Spiegel and Kavaler, 2002). These advocates included:

- **Edson Keith**, a successful hat merchant who sat on the board of Marshall Field, the department store.
- **Benjamin Lombard**, a successful farmer and businessman who created Illinois Liberal Institute (later, Lombard College), which ultimately closed during the Depression.
- **William Wrigley**, chewing gum industrialist and owner of the Chicago Cubs.
- **Victor Lawson**, owner of the *Chicago Daily News*. He also funded the Daily News Sanatorium, a 350-bed hospital entirely run by

homeopathic physicians. It was located in Lincoln Park on the shore of Lake Michigan.
- **Robert Sanderson McCormick**, owner of the *Chicago Tribune*.
- **Van H. Higgins**, a Superior Court judge.

Other Americans

H. J. Heinz (1844–1919) was the founder of the H. J. Heinz Co., the international food company. He contributed to the erection of the Hahnemann monument in Washington, D.C. and contributed $10,000 toward a dormitory at Kansas City University (which had a Kansas City Hahnemann Medical College affiliated with it), as a memorial to his wife.

George Westinghouse (1846–1914) was founder of Westinghouse Electric and Machine Company, later simply called Westinghouse. He and his wife made many contributions to the homeopathic hospital in Pittsburgh. These included giving the hospital free gas for heating, and X-ray equipment just months after Wilhelm Roentgen invented the first X-ray machine. They also donated to the creation of the Hahnemann monument in Washington, D.C.

Robert Pitcairn (1836–1909) was vice president of the Pennsylvania Railroad and a close friend of George Westinghouse and Andrew Carnegie.

John Pitcairn (1841–1916) was founder of Pittsburgh Plate Glass, which produced 65 percent of the plate glass used in the United States in 1900. Today, it is called PPG Industries, a $10-plus billion company. Pitcairn was the primary donor to the Post-Graduate School of Homeotherapeutics in Philadelphia, which was considered the best homeopathic school in the United States during its ten-year existence between 1890 and 1900, with **James Tyler Kent, MD**, as its leading teacher. In the first four years of the school's existence, its teaching clinic provided free care to more than 36,000 patients. Pitcairn was the president of the school. Pitcairn was also a leading advocate of the scientist-spiritual leader Emanuel Swedenborg, and is credited for introducing Dr. Kent to Swedenborgian thought (see Chapter 13, Clergy and Spiritual Leaders, for more details about Swedenborg).

Andrew Carnegie (1835–1919) was founder of Carnegie Steel Company, which later became U.S. Steel. He was the second wealthiest American (second to J. D. Rockefeller). Earlier in his career, he was an advocate for homeopathy, and in 1876, he was listed as a life trustee in the annual report of the Homeopathic Hospital and Dispensary in Pittsburgh, due to a large contribution he made. The fact that he lived next door to the Pitcairn family probably led to his interest in homeopathy, though Carnegie's interest in and support for homeopathy was not significant, especially as compared with most others listed in this chapter. Later in his life, the Carnegie Foundation worked closely with the American Medical Association in attacking homeopathy and supporting conventional medicine of the day. It is unclear how much of a role Carnegie himself played in this effort because he was 75 years old when his foundation issued the anti-homeopathy Flexner Report.

Phoebe Hearst (1842–1919) was the wife of Homestake Mining Company founder George Hearst and mother of William Randolph Hearst, the newspaper magnate. She served on the board of directors of the Hahnemann Medical College of the Pacific from 1882 until 1908, and provided significant funding for the establishment of the Hahnemann Hospital in San Francisco. She was also a Life Member of the Fabiola Homeopathic Hospital and Free Dispensary in Oakland, California (more details about this hospital are provided later in this chapter; Hearst papers).

Daniel B. Wesson (1825–1906) partnered with Horace Smith in the early 1850s to develop the first repeating rifle, the Winchester rifle. He and his wife gave their family home to be used to create the Hampden Homeopathic Hospital at Springfield, Massachusetts (Proceedings, 1901, 264).

Samuel F. B. Morse (1791–1872) invented the first electric telegraph and developed the signaling alphabet that became the Morse code. He was a homeopathic patient.

Peter Fennimore Cooper (1791–1883) was an American industrialist and founder of the Canton Iron Works near Baltimore, where he manufactured the first steam-powered railroad locomotive, called Tom Thumb. He was a homeopathic patient.

John H. Patterson (1844–1922) was founder of National Cash Register (NCR), a very progressively run company. In 1893, in response to the problem of sweatshops, Patterson constructed the first "daylight factory" buildings with floor-to-ceiling glass windows that let in light and air. In 1903 he hired H. H. Herman, MD, to run NCR's clinic for its employees. Although Dr. Herman was trained at a conventional medical school, he became a homeopathic doctor after a couple of years of working at the NCR clinic.

Henry Oliver (1840–1904) was founder of Oliver Iron Mining Co., a wholly owned subsidiary of U.S. Steel. He was one of the financial contributors to the famous Shadyside Hospital, a homeopathic hospital in Pittsburgh (now a part of the University of Pittsburgh Medical Center and no longer homeopathic).

Myron T. Herrick (1854–1929) was governor of Ohio and ambassador to France under two U.S. presidents. He served on the board of trustees of a homeopathic hospital in Cleveland.

European Patrons

Even before Samuel Hahnemann, MD, experimented with and later developed homeopathic medicine, he was an honored physician, chemist, and translator. Hahnemann received personal instruction in orthodox medicine of his day under the physician to the Austrian emperor, **Freiherr Von Quarin**. He then became the physician to some German and Austrian royalty.

Hahnemann also made some important discoveries in chemistry that were regularly used by pharmacists of his day, and his four-volume set of books, *The Pharmaceutical Lexicon,* became one of their important textbooks. Some historians of science assert that Hahnemann's role in the history of science was considerable, "far outstripping any of his numerous, even chemical contemporaries," and he would have become a historically renowned chemist if he had continued in this field (Von Lippman, 1953, 298).

After Hahnemann began to develop the homeopathic system, he achieved much notoriety among royalty, and his patrons included Prince Ferdinand of Anhalt-Kothen, the Duke of Meiningen, the Grand Duke of Baden, and many others. Homeopathy actually became so popular among German monarchs and government officials that it was a matter of good taste to be treated by a homeopathic doctor. This popularity increased further when two famous war heroes from Germany and Austria, Count Karl von Schwarzenberg and Field Marshall Johann Joseph von Radetzky, underwent much publicized and successful homeopathic treatment. Two of Germany's most famous authors of that time, Johann Wolfgang von Goethe and Jean Paul Friedrich Richter, wrote about these successes, along with their appreciation for homeopathy and their concern about the attacks against it from orthodox doctors.

Samuel Hahnemann, MD, was married and had eleven children. After his wife's death in 1830, he maintained an active practice in Germany until 1834, when he was 79 years old, at which time he met a 34-year-old French woman, with whom he fell madly in love. He soon moved to her home in Paris. His new wife, Melanie d'Hervilly, was an artist, a poet, and an intellectual whose friends were the elite of Paris. Because of Hahnemann's considerable reputation throughout Europe at that time, it was not long before his Parisian practice included many of Europe's social elite, especially members of the French and British upper and professional classes—nobles, clergy, military officers, and doctors.

Hahnemann's practice in Paris included many members of France's elite, including **Honoré de Balzac** (1799–1850, French novelist and playwright who is considered a founding father of realism in European literature), **Nicolo Paganini** (1782–1840, composer and virtuoso violinist), **Pierre-Jean David** (1788–1856, also known as David d'Angers, a highly respected sculptor who created a sculpture of Hahnemann), **Jacques Claude, comte de Beugnot** (1761–1835, French politician before, during, and after the French revolution), and **Philippe Musard** (1761–1859, who led one of the most popular orchestras of that time and was one of

Europe's most popular musicians, and who referred many members of his orchestra to Dr. Hahnemann).

Many members of the British aristocracy sought Hahnemann's care as well, including **Baron Mayer Amschel de Rothschild** (1818–1874, banker and financier, who sought care for his arthritis and neuralgia), **Lord Elgin** (1811–1863, an aristocrat who later became governor of Jamaica and, still later, governor of Canada), **Lady Kinnaird** (of Scotland's aristocracy), **Countess of Hopetoun** (also a Scottish aristocrat), **Lord Capel, Lady Belfast, Lady Drummond**, and the **Duchess of Melford** (Handley, 1997, 20–22).

Henry William Paget, known as the First Marquess of Anglesey and the Earl of Uxbridge (1768–1854), was a British military leader, politician, and titled aristocrat. He is primarily remembered today for leading the British cavalry as general in the Battle of Waterloo (1815). One of the last cannon shots in this battle hit Paget in the leg, leading to its amputation. He suffered with extreme pain for twenty-one years, until he was treated by Hahnemann in 1836.

Hahnemann also provided treatment to **William Leaf**, one of London's most wealthy merchants. Leaf had suffered from chronic disease for many years until Hahnemann completely cured him. The merchant decided to devote his great resources to the promotion of homeopathic medicine; he induced Dr. Paul Curie (1799–1853), a respected Parisian homeopath, to come to London to start a homeopathic hospital and a dispensary for the poor.

The **Tate family** (leading seller of sugar and founder of the famed Tate Gallery in London) and the **Wills family** (leading seller of tobacco) paid for and built the Liverpool and Bristol homeopathic hospitals that still exist (and thrive) today. And the **Cadbury** and **Rowntree** families (both leading sellers of chocolate) paid for and built homeopathic hospitals in Birmingham and York, respectively.

Ultimately, there was both good and bad news about homeopathy's connection to British aristocracy. Homeopathy's popularity in England tended to be largely confined to fashionable spa towns (such as Buxton, Leamington, Harrogate, Bath, and Malvern), to the wealthy coastal resorts (such as Eastbourne, Brighton, and Bognor Regis), and to London and southern England in general. Distinct from botanical medicine, which was popular in northern, industrial cities, homeopathy never really developed much usage among working-class people. Therefore, when the aristocrats went into significant decline after 1890, homeopathy did not have enough support from the masses to maintain its popularity (Cannadine, 1996, 88–181).

Robert Bosch

Robert Bosch (1861–1942) deserves a separate listing from other European corporate leaders and philanthropists due to his considerable interest in and support for homeopathy.

Bosch was founder of Robert Bosch GmbH, the large manufacturer of auto parts, appliances, and power tools in Germany. Besides creating quality products, the Bosch company has had a long history of providing a healthy work environment with good ventilation and lighting for its employees, and it was the first company in Europe to establish the eight-hour workday (rather than ten or twelve hours).

Bosch grew up in southern Germany in an area that was previously called the Kingdom of Württemberg. Queen Olga of Württemberg (1822–1892), a Russian princess, married Charles I, who became the king of Württemberg. Queen Olga, most of the aristocracy, and even most of the surrounding rural population in this area became strong advocates for homeopathy in the late 1800s.[104] Only the local university remained resistant and closed its doors to teaching homeopathy or to having dialogue with homeopathic doctors.

Bosch grew up using homeopathic and natural medicines. As an adult, Bosch's physician and homeopath was **Dr. Heinrich Goehrum**, who was also a very close confidant to him for more than fifty years. Bosch liked the fact that Goehrum had a special appreciation for homeopathy but was also interested in the broad field of natural medicine and environmental health.

Very committed to creating a homeopathic hospital, Bosch spent many decades and millions of German marks to make it a reality. The Robert

Bosch Hospital was finally opened in 1940 in Stuttgart. Bosch insisted that "homeopathy is preferable for internal illnesses" and for chronic diseases, though he also asserted that any proven treatment should be a part of this hospital (Heuss, 1994, 510). Bosch was indignant about the unjust way homeopathy was treated by conventional physicians, especially when they suggested that homeopathy was unproven or was superstition.

On his 80th birthday, Bosch was conferred an honorary doctorate of medicine by the medical faculty of the University of Tübingen. He was heartened to find that this medical school was finally beginning to appreciate homeopathic and natural medicine.

Today, the Robert Bosch Foundation is one of the largest German charities associated with a private company. The foundation funds projects involved in health and science, education and society, and international relations. Its institute for the history of medicine houses many of the original papers and ephemera of homeopathy's founder, Dr. Samuel Hahnemann.

Where Did the Money Go?

This question deserves the attention of serious historical scholars. There are some important historical people and events as well as facts and figures that can help us to understand what happened to the financial support that once existed for homeopaths and for homeopathy. The bottom line is that there was no one single reason that an enormous amount of money was lost or that the wealthy classes of people reduced or lost their interest in homeopathy. Below are some stories along with some reasons that this occurred.

To understand how and why the number of homeopathic physicians and homeopathic hospitals decreased so dramatically in the twentieth century and how and why so much financial support for homeopathy disappeared, it is necessary to learn something about the power of the AMA and its members' insidious attacks on homeopathy and homeopaths. Previous chapters have detailed the vigorous and harsh attacks in the nineteenth century, but the AMA learned new and more effective tactics in the next century.

History reveals that the AMA was dictatorially led for the first half of the twentieth century by George H. Simmons, MD (1852–1937), and his protégé, Morris Fishbein, MD (1889–1976). Simmons and Fishbein both served as general manager of the organization and as editor of its journal, the *Journal of the American Medical Association* (*JAMA*). While it is certainly true that these two leaders provided substantial benefit to the organization and to medical doctors, their methods of doing so have been severely criticized, with some historians referring to them as "medical Mussolinis" (Beale, 1939).

When George H. Simmons began in 1899 what became a twenty-five-year reign as head of the AMA, it was a weak organization with little money and little respect from the general public. The advertising revenue from the medical journal was a paltry $34,000 per year. Simmons came up with the idea to transform the AMA into a big business by granting the AMA's "seal of approval" to certain drug companies that placed large and frequent ads in *JAMA* and its various affiliate publications. By 1903, advertising revenue increased substantially, to $89,000, and by 1909, *JAMA* was making $150,000 per year. In 1900, the AMA had only 8,000 members, but by 1910, it had more than 70,000. This substantial increase in advertising revenue and membership was not the result of new effective medical treatments, for there were virtually no medical treatments from this era that were effective enough to be used by doctors today or even just a couple of decades later.

Some critics of the AMA have called their seal-of-approval program a form of extortion because the AMA did no testing of any products (Ausubel, 2000). When George Abbott, owner of a large drug company, Abbott Biologicals (known today as Abbott Laboratories), did not provide "blackmail" money to the AMA and when none of his products were granted AMA approval, Abbott went on the offensive. He arranged for an investigation of the AMA president that revealed that Simmons had no credible medical credentials, that he worked primarily as an abortion doctor for many years, and that he had had sex charges brought by some of his patients as well as charges of negligence in the deaths of others.[105]

After this meeting, the drugs made by Abbott Laboratories were regularly approved, and the company was not required to place any ads.

Simmons was shrewd enough to have the AMA establish a Council on Medical Education in 1904. This council's mission was to upgrade medical education—a worthy goal. The formation of the council seemed a good idea for homeopaths because surveys in *JAMA* itself had consistently shown that the graduates of the conventional medical schools failed the medical board examinations at almost twice the rate of graduates of homeopathic colleges (Robins, 2005, 76). However, the AMA developed guidelines to give lower ratings to homeopathic colleges. For instance, just having the word "homeopathic" in the name of a school had an effect on the rating because the AMA asserted that such schools taught "an exclusive dogma."[106]

In 1910, the same year that the Flexner Report was published, the AMA published "Essentials of an Acceptable Medical College" (Report of the Council, 1910), which echoed similar criteria for medical education and a disdain for nonconventional medical study. In fact, the AMA's head of the Council on Medical Education traveled with Abraham Flexner as they evaluated medical schools. The medical sociologist Paul Starr wrote in his Pulitzer Prize-winning book: "The AMA Council became a national accrediting agency for medical schools, as an increasing number of states adopted its judgments of unacceptable institutions." Further, he noted: "Even though no legislative body ever set up ... the AMA Council on Medical Education, their decisions came to have the force of law" (Starr, 1982, 121).[107] With the AMA grading the various medical colleges, it became predictable that the homeopathic colleges, even the large and respected ones, would eventually be forced to stop teaching homeopathy or die.[108]

In 1913, Simmons and the AMA went on the offensive even more strongly by their establishment of the "Propaganda Department," which was specifically dedicated to attacking any and all unconventional medical treatments and anyone (MD or not) who practiced them. In this same year, Simmons hired Morris Fishbein, MD, as a publicity man for the AMA.

In 1924, Simmons was forced out of the AMA due to the many scandals around him, and he took home all his personal files and burned them (Fishbein, 1969, 93), though Simmons was again wise enough to have trained his replacement, Morris Fishbein. Fishbein's specialty was publicity and the media, and he used the media to attack anyone who provided a real or perceived threat to conventional medicine. Besides severe attacks against anyone who practiced unconventional medical treatments, Fishbein and the AMA were also initially extremely antagonistic to those conventional medical doctors who supported pre-paid health insurance.[109]

Fishbein was a medical doctor who never practiced medicine. He was, however, an effective advocate for conventional medicine and a vocal critic of unconventional treatments. Shortly after he became head of the AMA, he wrote several books sharply critical of "medical quackery." He called chiropractic a "malignant tumor," and he considered osteopathy and homeopathy "cults." While Fishbein certainly provided benefit to the general public by warning them about some of the medical chicanery that existed at the time, he lumped together everything that was not taught in conventional medical schools and considered all such modalities quackery.[110] When one considers that the vast majority of medicine practiced in that era was inadequately tested and dangerous to varying degrees, Fishbein's obsessive fight against certain treatments provided direct benefits to the physicians he was representing.

Fishbein's frequent and strident attacks on "health fraud" were broadcast far and wide, in part through his own newspaper column, syndicated to more than 200 newspapers, as well as a weekly radio program heard by millions of Americans. His influence on medicine and medical education was significant, and it is surprising how few medical history books mention his influence or his questionable tactics. *Time* magazine referred to him as "the nation's most ubiquitous, the most widely maligned, and perhaps most influential medico" (June 21, 1937).

There are also numerous stories about Fishbein's efforts to purchase the rights to various healing treatments, and whenever the owner refused to sell such rights, Fishbein would label the treatment as quackery (Ausubel, 2000). If the owner of the treatment or device was a doctor, this doctor would be attacked by Fishbein in his writings and placed on the AMA's quackery list. And if the owner of the treatment or device was not a doctor, it was common for him to be arrested for practicing medicine without a license or have the product confiscated by the Food and Drug Administration (FDA) or the Federal Trade Commission (FTC). Although Fishbein denied these allegations, he and the AMA were tried and convicted of anti-trust violations for conspiracy and restraint of trade in 1937. Further, Fishbein wrote numerous consumer health guides, and his choice of inclusion for what works or what doesn't work was not based on scientific evidence.

Fishbein extended Simmons's idea for the AMA seal of approval to foods, and by including a significant amount of advertising from food and tobacco companies, he was able to make the AMA and himself exceedingly rich. In fact, under his reign, the tobacco companies became the largest advertiser in *JAMA* and in various local medical society publications. In fact, Fishbein was instrumental in helping the tobacco companies conduct acceptable "scientific" testing to substantiate their claims. Some of the ad claims that Fishbein approved for inclusion in *JAMA* were: "Not a cough in a carload" (for Old Gold cigarettes), "Not one single case of throat irritation due to smoking Camels," "More doctors smoke Camels than any other cigarette," "Just what the doctor ordered" (L&M cigarettes), and "For digestion's sake, smoke Camels" (because the magical Camel cigarettes would "stimulate the flow of digestive fluids").

By 1950, the AMA's advertising revenue exceeded $9 million, thanks in great part to the tobacco companies.

Coincidentally, shortly after Fishbein was forced out of his position in the AMA in 1950, *JAMA* published research results for the first time about the harmfulness of tobacco. Medical student Ernst Wynder and surgeon Evarts Graham of Washington University in St. Louis found that 96.5 percent of lung cancer patients in their hospitals had been smokers. Very shortly after the AMA withdrew its seal of approval for Morris Fishbein, he became a high-paid consultant to one of the large tobacco companies.

The following seemingly disparate stories of further attacks from conventional physicians, infighting among homeopaths, lost opportunities, natural disasters, and economic depressions help us to understand how homeopathic medicine went into sharp decline in the early and mid-twentieth century.

The first hospital in Cleveland was founded in May 1856, by Seth R. Beckwith, MD, a railroad surgeon and respected homeopath. Being liberal-minded, Dr. Beckwith wanted the hospital to have homeopathic and allopathic doctors, and he invited both homeopathic and allopathic doctors to treat patients in this hospital. However, by 1868, the allopaths insisted that they didn't want any homeopaths in the hospital, and they actually passed a resolution stipulating that no homeopaths were allowed to practice there. Rather than fight, the homeopaths decided to create their own separate hospital, but in the process, they handed over the entire hospital and its furnishings and equipment to the allopaths.

D. H. Beckwith, MD, Seth's son, who was also a homeopath, called the allopaths "narrow-minded, illiberal and unprofessional." Beckwith insisted that history record the allopaths' resolution to prohibit homeopaths from practicing in the hospital that they had created and the fact that the allopaths actually stole the hospital from the homeopaths. Beckwith wanted a historical record of this resolution because he predicted that in fifty years the medical community would deny that this happened (it may require 150 years before a real apology is extracted!) (Beckwith, 1903, 199).

The homeopaths purchased a new building, and it became the Cleveland Protestant Homeopathic Hospital, opening in 1868. The new hospital provided both free care for the poor and paid care for others who could afford it. Patients of all colors and creeds were allowed. Each patient could choose the clergy of choice, though no clergy were allowed to proselytze in the hospital.

A $10 million project was planned and developed for Chicago in 1928. The Medical Center for Hahnemann Institutions of Chicago had already purchased almost an entire square block in downtown Chicago, but this project and all of its money was lost as a result of the Depression (Suits, 1985, 29–30).

Several other homeopathic hospitals were forced to close during the Depression. A group of eighteen women founded Fabiola Homeopathic Hospital and Free Dispensary in Oakland, California, in 1857. Its bylaws stipulated that the management of the hospital must reside only in a woman's hands and that there must always be women physicians as staff doctors. This hospital provided free and reduced-rate care for fifty-six years. Due to the difficult economic times during the Great Depression, it was forced to close. Ultimately, the land was sold to Merritt Hospital, which today resides but a few blocks from Fabiola Hospital's original site. On the day that Fabiola Hospital closed, the *Oakland Tribune* headline eulogized, "Fabiola Ends Experiment in 'Feminism'" (October 16, 1932).

The Hahnemann College of the Pacific had just built a new hospital, and it opened on April 10, 1906, just shortly before the San Francisco earthquake on April 18, 1906. The hospital was devastated.

Anna T. Jeanes was the daughter of Isaac Jeanes, a very successful shipbuilder. Her older brother was **Jacob Jeanes, MD** (1800–1877), a co-founder of the American Institute of Homeopathy and of the famed Hahnemann Medical College (of Philadelphia). The entire family supported homeopathic colleges and hospitals in Pennsylvania. In fact, Mrs. Isaac Jeanes, Anna T. Jeanes, and numerous other family members were honorary members of the Hahnemann Medical College for donating more than $100,000. When the older brother Jacob died, the family fortune went to Anna.

Ms. Jeanes was a Philadelphia Quaker philanthropist who sought to improve community and school conditions for rural African Americans. In 1907 she donated $1 million to Booker T. Washington's Tuskegee Institute for the creation of a fund to hire black teachers as supervisors in African American schools and to improve black communities. Later this trust was merged with the Slater Fund to create the Southern Education Foundation, which may have done more for the education of black Americans than any other effort.

Sadly, the General Education Board (part of the Rockefeller group of associations, and covered in the above discussion) distributed this fund and other large trusts given by Anna T. Jeanes. Although the money designated for the education of underprivileged black Americans was put to very good use, the money that she left for health and medical care went to the creation of a conventional medical hospital, the Jeanes Hospital of Philadelphia. Because homeopathy's greatest antagonist, Frederick T. Gates, was in charge of the purse strings for the General Education Board, once again, no money was granted to any homeopathic institution. The Jeanes Hospital still exists today. It is a part of the Temple University Health System, and has nothing to do with homeopathy.

Homeopaths not only had to withstand the serious and frequent attacks against them from orthodox physicians and institutions, but they also had to withstand the inevitable infighting that occurs in every profession, especially because there were different schools of thought and practice within homeopathy and also simply because personalities in the homeopathic profession encouraged it.

The drama that occurred in Ohio was somewhat common. Hamilton Fiske Biggar, MD (1839–1926), was a respected homeopath in Cleveland who became the homeopath to J. D. Rockefeller (see above for details). In the 1880s the Cleveland Homeopathic Hospital Society, the organization that operated the Cleveland Homeopathic Hospital College, allowed any medical doctor or medical student to become a member upon simply paying a $5 membership fee. Dr. Biggar paid the membership for many medical students in exchange for their votes on specific issues with which the society dealt. In so doing, he was able initially to have a domineering effect upon the organization, until several members quit and started a new college and hospital next door to the original one (Kimmel, 1949).

After several years, the old college got Dr. Biggar to resign, and the two colleges reunited in 1898. In 1904, Biggar approached the Hospital College "to aid the college in any way possible," but because of problematic previous experience, no effort was made to accept his involvement, even though it was known that he could have brought much of Rockefeller's support to the school. Sadly, there is no evidence that Biggar did anything to encourage Rockefeller to provide any significant support to homeopathic colleges, hospitals, or organizations after the turn of the century.

Although Rockefeller expressed concern about the infighting among the homeopaths, he seemed to have little idea that at least some of the infighting resulted from his own personal physician.

William Wrigley (1861–1932), of chewing gum and Chicago Cubs' Wrigley Field fame, was a major advocate for homeopathy. His personal homeopath was **Julia Clark Strawn, MD**, an 1897 graduate of Hahnemann Medical College in Chicago. She sought to obtain his financial support for various homeopathic causes, but he declined, not because he didn't appreciate homeopathy but because he felt that the homeopathic colleges were not teaching "real" homeopathy. Instead, the homeopathic colleges had been forced to teach so much conventional physiology and pathology in order for their graduates to pass the state medical exams that they were not teaching homeopathy in adequate depth or breadth (Kirschmann, 2004, 153).

Wrigley was also concerned about the infighting in homeopathy. Some homeopaths were partial to highly individualized treatment of the person with highly potentized doses of medicine, while others preferred somewhat individualized treatment determined more by pathological diagnosis and usually relying on lower-potency medicine. Some homeopaths were "purists," preferring only to prescribe homeopathic medicines, while others used homeopathic medicines in conjunction with various conventional and other therapies.

A prominent dentist in Seattle, Washington (Dr. Hill) bequeathed $100,000 for the teaching and perpetuation of homeopathy in the state of Washington, but his heirs sought to break the will and were successful in doing so (Bryant, 1929, 19).

Historian Anne Taylor Kirschmann tells one sad story of major missed opportunities for support of homeopathy by wealthy patients in her impressive book, *A Vital Force: Women in American Homeopathy* (2004). Kirschmann describes the work of **Mary Ware Dennett** (1872–1947), who was hired to raise money for the American Foundation for Homeopathy (AFH), an organization of physicians and consumers who planned to work together to establish a major research center and hospital, to create a post-graduate school to teach homeopathy, and to develop a network of local lay organizations to educate the public about homeopathy. In her efforts to raise money, she contacted many leading homeopaths who were known to have wealthy patients. She was shocked and disappointed that most homeopaths chose not to cooperate with her. Some homeopaths asserted that only the American Institute of Homeopathy (an organization of medical doctors only) should be doing this work. Many women homeopaths incorrectly assumed that the AFH was anti-women and that it was affiliated with the New York Homeopathic Medical College, which did not admit women until 1941. The fact that three of the seven members of the board of trustees were women seemed to go unnoticed. Despite valiant efforts on the part of Dennett to raise money for homeopathy, she quit two years later due to lack of success.

Another factor that led to the decline of homeopathy was the guise of cure that many conventional drugs provided. In the late 1800s and early 1900s, when aspirin began to be marketed as a "wonder drug," conventional medicine was finally able to show the world that one of its drugs provided a real benefit of pain relief, with only minor side effects. Although aspirin didn't provide any real healing effect, it did relieve pain for many people in a relatively consistent manner, and such pain relief was a blessed discovery.

The discovery and manufacturing of insulin in the 1920s promoted the next big and beneficial effects of a conventional drug that literally saved lives (including that of my own father). In the 1940s, the discovery of penicillin heralded the antibiotic revolution—again, a great contribution to medical care.

Although each of these discoveries also had a dark side, the benefits that they provided far outweighed their problems, and the sense that "scientific medicine" was the new frontier gave the world the belief that conventional drugs and modern science were our salvation. The movement toward conformity with modern life of the 1950s nearly wiped out the entire field of natural medicine because "scientific medicine" seemed to be "proven," even if the results were short-lived. In the 1960s and 1970s the seeds of a new cultural revolution were planted, and its fruits are still ripening.

Modern Day Corporate Leaders and Philanthropists

Henry Samueli (1954–) is co-founder, chairman, and chief technology officer of the Broadcom Corporation, a leading supplier of integrated circuits for broadband communications in computer and telecommunications networking. Samueli received his BS, MS, and PhD from the University of California at Los Angeles (UCLA) and has been a professor of electrical engineering there since 1985. In 1999, due to tremendous financial success from his work at Broadcom, he donated $30 million to UCLA, where the school of engineering is now named after him. He also donated $20 million to the University of California at Irvine (UCI), the largest gift that this university has ever received. Its school of engineering is also named after Samueli.

Susan Samueli (1950–) has had a longstanding interest in alternative health care, having extensively studied and practiced with homeopathic medicine and Chinese herbs in the treatment of various chronic and acute illnesses. Henry and Susan Samueli have donated $5.7 million to UCI's medical school to support research to bridge the gap between conventional and alternative medicine; their gift created the Susan Samueli Center for Integrative Medicine. The Samuelis have also made significant yearly contributions to the Samueli Institute of Information Biology (www.siib.org). This organization has created an internationally prestigious network of researchers who have conducted and published high-quality scientific studies on homeopathic medicine, other selected natural therapies, and the characteristics of healing environments.

When interviewed recently, Susan Samueli asserted:

> Homeopathy has been a great gift to my family and me. I owe the health and well-being of the people I love to this viable alternative to standard medicine. It is my hope that in my lifetime, the science behind homeopathy will be discovered so that this form of medicine will be given the credibility and respect that it deserves. I feel blessed that I've been given the opportunity to fund institutes that are able to conduct rigorous scientific research so that one day there

will no longer be questions as to the viability of homeopathy. (Samueli, 2006)

Nancy Davis (daughter of Marvin Davis, the billionaire former owner of Twentieth Century Fox, Pebble Beach, the Beverly Hills Hotel, and the Denver Broncos NFL team) is a philanthropist and health advocate.

Ms. Davis was first introduced to alternative medicine when Jason, her youngest son, was 5 years old. He had missed school several days each week for a three-year period due to chronic ear pain. He also suffered with various gastrointestinal problems as a result of recurrent antibiotic use. After seeking the care of six different physicians, Nancy decided to go to a homeopathic doctor, even though she was quite skeptical of this method. The homeopath conducted a detailed interview of Jason and his mom to discover what specific symptoms he was experiencing. The homeopath was not simply interested in knowing the specific and unique ear pain he had and all of the features of his digestive discomfort, but he also inquired about whatever other common and rare symptoms he had. Further, he inquired about Jason's personality. This homeopathic interview process was conducted to help the homeopath find a "constitutional medicine," that is, a homeopathic medicine to match the unique syndrome of body and mind symptoms that Jason was experiencing. Much to Nancy's surprise, Jason had no further earaches after that first homeopathic prescription.

At age 33, Nancy Davis was diagnosed with multiple sclerosis. She suffered from many of the common symptoms of MS for ten years until she began taking homeopathic medicines. Since then, she has relied on homeopathic medicines and doesn't take any conventional drugs for MS. She told a *USA Today* reporter:

> I've been doing amazingly well with my MS by using a more homeopathic approach. The ABC drugs [the conventional ones] are great for some people, and I'm glad we have them as options. But I don't take them. Many doctors argue with me about my decision. And just as many doctors ask me

what it is I'm doing to stay so healthy. (Morgan and Shoop, 2004)

Nancy wrote an important health book called *Lean on Me* (2006), an autobiographical description of her personal health journey in which she provides ten steps to move beyond the diagnosis of whatever disease you may have and how to take back your life. Although Nancy acknowledges that homeopathic and alternative medicine may not be appropriate for everyone, it certainly has benefited her greatly. Besides receiving homeopathic constitutional medicines that are individually prescribed to strengthen her overall immune and defense system, she also has learned how to use select homeopathic medicines to treat common acute ailments in herself and her family.

Nancy is a particularly strong advocate for *Oscillococcinum,* a well-known and well-researched homeopathic medicine that has consistently been found to be effective in treating people with the flu or flu-like symptoms. Nancy prefers taking it as soon as she thinks that she has been exposed to someone who is contagious, and she always brings it on an airplane, just in case. As she said recently, "*Oscillococcinum* is my major drug of choice, and not everyone will agree with me because some people don't like homeopathic medicine." Davis continued, "All I can say is that I am living proof that it has made my health 100 percent better" (Morgan and Shoop, 2004).

References
American Institute of Homeopathy, *The Hospitals and Sanatoriums of the Homeopathic School of Medicine.* Washington, D.C., 1916.
Ausubel, K. *When Healing Becomes a Crime.* Rochester: Healing Arts, 2000.
Barry, J. M. *The Great Influenza: The Epic Story of the Deadliest Plague in History.* New York: Penguin, 2004. (Despite this book's scholarship on various topics, the author displays ignorance of homeopathy in referring incorrectly to Samuel Hahnemann, MD, and his book as "The New Testament of Homeopathic Medicine." Giving this religious name to a book published as *Organon of the Medical Art* seems to be evidence of bias and ignorance.)
Beale, M. A. *Medical Mussolini.* Washington, D.C.: Columbia, 1939.
Beckwith, D. H. History of the Cleveland Homeopathic Hospital, *Cleveland Medical and Surgical Reporter,* May 1903, p. 309.

Benison, S., and Rivers, T. *Reflections on a Life in Medicine and Science.* Cambridge: MIT Press, 1967.
Berliner, H. *A System of Scientific Medicine: Philanthropic Foundations in the Flexner Era.* New York: Tavistock, 1985, pp. 101–127.
Bittinger, Rev. B. F. *An Historic Sketch of the Monument Erected in Washington City.* Washington, D.C.: American Institute of Homeopathy, 1900. (The history of the Hahnemann monument.)
Boston references:
  Homeopathic Medical Society, *Boston Daily Globe,* Oct. 10, 1872
  Annual Meeting, *Boston Daily Globe,* Jan. 12, 1877
  Homeopathy's Growth, *Boston Daily Globe,* Jan. 16, 1885
  Homeopathic Hospital Work, *Boston Daily Globe,* Jan. 23, 1895
Brown, E. R. *Rockefeller Medicine Men: Medicine and Capitalism in America.* Berkeley: University of California Press, 1979, pp. 135–191.
Bryant, C. P. Homeopathy in the Far Northwest, *The Homeopathic Survey,* April 1929.
Cannadine, D. *The Decline and Fall of the British Aristocracy.* London: Routledge, 1996.
Chernow, R. *Titan: The Life of John D. Rockefeller, Sr.* New York: Vintage, 1998.
Chesney, A. M. *The Johns Hopkins Hospital and the Johns Hopkins University School of Medicine: A Chronicle.* Vol 3: 1905–1914. Baltimore: John Hopkins University Press, 1963, pp. 175–214.
Coulter, H. L. *Divided Legacy.* Vol. III: The Conflict Between Homoeopathy and the American Medical Association. Berkeley: North Atlantic Books, 1973.
Davis, N. *Lean on Me.* New York: Fireside, 2006.
Dewey, W. A. Homeopathy in Influenza—A Chorus of Fifty in Harmony, *Journal of the American Institute of Homeopathy,* May 1921, 14(2):1038–1043.
Enstam, C. H. What Homeopathy Can Do for You, *Homoeopathic Recorder,* April 1943, 58(10):487–492.
Fishbein, M. *Morris Fishbein, MD: An Autobiography.* New York: Doubleday, 1969.
Flexner, A. *Report on Medical Education in the United States and Canada.* New York: Carnegie Foundation, 1910.
Frass, M., Dielacher, C., Linkesch, M., et al. Influence of potassium dichromae on tracheal secretions in critically ill patients, *Chest,* March 2005, 127:936–941.
Haehl, R. *Samuel Hahnemann: His Life and Work* (2 vols.). London: Homeopathic Publishing Co., 1922 (reprinted New Delhi: B. Jain, no date).
Handley, R. *In Search of the Later Hahnemann.* Beaconsfield, UK: Beaconsfield Publishers, 1997.
George and Phoebe Apperson Hearst papers, 1849–1926. Online Archive of California, UC-Berkeley Bancroft Library, microfilm reel 75.
Hertzog, L. High Spots of Ohio Homeopathic History, 1890–1949, *Ohio State Medical Journal,* December 1949, 45:1189–1195.
Hiatt, M. D. Around the Continent in 180 Days: The Controversial Journey of Abraham Flexner, *Pharos,* Winter 1999, pp. 18–24.
Homeopathic Lives, *Monthly Homeopathic Review,* September 1, 1879, p. 579.

Hospitals and Sanatoriums of the Homoeopathic School of Medicine. Washington, D.C.: American Institute of Homoeopathy, 1916. (An online copy of the photos from this book and other sources is available at www.homeoint.org.)

Heuss, T. *Robert Bosch: His Life and Achievements.* New York: Henry Holt, 1994.

Kaufman, M. *Homeopathy in America: The Rise and Fall of a Medical Heresy.* Baltimore, Johns Hopkins University Press, 1971.

Kimmel, B. B., MD. A Historical Sketch of Huron Road Hospital, *Journal of the American Institute of Homeopathy,* 1949:, 42:3–8.

Kirschman, A. T. *A Vital Force: Women in American Homeopathy.* Piscataway: Rutgers University Press, 2004.

Leslie, S. W. *Boss Kettering.* New York: Columbia University Press, 1983.

Lydston, G. F. *How Simmons, "Our Peerless Leader," Became a Regular.* Self-published, 1909.

McCann, T. A. Presidential Address. Journal of the American Institute of Homeopathy, October 1921, 14(4).

McDowell, E. What's New on the Business Bookshelf: *Boss Kettering* and *Inventions, New York Times,* June 26, 1983. (A book review of *Boss Kettering.*) Available at http://query.nytimes.com/gst/fullpage.hjtml?res=9B02E2D8133BF935A15755C0A9 65948260

Medical and Surgical Record, Editorial, 1889, 1(6):151.

Mendenhall Papers, 1851–1951, Worcester Polytechnic Institute, George C. Gordon Library, Box 21, folder 3, June 14, 1920.

Morgan, J., and Shoop, S. A. Hollywood philanthropist "babies" her MS, *USA Today,* May 13 2004. Available at www.usatoday.com/news/health/spotlighthealth/2004-05-11-davis-ms_x.htm

Morrell, P. *British Homeopathy During Two Centuries.* Available at http://homeoint.org/morrell/british/patronage.htm (A research thesis submitted to Staffordshire University for the degree of Master of Philosophy, June 1999.)

Morrell, P. A Brief History of British Lay Homeopathy, *The Homoeopath* 59, October 1995. Revised version at http://homeoint.org/morrell/articles/pm_lay.htm

Mullins, E. *Murder by Injection: The Story of the Medical Conspiracy Against America.* Stauton, Va.: National Council for Medical Research, 1988. Available at www.thespectrumnews.com/papers/S0401.pdf (pp. 22–39 in the file)

Murphy, N. A History of Huron Road Hospital, Centennial edition of *Today Magazine* (bulletin of Huron Road Hospital), 1974.

Nevins, J. D. *Rockefeller: The Heroic Age of American Enterprise.* Vol. II. New York: Charles Scribner, 1940.

Ohio State University, College Prospectus, College of Homeopathy (1914–1922), pp. 439–446.

Osler, Sir W. On Full-Time Clinical Teaching in Medical Schools. *CMAJ* (Canadian Medical Association Journal), 1962, 87(6):762–765.

Our Colleges and State Medical Licensing Boards, *New England Medical Gazette,* July 1913, pp. 372–376.

Proceedings of the Massachusetts Homoeopathic Medical Society, 1901, p. xv.

Rand, J. P., Dewey W. A., and Hanchett, A. P. American Institute of Homeopathy, *Cleveland Medical and Surgical Reporter,* July 1903, p. 310.

Renner, J. The Full Bloom of Homeopathy in America, *Journal of the American Institute of Homeopathy,* March 1974, 67(1):37–42.

Report of the Council on Medical Education: The Essentials of an Acceptable Medical College, *JAMA,* 1910, pp. 1974–1975.

Roberts, H. A. A Letter is Answered, *Homoeopathic Recorder,* July 1938, 53(7):22–32.

Roberts, W. H. Orthodoxy vs. homeopathy: Ironic developments following the Flexner Report at the Ohio State University, *Bulletin on the History of Medicine,* Spring 1986, 60(1):73–87.

Robins, N. *Copeland's Cure.* New York: Knopf, 2005.

Rockefeller Foundation Archives, Frederick T. Gates Collection. Box 2, Folder 33, letter of May 19, 1911.

Rothstein, W. *American Physicians in the Nineteenth Century.* Baltimore: Johns Hopkins University Press, 1972.

Samueli, S. Personal communication, May 30, 2006.

Schellenger, Harold, Interview with. November 6, 1984. Ohio State University Archives. Available at http://library.osu.edu/sites/archives/manuscripts/oralhistory/schellenger.htm

Spiegel, A. D., and Kavaler, F. The Role of Abraham Lincoln in Securing a Charter for a Homeopathic Medical College, *Journal of Community Health,* 2002, 27(5): 357–380.

Starr, P. *The Social Transformation of American Medicine.* New York: Basic Books, 1982.

Suits, A. *Brass Tacks: Oral Biography of a 20th Century Physician.* Ann Arbor: Halyburton, 1985.

Sullivan, J. *The History of New York State.* New York: Lewis Historical Publishing Company, 1927.

The Gift That Grew: The History of the Genesee Hospital (1889–1965), 1965.

Von Lippman, E. O. *Beitraege zur Geschichte der Naturwissenschaften und der tecnik* (Contribution to History of Science and Technology). Zweiter Band. Weinheim: Verlag Chemie, 1953 (cited in Coulter, H. L. *Divided Legacy: A History of the Schism in Medical Thought,* volume II: Progress and Regress: Van Helmont to Bernard, Berkeley: North Atlantic Books, 1977).

Ward, J. Why I Am a Homeopathic Physician, *Pacific Coast Journal of Homeopathy,* May 1900, 8(5):99–108.

Wershub, L. P. *One Hundred Years of Medical Progress: A History of the New York Medical College, Flower and Fifth Avenue Hospitals.* Springfield: Charles C. Thomas, 1967.

Winston, J. *The Faces of Homoeopathy.* Tawa, New Zealand: Great Auk, 1999.

Young, R. McP. *Boss Ket: A Life of Charles F. Kettering.* New York: McKay, 1961.

CHAPTER 12

The Royal Medicine:
Monarchs' Longtime Love for Homeopathy

The love of homeopathy by the British royal family is well known today, in part because Queen Elizabeth II is patron of the Royal London Homoeopathic Hospital[111] and because Prince Charles has taken an active role in his support for homeopathic and "complementary" medicine.

What is less well known is the love for homeopathy by so many other monarchs of yesterday. When one considers that these members of royalty had access to the best of available medical treatment and that there were certainly implications of their choice of less orthodox methods, the large number of monarchs who chose homeopathy represents a significant statement about the value they found in this medical system.

In 1842, an astonishing number of seventy-seven homeopathic physicians were on record to have served as personal physicians to monarchs and their families (Everest, 1842, 200–203).

British Monarchs

The British royal family has had a longtime and deep appreciation for homeopathic medicine, ever since **Queen Adelaide** (1792–1849), wife of King William IV, first made public her special interest in this "new medicine" in 1835. Other British aristocrats shared the queen's interests, including the Marquess of Anglesey who crossed the British Channel to go to Paris for treatment by the founder of homeopathy, Dr. Samuel Hahnemann.

In 1830, the Earl of Shrewsbury (1791–1852) had asked Hahnemann for the name of a homeopath who could come to England to be his doctor, and Hahnemann suggested **Dr. Francesco Romani** (1785–1854) of

Italy. Dr. Romani's cures were so remarkable that he soon created a sensation in London and its surrounds. Queen Adelaide heard about this new medical system from his good work. However, the cold climate didn't suit the Italian homeopath, and he returned home just one year after his arrival (Granier, 1859).

Queen Adelaide had been suffering from a serious malady that the court physicians couldn't cure. The queen called for the services of one of Hahnemann's oldest and most faithful colleagues, **Dr. Johann Ernst Stapf** (1788–1860), who cured her, creating the first of many supporters of homeopathy from British royalty. The British homeopath to the titled Marquess of Anglesey, **Dr. Harris Dunsford** (1808–1847), wrote a book on homeopathy that was dedicated, with permission, to Queen Adelaide (Dunsford, 1842). This dedication made public her interest in and her appreciation for homeopathy. She was instrumental in helping to establish homeopathy's early popularity, especially among the upper classes in England.

Various kings and queens of Great Britain since Queen Adelaide have openly sought medical care from homeopathic physicians. Princess May, who later became **Queen Mary** (1865–1953), wife of King George V, headed the fundraising efforts to move and expand the London HomoeopathicHospital. **King George V** (1865–1936) was appreciative of homeopathy because it provided him with the real practical benefit of treating his seasickness whenever he suffered from it.

King Edward VII (1841–1910) carried on the homeopathic tradition and was a close drinking and eating partner of **Dr. Frederick Hervey Foster Quin** (1799–1878), the first British physician to become a homeopath. Edward's daughter, Maud (1869–1938), married King Haakon VII of Norway, and both sought the homeopathic care of Sir John Weir, MD (see below).

King Edward VIII (1894–1972), known as Prince Edward, Duke of Windsor, after his abdication in 1936, carried his homeopathic medicines in powder doses in his pocket. His brother, **King George VI** (1895–1952), also had a special love for homeopathy. He even named one of his prize racehorses Hypericum, after a homeopathic medicine for injuries. He was

The Royal Medicine

known to be an expert user of homeopathic medicine himself, and he formally granted the use of the royal title to the London Homoeopathic Hospital, now called the Royal London HomoeopathicHospital. Today's **Queen Elizabeth II** (1926–), King George VI's daughter, who ascended the throne in 1952, is patron to this important hospital, which underwent a $35 million refurbishing in 2005.

The most famous homeopath to royalty was **Sir John Weir** (1879–1971), who served six monarchs: King Edward VII, George V, Edward VIII, Duke of Windsor, George VI), Elizabeth II, King Gustav V of Sweden (1858–1950), and King Haakon VII of Norway (1872–1957).[112]

The early growth of homeopathy in Britain in the mid-1800s became possible in large part through royal support and British aristocracy. The first British homeopath to British royalty, Dr. Quin, was a son of the Duchess of Devonshire (1765–1824), and thus himself an aristocrat. When Quin began his full-time homeopathic practice in London in 1832, he primarily treated members of his own noble class. During the mid-1800s, poor people could not usually afford treatment from doctors and instead tended to use the services of herbalists and apothecaries for their health care.

Another reason that the British royalty embraced homeopathy is that its approach of individualized treatment for each person seemed to give them the real sense that they would not be given medicines that would be prescribed for just anybody (Morrell, 1999). This premise of individualization of treatment is an integral part of homeopathy, and it makes sense to educated classes of people.

The fact that the royals have been Christians has probably also helped link them to homeopathy in subtle ways. Homeopathy has had a solid history of support from the clergy in both Europe and the U.S. (see Chapter 13, Clergy and Spiritual Leaders, for more details on this subject). A board of governors, primarily composed of clerics and bankers and a few titled persons and minor aristocrats, headed most of the homeopathic dispensaries for the poor. This was a consistent pattern in Europe and America.

Not only did British royalty express their support for homeopathy by going to homeopaths and openly encouraging others to do so, they also put their money where their beliefs lay. Many British royalty were patrons to homeopathic organizations and hospitals. HRH Princess Adelaide (the Duchess of Teck) (1880–1940), the Lord Mayor of London, Sir George Wyatt Truscott (1860–1940), the Duchess of Hamilton and Brandon (1865–1940), Lord Cawdor (1870–1914), Lord Robert Grosvenor (1801–1893), the Earl of Wemyss and March (1857–1937), and the Earl of Donoughmore (1875–1944) were but some of a long list of royal patrons to homeopathy.

Others included: the Dukes of Beaufort, Dukes of Cambridge, Earl of Essex, Lord Gray of Gray, Viscount Malden, Lord Ernle, Earl of Kintore, Earl of Kinnaird, the Lords Paget, Dukes of Sutherland, Earls of Dudley, Lord Leconfield, Earl of Wilton, Earl of Albermarle, Viscount Sydney, Lady Radstock, Duke of Northumberland, Earl of Scarborough, Earl of Dysart, Marchioness of Exeter, Countess Waldegrave, Countess of Crawford and Balcarres, Lord Headley, Earl of Plymouth, Lord Calthorpe, Earls of Shrewsbury, Lord Horder, Lord Gainford, Lord Moynihan, Lord Ernle, Lord Ampthill, Lord Home, Viscount Elibank, and the Earls of Lichfield. One can also add numerous knights, barons, military officers, and clerics to this already impressive list.

Sir Henry Tyler (1827–1908) was another titled and rich patron to homeopathy. He not only personally contributed large amounts of money for the expansion of the London Homoeopathic Hospital, but his daughter, the later famed **Dr. Margaret Tyler** (1857–1943), became an influential homeopathic doctor in London. She authored *Homoeopathic Drug Pictures,* a book that is still popular among practicing homeopaths, and she was the editor of a leading journal simply called *Homoeopathy.*

It is not surprising that homeopathy in nineteenth-century England came to be called the "rich-man's therapy."

Other European Monarchs

Various monarchs throughout Europe were not simply patients of homeopaths; they were also advocates for this system of medicine. Because European royalty usually do not have a history of expressing advocacy without obvious and strong reasons, it is important to ask why so many European monarchs were so supportive of homeopathic medicine. The most obvious reason was that it was extremely effective for them, and, compared with conventional medicine of that day, it was considerably safer than the strong drugs, debilitating bleedings, and use of leeches.

It has been theorized that the British royals (House of Windsor) learned about homeopathy from the German royals, who were all particularly strong advocates of this medical system that was originally founded by a German physician, Samuel Hahnemann, MD. The German kings sought homeopathic care from Dr. Hahnemann and his disciples. Thus, when Queen Victoria (1819–1906) married a German, Prince Albert of Saxe-Coburg and Gotha (1819–1861), the German royals' interest in homeopathy began to develop even more popularity among British royalty, though Queen Victoria herself was not a vocal supporter of homeopathy.[113]

It should also be noted that the Belgian royalty were also advocates of homeopathy. Prince Leopold, who later became **King Leopold I**, sought the homeopathic care of Dr. Quin.[114] Royalty from other countries soon also began to seek out homeopathic physicians and even became advocates of this new, safer system of medicine.

Even before Quin became a homeopath, he was a highly respected physician to various royalty. Dr. Quin was even called to become personal physician to Napoleon Bonaparte, though the day before Quin was to attend him, Napoleon died.

France

There is some evidence and some significant controversy about Emperor **Napoleon Bonaparte**'s (1769–1821) interest in homeopathy. To provide historical context, it is useful to note that when Napoleon's army retreated from Russia in 1812, as typhus ravaged his soldiers, news of the successes of homeopathy in treating this epidemic spread throughout Europe. In fact, Hahnemann and homeopathy's first notoriety resulted from successful treatment of people suffering from typhus during this time (Wells, 1879; Coulter, 1977, II, 315). Napoleon's next battle and serious loss took place in 1813 in Leipzig (Germany), where Hahnemann lived at the time. Napoleon's army was defeated by an Austrian army led by General and Prince Karl Phillip von Schwarzenberg (1771–1820), who later became Hahnemann's patient and a supporter of homeopathy.

Richard Haehl, MD, the leading biographer of Hahnemann, noted that Napoleon was treated by a homeopath some time after the Battle of Leipzig and had such a positive experience that he expressed extremely strong appreciation for this system of medicine. Haehl wrote:

> When Napoleon was treated by Dr. [J. P.] Maragnot on the isle of Elba by the homeopathic system for a dangerous form of pityriasis (a skin disease) and the Emperor regained his health, he made his physician acquaint him with the meaning and advantages of the new art of healing, and called it "the most beneficent discovery since the invention of the art of printing." (Haehl, 1922, II, 159; also Ewers, 1826, 155; Baumann, 1857, 15;, Krauss, 1925)

Haehl further reported that Napoleon planned, in 1813 upon his return to France, "to have homeopathy taught in all the medical schools of his kingdom"—but he never returned to power in France. However, Haehl also reported that Hahnemann wrote, on October 17, 1825, that he was suspicious of the accuracy of this reporting and described this information as "improbable, such palpably invented tales, which are utterly devoid of proof"[115] (Haehl, 1922, II, 142). None of the leading biographies of Napoleon make similar reference to his interest in or experience with homeopathy, and one would have to expect some references to homeopathy if these statements are true. There is much more evidence that Napoleon himself was primarily treated by orthodox physicians of his day and that their medical treatments hastened his death from stomach cancer[116] (Lugli, et al., 2007).

In a book published as a memorial to Constantine Hering, MD (1800–1880), Hering's opposition to courting favor with government leaders was described. He preferred to have his own cause slighted than introduced by force, which is what nearly happened when Napoleon read

Hahnemann's *Organon* (the first book describing the homeopathic science and art, initially published in 1810) before his march into Russia in 1812. However, speaking after the fact, Hering was glad that Napoleon was overthrown because Hering considered any restraint upon the arts and sciences as odious as the loss of personal liberty (Hering, 1880, 86–87).

There is much more evidence about Charles Louis Napoleon Bonaparte (aka **Napoleon III**) (1808–1873) and his special interest in and appreciation for homeopathy.[117] Napoleon III was Napoleon I's nephew, and he served as the president of France during 1849–1852 and then emperor until 1870. Napoleon III received homeopathic treatment from **A. J. Davet** (1797–1873), one of Hahnemann's early students of "pure" homeopathy. Dr. Davet was decorated with the Knight's Cross of the Legion of Honor by Napoleon III for his homeopathic treatment of the emperor. Italian by birth and French by adoption, Davet became physician to the ambassador to Italy and to the Italian prime minister (Hunt, 1863; Bradford, 1897).

Napoleon III also received homeopathic treatment from **Dr. Alexandre Charge** (1810–1890), who had gone to the south of France to treat villagers during a major cholera epidemic (Haehl, 1922, II, 463; Payne, 1855, 27). For the exceptional care that Dr. Charge provided during this epidemic, Napoleon III bestowed the Legion of Honor upon him. Records show that he treated 1,662 cases of cholera and had only forty-nine deaths (2.9 percent) in 1849, as compared with 10 percent or higher at other hospitals. Pope Pius IX also granted Dr. Charge the Order of St. Gregory the Great, "in consideration of the services he rendered during the cholera epidemic" (Hunt, 1863, 121).

Empress Eugenie (1826–1920), wife of Napoleon III, introduced homeopathic medicine to her husband. She sought care from her own homeopath, **Dr. Jules Bocco** (Hunt, 1863, 123), and in 1855, from **Dr. Clemens Maria Franz von Böenninghausen** (1785–1864), of Münster in Westphalia (Germany), whom Hahnemann considered to be one of his best students and most respected colleagues[118] (Haehl, 1922, I, 397).

In 1861, Eugenie took special pleasure in honoring **Count des Guidi**

(1769–1863), the first and oldest homeopathic physician in France, declaring, "You have rendered great service to humanity" (Vingtrinier, 1860).

On April 20, 1861, Napoleon III awarded the Knight's Cross of the Legion of Honor to von Böenninghausen. The eldest of von Böenninghausen's sons, Karl, ended up marrying the adopted daughter of Melanie Hahnemann (Samuel Hahnemann's second wife). With Melanie Hahnemann's connections to Napoleon III, she was able to get the emperor's permission to grant her new son-in-law the right to practice homeopathic medicine in Paris without taking the usual medical examination (Handley, 1990, 195).

Napoleon III also bestowed the Knight's Cross of the Legion of Honor upon **Dr. J. Mabit** (1781–1846). Dr. Mabit was head of a hospital in Bordeaux where he provided homeopathic and allopathic treatment, and upon comparing his results, he consistently found the superiority of homeopathic medicines (www.homeoint.org). Dr. Mabit was also a close friend of René Laënnec (1781–1826), who invented the stethoscope, and Dr. Mabit was the first doctor in Bordeaux to use this new technology.

The history of the **Bonaparte family**'s use of homeopathy was not always positive. The health crisis and ultimate death of Napoleon's 21-year-old niece, Bathilde Bonaparte, created a drama in the household and in the country. Bathilde was married to Louis Cambacérès, son of Jean-Jacques-Régis de Cambacérès, the lawyer, statesman, and author of the Napoleonic Code. Napoleon insisted that his niece see an allopath, Dr. Rayer, while the Cambacérès family insisted upon homeopathic treatment. When she died four months later, after repeated bloodlettings, the Cambacérès family and the homeopaths blamed the allopaths, and the allopaths blamed the homeopaths (Poulet, 1973; Poulet, no date).

Other members of the Bonaparte family owed their life to homeopathy. The half-brother of Napoleon III, Charles Auguste Louis Joseph (1811–1865), later made duc de Morny, contracted cholera in the 1850s but was saved by homeopathic medicines (*British Journal of Homeopathy,* 1854).

Napoleon Bonaparte's elder brother, Joseph Bonaparte (1768–1844), also sought care from a homeopathic doctor, **Dr. Jules Bocco**, when he served as king of Naples and king of Spain (Hunt, 1863, 123).

Even before Napoleon III came to power, **King Louis Philippe** (1773–1850), France's last king, was partial in some way to homeopathy. Upon Hahnemann's arrival in Paris, his French wife, Melanie, requested from the king and received permission through her friend, the minister of education, M. Guizot, for Hahnemann to practice homeopathy (Haehl, II, 345).

Russia

Homeopathy also became popular among several monarchs in Russia during its early history. Grand Duke[119] **Constantine Pavlovich Romanov** (1779–1831) openly patronized homeopathy by keeping **Dr. Jean Bigel** (1769–?), a homeopathic doctor, as his personal physician, as did the grand duchess (Bojanus, 1876). The grand duke was so pleased with the homeopathic treatment of his family that he insisted that Dr. Bigel also provide care for 500 sons of soldiers (Bojanus, 1876). Dr. Bigel became a significant advocate for homeopathy in Russia, authoring a popular book on the subject and then even translating into French one of Hahnemann's important books on chronic disease.

Two of Grand Duke Constantine's brothers, Grand Duke Mikhail and Emperor Nicholas I (1796–1855), also became interested in the new teaching. Emperor Nicholas, who later became **Czar Nicholas**, was known personally to influence many physicians to study it, and he never went into the country without his case of homeopathic medicines. But even the emperor, gifted with unequaled force of character, with an iron will, and with all of the power of his position, still could not, as Dr. Carl Frantz Von Villers said, break down "the Chinese wall by which the medical hierarchy surrounds its domain" (Historical and Statistical Report, 1876).

In 1841 a homeopathic hospital was established in Moscow, and in 1849, another hospital was built in Nizhniy-Novgorod (Russia's fourth largest city). Homeopathy developed even greater popularity during the next several decades due to support from Russian monarchs, as well as from Russian clergy (see Chapter 13, Clergy and Spiritual Leaders), enabling homeopathy to be practiced in the huge country's most remote corners.

Nicholas I married Alexandra Feodorovna (1798–1860), who previously was Princess Charlotte of Prussia. Empress Alexandra had enough appreciation for homeopathy that she commissioned a British homeopathic pharmacy, Ashton & Parsons, to make a special homeopathic medicine kit with her emblem. One of these kits, which sold on eBay in May 2006, bore the Romanov crest and the crown of Great Britain.

One of the daughters of Nicholas and Alexandra was Olga (1822–1892), who later became **Queen Olga** of Württemberg by marrying Crown Prince (later King) Karl of Württemberg in 1846. Queen Olga of Württemberg was a "true homeopath, and she let everybody know it" (Hoyle, 1913, 249). When she was vacationing at Lake Geneva, Switzerland, she broke her leg. She was so pleased with the homeopathic treatment she received from **Dr. Alfons Beck** that she insisted he come to St. Petersburg to be her personal homeopath. Dr. Beck stayed there for five years, until his own health led to his return to Switzerland (Schmidt, 1926). After Queen Olga's death, a British physician who visited Russia asserted that her support for homeopathy was "one reason why homeopathy has taken such a firm hold on this Kingdom, despite the severe and ever-present allopathic opposition of which many tales were told to me" (Hoyle, 1913, 249).

Shortly after Dr. Beck's return, another Russian princess sought his care for a serious condition of genital cancer that had spread to her rectum and breasts. She realized the difficult challenge her health posed, and she promised him additional payments for every month that she lived. She summoned him on New Year's day to give him a gift. Following the etiquette of Russian nobility, that the gift be placed on the ground and the recipient kneel to get it, she placed an exquisite golden cigarette case on the rug at her feet. Dr. Beck was a venerable old man at the time, and rather than kneel to pick it up, he replied, "Princess, I have never gone on my knees to receive a gift. Keep it for yourself and do not forget that I am your physician." The princess was so impressed by the dignity that Beck showed that she bent at his feet and offered it to him (Schmidt, 1926).

After **Czar Alexander II** (1818–1881), who was an advocate for homeopathy, was assassinated, a homeopathic hospital was erected in St. Petersburg and named after him. His predecessor, Emperor Alexander III, gave 5,000 rubles to the cause (Kotok, 2000). Some of the beds in the hospital were named after Emperor Nicholas, the Empress Maria Feodorovna, and Emperor Alexander III (Encyclopedia Britannica). In addition, donations from the minister of communications, the minister of the interior, and leading members of the imperial court supported the development of this homeopathic hospital. However, in 1918, shortly after the communists overthrew the Russian government, the hospital was turned over to conventional physicians.

The early history of homeopathy in Finland is directly linked with that of the Russian royalty. In 1809, Sweden was forced to grant its former province Finland to Russia. From this time until the Russian Revolution, Finland was under the control of the Russian empire.

In 1871, the governor general of Finland, **Count Nikolai Adlerberg** (1819–1892), invited a highly respected German homeopath, **Dr Eduard von Grauvogl** (1811–1877), to introduce homeopathy in Helsinki. Grauvogl accepted the invitation as long as he could bring a reliable pharmacist with him, a condition he was granted (Jütte, 2006, 31).

Czar Alexander II granted Dr. Grauvogl two sickrooms in the Helsinki military hospital to treat patients. Grauvogl also maintained a successful private practice, attracting patients from as far away as St. Petersburg. However, he soon complained about extreme hostilities from allopathic doctors and pharmacists who made his practice difficult. Grauvogl was concerned that only chronically ill patients were transferred to his homeopathic ward in the military hospital, which led to a higher mortality rate.

His benefactor, the governor general, fell seriously ill while they were traveling together on an inspection journey through the country, and Grauvogl was forced to devote his time entirely to the treatment of his important patient. He was quite aware of the consequences he would face if his homeopathic treatment was unsuccessful. As it turned out, the governor general did recover, and the czar bestowed the Order of St. Anne on Grauvogl. Sadly, Grauvogl continued to experience great hostility from his antagonists, and he chose to return to his Munich home just two years later (Jütte, 2006, 32).

Germany

Even before Hahnemann developed homeopathy, he was respected enough as a physician to serve German royalty. In 1797, he was physician to Duke Ernst of Gotha and Georgenthal (Haehl, 1922, II, 125).

Hahnemann's mother country granted him and homeopathy much support. Wherever he lived in Germany, Hahnemann was able to obtain special permission from the local ruling government to practice homeopathy and dispense his own medicines, a privilege rarely granted due to the strong antagonism from local apothecaries.

In 1822, Hahnemann was honored by **Ferdinand, Duke of Anhalt** (a region in Germany in which Hahnemann resided while living in Köethen), who named him to be "Hofrath," a special distinction given to leading members of society (Haehl, 1922, II, 132).[120]

Hahnemann's nephew, **Dr. C. Bernhard Trinius** (1775–1844), was a homeopath as well, and he became physician to the princess of Württemberg, as well as the duke of Coburg and Gotha (Haehl, 1922, II, 207).

King George V of Hanover (1819–1879) and his **Queen Alexandrine Marie** (1818–1907) received homeopathic care from **Dr. G. A. Weber**. The king honored him for the good care he provided (Hunt, 1863).

Dr. Gustav Kramer, a respected German homeopath, became physician to the Grand Duke of Baden, a state in Germany (Haehl, 1922, II, 199–200).

Dr. Anton Schmit, another homeopath, was personal physician to the Duchess of Lucca (Haehl, 1922, II, 243).

Dr. Bernhard Baehr (1828–?), royal medical counselor and private physician to **King George V** of Hanover (1819–1878), speedily gained a reputation due to his thorough and scientific *Treatise on Digitalis purpurea in its Physiological and Therapeutical Actions,* for which homeopathic physicians awarded him an honorary prize (Granier, 1859).

G. A. H. Muhlenbein, MD, was physician to William VIII, Duke of

Brunswick. Dr. Muhlenbein initially practiced allopathy but then became a homeopath. He wrote:

> I have been a Doctor in medicine for fifty years, during the first thirty-three of which I practiced Allopathically.... but I assure you that I owe daily oblations to my Creator for an allowance of sufficient years to become convinced of the Homeopathic truth. Indeed, it is only since I have practiced Homeopathia that I have been satisfied of the utility of any system of medicine." (Everest, 1842, 196)

Due to the impressive curative care he provided, he was awarded the Knight of the Order of Guelph, an honor conferred by the British crown.

Homeopathy did not get support in every part of what we know today as Germany. For instance, in what was once the kingdom of Bavaria (where Munich is the capital), homeopathy was declared a faddish cure by a high ministry of war and its practice was forbidden in military hospitals. Support for homeopathy from the military in other regions, however, was much more positive. At that very same time, the ministry of war in the principality of Hessen ruled that no doctor should be hired for the military unless he was also a homeopath (Baumann, 1857).

Austria

The history of homeopathy in Austria is of particular interest and significance because homeopathy and homeopaths experienced some of the strongest attacks in this country, though later, it also experienced its greatest successes and general acceptance.

One of the earliest experiences that Austrian royalty had with homeopathy is typical of the many controversies that occurred in this country. The head of Austria's army against Napoleon was General and Prince **Karl Phillip von Schwarzenberg** (1771–1820). General von Schwarzenberg was successful against Napoleon in the famous 1813 battle at Leipzig, a German city where Hahnemann lived at the time. The general did not receive homeopathic treatment at this time nor after experiencing a stroke in 1817. However, when he had his second stroke in 1819, he sought homeopathic treatment from Dr. Hahnemann. After initial homeopathic treatment, Dr. Hahnemann visited the general and was shocked to find another doctor bloodletting him. Because of this problem and because the general chose not to stop his vigorous consumption of alcohol, Hahnemann withdrew from being his physician. Shortly afterward, the general died, and the conventional physicians and apothecaries blamed Hahnemann for the death.

The German literary great, Johann Wolfgang von Goethe, was extremely critical of conventional medicine of that day and of doctors' efforts to restrict access to homeopathic treatment. On May 5, 1820, he wrote: "In this place a curious game is being played by refusing and damming up innovations of every kind. E.g., nobody is allowed to practice by Hahnemann's method" (Haehl, 1922, I, 113).

Francis I (1792–1835), emperor of Austria, actually prohibited the practice of homeopathy from 1819 until 1835. In 1828, he ordered that an experiment be made with homeopathic treatment over a sixty-day period. In spite of the fact that only one of the forty-three patients treated in the hospital died and that all nine patients with serious inflammatory diseases were cured with homeopathic medicine, Professor Zang, one of the conventional doctors who oversaw the experiment, asserted, "It is wonderful what nature can accomplish" (Haehl, 1922, II, 493). Although the prohibition against homeopathy was not withdrawn until the new emperor took over the country several years later, Austria's Archduke Johann appointed a homeopath as his personal physician shortly after this experiment.

After the death of Francis I in 1835, homeopathy experienced unprecedented growth. In fact, several of Austria's royalty became practitioners of homeopathy. Patients came in crowds to Count Gustav Auersberg on account of his successes in homeopathic treatment. **Princess Wilhelmina Auersberg**, renowned for her benevolence, went from cottage to cottage in her estates in Bohemia, giving her needy tenants the benefits of homeopathic treatment. In Zleb, in Bohemia, she established a hospital with twelve beds for poor peasants, attended by her physician, Dr. Kohout. In 1846, **Countess Harrach** also founded a homeopathic hospital for the poor in Nechanitz, in which 404 patients were treated during the first three years (Mueller, 1876).

Count de Fickelmont, Austrian ambassador to His Majesty the King of the Two Sicilies (part of Italy), then at Vienna, wrote a letter very supportive of homeopathy to General Luigi Caraffa, who himself was a friend of homeopathy. The count wrote:

> The system [homeopathy] has passed through the trial to which it was submitted with the most brilliant success. That explains why its opponents put every difficulty in the way of the publication of the report. I found since my last journey to Vienna that homoeopathy had made immense progress. The consequence will be that no one can refuse to believe the evidence of facts. The patients cured are a speaking proof that must of necessity make converts. (Granier, 1859, 69)

The new medicine continued to spread throughout the empire. People of rank gave it their support, the rich assisted with their means, and many heads of scientific societies favored its dissemination.

In the 1840s, some observers noted that homeopathy was practiced more in Austria than in any other European country. There were hospitals and dispensaries everywhere, and homeopaths were nearly as numerous as conventional doctors (Hunt, 1863). The University of Vienna and the military academy had professors of homeopathy. Medical students could choose between the systems. Still further, the Duke of Batthyanny of Fkervar, Vienna, and Stein-am-Anger had his own homeopath, **Dr. H. Rosenberg** (Haehl, 1922, II, 496).

Homeopathy's popularity in Austria grew even more as a result of the remarkable cure of Field Marshall Radetzky. **Joseph von Radetzky** (1766–1858) was a nobleman and Austrian general, immortalized by Johann Strauss's *Radetzky March*. The emperor appointed Radetzky his field marshall in charge of the Austrian army in 1836, when Radetszky was 70 years old. In 1841, he suffered from a tumor in the orbit of his right eye. Radetzky being a favorite of his, the emperor insisted that he be seen by two professors of ophthalmology, Francisco Flarer and Friedrich Jaeger;[121] both asserted that he was incurable.

Radetzky then sought the care of a homeopathic doctor, **Dr. J. Christophe Hartung** (1779–1853), a colleague and early student of Hahnemann. Within six weeks, Radetzky was completely cured (Clarke, 1905, 103–106).

As with many cures resulting from homeopathic treatment, conventional physicians and apothecaries questioned the authenticity of the ailment and the cure. Fifteen years after Field Marshall Radetzky was cured, a conventional medical journal raised questions, but the field marshall responded forcefully, asserting real value to the homeopathic treatment he received.

Italy

Homeopathy was introduced into Italy and to the Italian monarchs as a result of the Austrian occupation of Naples. Austria's head army commander was **Baron Francis Koller**, who was a devoted follower of Hahnemann. When he first arrived in Naples in 1822, he sent for his personal homeopathic doctor, **Dr. George Necker**. Necker lived and practiced in Naples for four years, during which time he convinced three leading Italian physicians of the power and value of homeopathic medicines; these were Doctors Francesco Romani, Giuseppe Mauro, and Cosmo Maria de Horatiis (Mitchell, 1975, 72).

In addition to his private practice, Dr. Necker, in May 1823, opened a dispensary for the poor, in which he was always assisted by Dr. Romani and sometimes by Doctors Smicht and Kinzel. In 1824, the queen of Naples sent Necker to Rome to take professional charge of her sister, Maria Louisa of Bourbon, then queen of Etruria and mother of the reigning Duke of Lucca, Carlo Lodovico. Dr. Necker was appointed physician to the Duke of Lucca (in Tuscany) and his court,[122] a position that he held until 1847 (Homeopathy in Italy, 1876).

The three Italian doctors who became Dr. Necker's homeopathic colleagues were some of Italy's finest doctors. **Dr. Francesco Romani** had the reputation in Naples and abroad of being a learned physician and distinguished intellectual and poet. England's Lord Shewsbury even brought him to his estate to be his personal homeopath in 1831, making Dr. Romani the first homeopath to practice in England. Dr. Romani was the personal homeopath to the Queen Dowager of Naples (Atkin, 1853). **Dr. Giuseppe Mauro** was a distinguished practitioner and private physician of Prince Ruffo, minister of the royal house of Bourbon. **Dr. Cosmo Maria de Horatiis** was the alternate of the famed anatomist, Antonio Scarpa, in the chair of surgery of the Athenaeum of Ticino, which some historians suggest was an honor far transcending any that the kings of the earth could bestow. He was also surgeon-in-chief of the Neapolitan army, inspector-general of the military hospitals, private physician to the hereditary prince, the Duke of Calabria, afterwards Francis I, then physician to this king, and subsequently professor of clinical surgery at the University of Naples. Dr. Horatiis was the first translator of Hahnemann's writings into Italian (Homeopathy in Italy, 1876).

Of additional significance, in 1828, Dr. Romani converted to homeopathy his countryman, **Dr. Count Sebastiano de Guidi**, who subsequently held eminent positions at three French universities, as a professor of mathematics and then of medicine. The cure of his wife's serious health problems led him to become the first, and later the oldest, practicing homeopath in France; he is considered the father of homeopathy in France (www.homeoint.org).

The first homeopath to establish a practice in Rome was **Settimio Centamori, MD**, in 1826. He was known to successfully treat many people who suffered from cholera, though in 1837 he did not succeed in treating the rector at St. Peter's, who was dying of cholera. Several conventional physicians accused him of poisoning the prelate, though his reputation wasn't significantly affected. In fact, he became physician to the Duke of Lucca, and in 1842 he married French royalty, Charlotte Bonaparte, the niece of Napoleon I.

King **Vittorio Emmanuel** (1820–1878) of Sardinia, now a part of Italy, also sought out homeopathic treatment (Hunt, 1863).

Spain

The monarchs of Spain also appreciated homeopathy. In 1829, the king of Spain, **Ferdinand VII** (1784–1833), married Donna Maria Cristina, who was the daughter of the king of Savoy (which in 1860 became a part of France). The wedding took place in Madrid, and one of the guests was the king of Naples, Ferdinand II, who brought with him his homeopathic doctor, Dr. Horatiis. Initially, homeopathy didn't spread rapidly, in large part because of a civil war that dominated Spain until 1840. **Dr. Don Andrés Marino**, one of Madrid's most respected conventional physicians, who became a homeopath, was made honorary physician to the queen of Spain (History of Homeopathy in Spain, 1876).

The Spanish monarchs developed a particularly deep appreciation for homeopathy once they were introduced to **Dr. José Nuñez** (1805–1879), who studied homeopathy with Hahnemann himself. Nuñez returned to Spain in 1844 after studying and practicing in France, and he continued his practice with such zeal and brilliant results that he received admiration of all, except the allopathic doctors. Eventually, his growing reputation carried Dr. Nuñez into the palace of **Queen Isabelle II** (1830–1904), and he remained one of the physicians of the bedchamber until the revolution in 1868. The queen rewarded him with the title of Marquis of Nuñez as well as the Grand Cross of Charles III and the Civil Order of Beneficencia.

In 1850 an allopathic medical journal bemoaned the fact that a royal ordinance granted two chairs of homeopathy in a Spanish university "because the orthodox practitioners foolishly consented to an experimental trial of the system" (*L' Union Medicale*, 1850). Sadly, other medical societies rarely chose to give homeopaths a fair trial.

The prince of Spain and Portugal, the **Infante Don Sebastian Gabriel** (1813–?), was cured of a very serious illness by another homeopath, **Dr. Tomás Pellicer, Sr.**, who was named first physician of the bedchamber and was honorary physician to the queen. Like Dr. Nuñez, he was awarded Knight of the Order of Charles III and the Grand Cross of Isabella the Catholic; these orders were also bestowed upon Dr. Don Andrés Marino, the royal family's first homeopath. The support for homeopathy by Spain's royal family was even more marked after the 1868 revolution that sent them into exile. The Infante Don Sebastian appointed **Dr. Joaquin Pellicer, Jr.** as second physician of the bedchamber, and in Paris, Her Majesty Queen Isabella II chose a highly respected French homeopath, **Dr. Leon Simon**, to take charge of her health (History of Homeopathy in Spain, 1876).

Prussia

In the nineteenth century, the country of Prussia existed in the area that today is northeastern Germany, northern Poland, eastern Russia, and Lithuania. The last capital of Prussia was Berlin. As in many countries in Europe, doctors could prescribe homeopathic medicines or conventional drugs, but they were not always allowed to dispense them. They were required by law to have pharmacies (called apothecaries at that time) sell the prescriptions. However, because apothecaries were required to charge for drugs based on the amount sold, they could not make much money selling homeopathic medicines because the doses were so small. Due to the economic hardship of making and selling homeopathic medicines, many apothecaries sold fraudulently made homeopathic medicines.

As a result of these problems, Hahnemann and many homeopaths sought to make their own medicines, and they were sometimes arrested for these actions. However, Hahnemann and his colleagues asked their royal patients for special dispensation, and were ultimately granted it—in Württemberg, Prussia in 1829 and in Hessen in 1833. The struggle in the entire country of Prussia ended when **King Friedrich Wilhelm IV** (1795–1861) gave authorization in 1843 to homeopaths to dispense their medicines (Kotok, 1999, note 183).

In 1842, King Friedrich Wilhelm IV wrote the following letter to his homeopath, **Dr. Matthias Marenzeller** (1765–1854):

> I am grateful to you for the confidence with which you, in your letter of October 14th, recommend the homeopathic method to my protection, and I attach no small value to the recommendation of this important subject by a man who, like you, has practised homeopathy with success through a

whole generation. I shall willingly continue, as I have begun, to give the system every help that might aid in its development. I have already sanctioned the erection of a homeopathic hospital and have promised the necessary funds from the State Treasury, and I intend to permit homeopathic practitioners to dispense medicines themselves under certain conditions, and negotiations are still going on this point. (Ameke, 1885)

Earlier, homeopathy in Prussia also benefited from the patronage of **Princess Friedricka** (1767–1820), who appointed one of Hahnemann's earliest physicians, **Dr. Julius Aegidi** (1795–1874), as her personal physician. Sadly, significant harassment and legal threats to Dr. Aegidi's life and practice forced him to resign after four years (Haehl, 1922, II, 201, 207). Luckily for the princess, another of Hahnemann's senior physicians, **Dr. George Heinrich Gottleib Jahr** (1800–1875), accepted this position in Aegidi's place.

Because of the sensational results that these homeopaths experienced, the Royal Prussian Hofrath Nordmann of Muhlhausen from the district of Erfurt, wrote to Hahnemann to recommend a homeopath for his district and himself (Haehl, 1922, II, 203).

The Netherlands and Other European Countries

The Dutch royalty's interest in homeopathy started with **King William I** (1772–1843), who was known to be under the care of a homeopathic physician in Brussels, **L. J. Varlez, MD**. Later, **King William III** of the Netherlands (1817–1890) also had a homeopathic doctor, **Professor Everhard**.

Dr. Joseph Attomyr (1807–1856) was an early student of Hahnemann's, and Hahnemann particularly appreciated his brilliance in writing responses to the doctors and apothecaries who wrote ill-informed articles attacking homeopathy. Dr. Attomyr later became personal physician to **Count Czaky of Zips** (today called Spiš), previously in Hungary but today an administrative county in Poland. Later in his life, he became personal homeopath to the Duke of Lucca in Tuscany, Italy.

Dr. H. Rosenberg was the personal homeopathic physician to the **Duke of Batthyany of Stein-am-anger** (today called Szombathely, a county administrative city in Hungary). Dr. Rosenberg introduced several medicines to homeopathy, including *Vinca minor,* an important medicine in cancer (and from which conventional drug companies make a popular chemotherapeutic drug called Vincristine).

In Hungary, **Viceroy Joseph** patronized homeopathy and warmly encouraged its progress. In 1844, the two houses of the states of Hungary unanimously agreed to establish a homeopathic hospital and a university chair in the capital city. Three homeopathic pharmacies opened shortly afterward, and the homeopathic movement, supported by the higher classes, grew throughout Hungary.

In much the same way that homeopathy became popular in the German states, homeopathy in the Czech Republic owed its acceptance in the first half of the nineteenth century to its efficacy during the cholera epidemics in the 1830s and 1840s. After this, homeopathy had influential supporters, especially members of the aristocracy, who consulted homeopathic physicians. The Princes Windischgrätz and Lamberg zu Zusiowitz as well as Princess Wilhelmine Auersperg were all known to have homeopaths as their personal physicians (Jütte, 2006, 60). This princess was even known to be the benefactor to a small homeopathic hospital in her hometown.

Other Monarchs

Amazingly enough, homeopathy's popularity among royalty extended far beyond Europe. **E. Cook Webb, MD**, arrived in Hawaii on May 17, 1880. He was previously chief of staff of the Homeopathic Hospital on Ward Island in New York, a highly respected and very large hospital with more than 1,800 beds. He developed a popular homeopathic practice in Hawaii shortly after his arrival, including the royal family of Hawaii (Smith, 2002).

George Henry Martin, MD (1859–1944), graduated from the homeopathic medical school at Boston University, in 1881. In 1882 he arrived in Hawaii and soon became homeopath to **King Kalakaua** (1836–1891), the last reigning king of the kingdom of Hawaii. Dr. Martin moved to

California in 1887, where he practiced and taught homeopathy for fifty-seven more years.

Queen Liliuokalani (1838–1917), the last monarch of the Kamaka'eha family of the kingdom of Hawaii, was known to receive homeopathic treatment from **Charles F. Nichols, MD** (1846–1915). Nichols was a Harvard graduate who was invited to visit by Chief Justice Elisha H. Allen of Hawaii. He developed a good reputation for his successful treatment of people with leprosy and other diseases, which impressed the Hawaiian royalty (Mamiya Medical Heritage Center, 2005). Although Dr. Nichols only spent two years in Hawaii, his good work was so appreciated that he became an adopted member of the Hawaiian Society of Mission Children.[123]

Attacks on Royal Support for Homeopathy

Perhaps the strongest body of evidence showing the powerfully positive influences that royal support for homeopathy was having on the growth and acceptance of homeopathy in the general population was the degree of anger and antagonism that such support generated from conventional physicians.

When Dr. Frederick Quin first began his homeopathic practice in London in 1827, the College of Physicians sent an order to him forbidding his practice of homeopathy. Quin ignored it, and within a short period of time, he became very popular among London's high society (Mitchell, 1975, 95).

Sir William Henderson, MD (1811–1872), was one of the early British physicians to become a homeopathic doctor. He not only was a professor of medicine at the University of Edinburgh (during 1832–1869) but also held the chair of pathology there. The editors at *The Lancet* were so outraged when he became a homeopath that they called for his resignation from the university.

Even the editor of *The London Medical Review* wrote: "I venture to say, there is scarcely a medical man in the kingdom who has not felt the influence of this 'delusion' of his professional income." He then expressed further consternation that "I fear that the 'delusion' is rather increasing than otherwise" (Nicholls, 1988, 136).

Attacks against homeopathy were quite common in the conventional medical journals of the day. Although the first case report about homeopathy ever published in *The Lancet* was actually positive (1843), rebuttals to this initial article were swift, strong, and frequent. The tone of the anti-homeopathy articles was consistently hostile or arrogantly amused. Shortly after Queen Adelaide expressed her interest in and support for homeopathy, a letter was published in *The Lancet* that doubted her intelligence because she was a woman:

> Her Majesty is still persevering in the homeopathic system, and she supposes that she derived advantage from it. Nothing, however, can be more absurd.... Her brother... sends her these invisible pills from Germany, and they are such atoms that a quill filled with them lasts her Majesty a couple of months. And [scurrilously] Her Majesty has also an extraordinary bottle [of homeopathic medicines] which she smells whenever she wants a movement in her royal bowels, and my correspondent tells me that the effect of smelling this bottle is so immediate that her Majesty is obliged to leave the room at a moment's notice. (Nicholls, 1988, 116)

The antagonism against homeopathy and homeopaths among conventional physicians was getting so strong that simply consulting with, or referring to, a homeopath became grounds for dismissal from any teaching position or professional organization. One doctor was reprimanded because he consulted with another physician who he didn't know was a homeopathic doctor; his antagonists asserted that he should have known.

The College of Physicians in England required its members to take an oath, which sadly and humorously smacks of what could have been the word of the French playwright Molière or another medical satirist. The first sentence of this oath was: "I engage not to practice any system or method (so called) for the cure or alleviation of disease of which the College has disapproved" (Pope, 1876).

The attacks against homeopathy were not limited to Britain or America. In the 1850s, the emperor of Russia banned its practice because his father had died after unsuccessful treatment by a homeopathic physician. This extreme action due to a single incident was typical of the strong anti-homeopathy prejudices that some people held, though during this same time, the father to Queen Adelaide of Britain, George I, Duke of Saxe Meininger, died as a result of excessive bloodletting by a conventional physician, yet no monarch outlawed this common and deadly medical practice of the day.

The emperor of Austria, Francis I (1792–1835), decreed that homeopathic practice was prohibited in 1819, though homeopathy continued to grow, in large part because of the clerical support it received (see Chapter 13, Clergy and Spiritual Leaders). This action was taken at the behest of the emperor's doctor, Dr. Stift, who had a lifelong antagonism against homeopathy. Information about homeopathy in newspapers and medical journals was even censored, though the various attacks against it and homeopaths were rarely, if ever, censored. Replies to the attacks were prohibited from being published.

In Prussia, an edict in 1831 prohibited homeopaths from dispensing their own medicines. Homeopaths were not even allowed to possess a household medicine chest, so common to all other medical practitioners. The police watched the homeopaths closely, as if they were criminals. An additional feature of this edict can help us understand the economic factors that led to this new law: Homeopaths were not allowed to refer patients to a specific (homeopathic) apothecary. Apothecaries of this day were obviously as powerful as the drug companies of today.

Royal Homeopathy Today

Her Majesty, Queen Elizabeth II (1926–), is an active supporter of homeopathy. She is patron of the Royal London HomoeopathicHospital, which was originally founded by Dr. Frederick Quin, the first "royal physician." Her personal homeopath is **Dr. Peter Fisher**, who is also the medical director of the Royal London HomoeopathicHospital as well as editor of the leading academic journal in the field, *Homeopathy* (originally called the *British Homoeopathic Journal*).

Until her death in 2002, at the ripe old age of 101, Her Majesty the Queen Mother, was the principal royal patron of the British Homeopathic Association. The Duke of Gloucester, formerly Prince Richard, remains royal patron of the association. Princess Alice, the late Duchess of Gloucester, was the patron of the Blackie Foundation Trust established in honor of Dr. Margery Blackie, the former royal homeopathic physician who served from 1969 until 1980. At present, Princess Alexandra, Lady Ogilvy, is patron to the Blackie Foundation Trust, and Mary, Duchess of Roxburghe, serves as one of the vice-presidents of this organization.

Prince Charles, the Prince of Wales (1948–), has been the most outspoken modern-day royal family member to advocate for what he has popularized as "complementary medicine."[124] In 1982, he became president of the British Medical Association, and made it his mission to get the medical community to understand the problems and limitations of orthodox medicine and to appreciate the contributions of various complementary therapies, including homeopathy.

In 1996, the prince established what is now called The Prince's Foundation for Integrated Health (FIH) and made a substantial contribution toward a £2 million endowment for the charity. In February 1996, he convened and chaired a seminar involving various health care professionals to discuss practical steps to improve communication and cooperation among all those concerned with the provision of health care. As a result, working groups were created to examine requirements for research and development, education and training, regulation, and the delivery of integrated care.

On May 28th, 1998, Prince Charles made a speech at a conference organized by FIH, in which he asserted: "I hope that we shall see an increase in research, not only into the effectiveness and safety of complementary and alternative therapies and how to improve their effectiveness, but also into what people want from their health care and why they turn in particular to less conventional care."

He went on to say: "It is not a question of orthodox medicine taking over or of complementary and alternative medicine diluting the intellectual rigor of orthodoxy. It is about reaching across the disciplines to help and to learn from one another." The prince added: "When I cast my mind back 15 years to the reaction that greeted my speech on the occasion of the BMA's [British Medical Association] 150th anniversary, it is encouraging that things have moved along the road enough to allow a conference like this to take place at all" (Prince Charles, 1998).

It is sad and somewhat strange that American and European media have often trivialized Prince Charles, despite his impressive intelligence, his longtime commitment to the health and welfare of the average person, and his important and even vital questioning of orthodox medical thinking and practice.

Prince Charles may be the most vocal royal proponent of homeopathic medicine, but he and the queen certainly are not alone. **Diana, Princess of Wales, Prince Andrew**, and **Sarah Ferguson, Duchess of York**, sought homeopathic care from **Jack Temple**, an unconventional homeopath who died in 2004 at age 86 (*Daily Telegraph*, 2004; Rayner and Paveley, 2001). Princess Diana was also a regular at the Hale Clinic, an "alternative and complementary medicine" clinic in London, which was opened by Prince Charles. Simone Simmons, an "alternative healer" and close confidante of Diana, confirmed what many others have known, that "Prince Charles only uses homeopathic and complementary medicines as Diana and the children did" (*Daily Mail*, 2005).

In 1997, Sarah, Duchess of York, made an unannounced trip to **Dr. Isaac Mathai**'s holistic health center in Bangalore, India. A reporter asked her: Now that you had holistic treatment, what is your perception about alternative healing methods? Sarah replied, "We were on the homeopathic system at home for a long time. My grandmother, who died in December (1996), was a homeopathic practitioner. As children, we were given *Arnica* for colds and other ailments." (*The Week*, 1997)[125]

References

Atkin, G. *The British and Foreign Homoeopathic Medical Directory and Record*. London: Aylott and Company, 1853.

Ameke, W. *History of Homœopathy: Its Origin; Its Conflicts.* 1885. Available at http://homeoint.org/seror/ameke/index.htm

Baumann, J. *The Old and New Therapy with/of Medicine According to the Writings of Others and According to Personal Experience for the Thinking Public.* German: Das alte und neu heilverfahren mit Medicin. Nadj den Schriffen Anderer und nach eigener Erfahrung.) Remmingen: Oscar Belsenfelder. 1857.

Blodi, F. C. Field Marshall Radetzky's Orbital Abscess, *Documenta Ophthalmologica,* 1989, 71:205–219.

Bojanus, Dr. C. Historical and statistical report of the rise, progress and present condition of homoeopathy in Russia, *Transactions of the World Homoeopathic Convention,* Philadelphia, 1876, Vol II.

Bradford, T. L. *Life and Letters of Samuel Hahnemann,* Letters to Schweikert. Philadelphia: Boericke and Tafel, 1895.

Bradford, T. L. *Pioneers of Homoeopathy.* Philadelphia: Boericke and Tafel, 1897.

British Journal of Homeopathy, 1854, 686 (letter from French medical correspondent). Quoted in Tyler, M. L., Lecture to Missionary Students, *Homeopathy,* April 1932, 1(4):126–134.

By Royal Appointment, *Health and Homeopathy,* Spring 1992.

Clarke, J. H. Homoeopathy Explained. London: Homoeopathic Publishing Company, 1905. (Reprinted New Delhi: B. Jain, no date.)

Cook, T. *Samuel Hahnemann: His Life and Times.* Wellingborough: Thorsons, 1981.

Coulter, H. L. *Divided Legacy: A History of the Schism in Medical Thought.* Vol. III: The Conflict Between Homeopathy and the AMA. Berkeley: North Atlantic Books, 1973.

Coulter, H. L. *Divided Legacy: A History of the Schism in Medical Thought.* Vol. II: Progress and Regress: J. B. Van Helmont to Claude Bernard. Berkeley: North Atlantic Books, 1977.

Daily Mail (UK), Diana's Confidante Talks about the "People's Princess," August 17, 2005. Available at www.dailymail.co.uk/pages/live/articles/webchats/webchat.html?in_page_id=1868&in_article_id=146641

Daily Telegraph (UK), Jack Temple (obituary), February 20, 2004.

Dunsford, H. *The Practical Advantages of Homoeopathy, Illustrated by Numerous Cases. Dedicated, by permission, to Her Majesty, Queen Adelaide.* Philadelphia: John Pennington. 1842.

Encyclopedia Britannica, Volume 13, Homoeopathy. Available at http://jcsm.org/Study Center/Encyclopedia_Britannica/HIG_HOR/HOMOEOPATHY_from_the_Greek _6pn.html

Everest, Rev. T. R. *A Popular View of Homeopathy.* New York: William Radde, 1842.

Ewers, F. W. *Bewahrte Heilmethod der Lausesucht u des Grindes, ...* (Translation: Tried and True Therapies for Eliminating Lice and Impetigo/mange/scabies). Ilmenau, 1826.

Forbes, Sir J. *Homoeopathy, Allopathy and 'Young Physic.'* New York: William Radde, 1846.

Granier, M. *Conferences Upon Homoeopathy: The Spread of Homeopathy.* London: Leath and Ross, 1859.

Haehl, R. *Samuel Hahnemann: His Life and Work* (2 vols.). London: Homeopathic Publishing Co., 1922. (Reprinted New Delhi: B. Jain, no date.)

Handley, R. *A Homeopathic Love Story: The Story of Samuel and Melanie Hahnemann.* Berkeley: North Atlantic Books, 1990.

Hering, C. *A Memorial to Constantine Hering* (Raue, C. G., ed.) Philadelphia: Globe, 1880.

Historical and Statistical Report of the Rise, Progress, and Present Condition of Homeopathy in Russia, *Transactions of the American Institute of Homeopathy,* 1876, vol. II.

History of Homeopathy in Spain and its Colonies, *Transactions of the American Institute of Homeopathy,* 1876, vol II, Part II.

Homoeopathy, Knight Grand Cross of St. Olav, March 1939, p. 96.

Homoeopathy in Italy, *Transactions of the American Institute of Homeopathy,* 1876, vol II, Part II.

Hoyle, E. P. International Council, *The Homeopathician,* June 1913, p. 249.

Hunt, W. F. The Condition of Homeopathy in Europe, *Transactions of the New York State Homeopathic Medical Society,* 1863, 118–123. (The author of this article graduated from Indiana Medical College, a conventional medical college, and later became a homeopath and professor of material medica, medical jurisprudence, and medical botany at the New York Homeopathic Medical College during 1859–1869. He also took an active role in creating asylums for the blind, the deaf, and the dumb, including the State Asylum for the Insane. He wrote the law that made care at these facilities free. Hunt's father was General George Hunt, a pioneer in the Indiana territory, and his great-grandfather was Jonathan Hunt of New Jersey, a colonel in the Continental Army (Wershub, 1967, 34).)

Jütte, R. *The Hidden Roots: A History of Homeopathy in Northern, Central and Eastern Europe.* Stuttgart: Institute for the History of Medicine, 2006.

Kotok, A. The History of Homeopathy in the Russian Empire until World War I, as compared with other European countries and the USA: Similarities and Discrepancies. PhD thesis submitted to the Senate of the Hebrew University of Jerusalem, November 1999. Available at http://homeoint.org/books4/kotok/index.htm

Kotok, A. The Alexander II Homeopathic Hospital in St Petersburg, *The Homeopath,* Autumn 2000, 79:8–11.

Krauss, J. Hahnemann and Hahnemann's Organon of Medicine, *The Homeopathic Recorder,* November 15, 1925, 40(11):481–497.

Lugli, A., Zlobec, I., Singer, G., et al. Napoleon Bonaparte's Gastric Cancer: A Clinicopathologic Approach, *Nature Clinical Practice Gastroenterology & Hepatology,* 2007, 4(1):52–57.

L' Union Medicale, 1850. Quoted in Progress of Homoeopathy in Spain, *Monthly Journal of Homeopathy,* 1850, issue 12.

Mamiya Medical Heritage Center (Archives of the Hawaiian Medical Library), 2005. Available at http://hml.org/mmhc/mdindex/nicholsc.html

Mitchell, G. H. *Homoeopathy.* London: W. H. Allen, 1975.

Morrell, P. British Homeopathy During Two Centuries. Available at http://homeoint.org/morrell/british/index.htm (A research thesis submitted to Staffordshire University for the degree of Master of Philosophy, June 1999.)

Mueller, M. L. History and Statistics of the Homoeopathic Hospitals of Austria, *Transactions of the American Institute of Homeopathy,* 1876, vol II.

Nicholls, P. A. *Homoeopathy and the Medical Profession.* London: Croom Helm, 1988.

Payne, W. E. *Address and Poem delivered before the Massachusetts Homeopathic Medical Society.* Boston: Otis Class, 1855.

Pope, A. C. The History and Details of British Legislation Affecting Practitioners of Homoeopathy, *Transactions of the American Institute of Homeopathy,* 1876, vol II.

Poulet, J. Approche de l'Homoeopathie, *l'Homoeopathie Francaise,* 1973, pp. 452–454.

Poulet, J. *Archives du Chateau de Montgobert, Les Bonaparte et l'homeopathie.* Montgobert: Le Club de Retz, no date.

Prince Charles. "Open-Minded" Healthcare. BBC Online. May 28, 1998. Available at http://news.bbc.co.uk/2/low/health/102246.stm

Rayner, G., and Paveley, R. Cherie health guru who believes MMR jab is unnecessary, *Daily Mail* (London), December 26, 2001.

Schmidt, P. Historical Sketch of Homeopathy in Switzerland, *Journal of the American Institute of Homeopathy,* February 1926, 19(2):164–170.

Smith, D. D. *Notable Psychiatrists in Hawaii Over the Past 150 Years,* Archives of the Hawaii Medical Library, July, 2002. Available at www.hawaiipsychiatric.org/HawaiiPsychiatric.data/Library/History/Hawaii%20Psychiatrists%20Hx.pdf

Vingtrinier, A. Chronique Locale [Local Chronicle], *Revue du Lyonnais,* 1860.

The Week, February 9, 1997. Available at www.soukya.com/theweek.html

Tyler, M. *Homoeopathic Drug Pictures.* London: Homoeopathic Publishing Company, 1942. (Reprinted New Delhi: B. Jain, no date.)

Wells, P. P. What Is Homoeopathy, and What Are the Possibilities and Duties of Its Practice? *The Organon,* July 1879, issue 3.

Wershub, L. P. *One Hundred Years of Medical Progress: A History of the New York Medical Colllege, Flower and Fifth Avenue Hospitals.* Springfield: Charles C. Thomas, 1967.

Young, N. *Napoleon in Exile: St. Helena (1815–1821).* London: Stanley Paul, 1915.

CHAPTER 13

Clergy and Spiritual Leaders: More than Prayer for Homeopathy

In Shakespeare's *Romeo and Juliet*, Friar Lawrence chooses the plant from which he will make Juliet's sleeping potion, and he tells us: "Within the infant rind of this small flower, Poison hath residence, and medicine power."

Although we do not today think about going to a clergyman to obtain medicinal treatment and may even laugh at the thought of it, in the not-too-distant past the clergy were often knowledgeable of various medicinal systems of healing and some were even practitioners.

Ever since the beginning of homeopathy in the early 1800s, some of its most active advocacy has come from the clergy, and not just any clergymen, but many of the most respected of that era. In 1838 the president of the New York State Medical Society lamented: "Some of the chief supporters of homeopathy and other kindred delusions are distinguished clergymen" (Coulter, 1973, III, 111).

This president expressed further concern, saying:

> If in any community there happens to be a practitioner of homeopathy, hydrotherapy, a "faith doctor," or a Mesmerizer [hypnotist], ten chances to one if the first person who employs him is not one of the reverend gentlemen above named, or, it may be, a Right Reverend himself. (Coulter, 1973, III, 111)

The serious interest in and support for homeopathy expressed by influential leaders in the Jewish and the Muslim communities raises the question of whether it is possible for homeopathic medicine to provide common ground between these two normally warring groups of people. One may wonder if the use of homeopathic medicines can be seen and understood as a way by which people of various religious backgrounds can find common ground on which to stand.

Biblical References to Homeopathic Principles

Homeopathy itself was not formerly systematized into a specific medical system until a German physician, Samuel Hahnemann, MD, performed his first experiments in the late 1700s and early 1800s. Still, long before Hahnemann, many physicians, healers, or simply curious and observant individuals discovered a basic principle of health and healing: that symptoms of illness are not just evidence of something "wrong" with the person but they represent efforts of the person's body and mind to defend against infection, poisons, or various stresses.

According to Hippocrates (the "father of medicine" and a leading medical historian), some physicians and healers used medicinal agents to "combat" symptoms, "fight" disease, or simply work antagonistically against a specific symptom. Distinct from this school of thought and practice were other early physicians and healers who sought to use medicinal agents that would nourish, nurture, or augment the body's own healing wisdom. These healers would use medicinal substances that actually might cause or mimic the symptoms that the sick person experienced, in order to initiate the healing process. Thus, instead of fighting against the sick person's symptoms, the healer would prescribe a plant, mineral, or animal substance that would mimic the wisdom of the body.

It seems that Moses had an innate sense of this latter medicinal school of thought. It probably sounds like a joke if one says or suggests that Moses was a homeopath, but the Bible does describe specific actions of Moses that certainly sound as though he was a homeopath.

One of the most familiar stories from the Bible is the description of Moses going to Mt. Sinai to talk to God. He was gone longer than the Israelites had expected, and they became impatient, and their belief in Moses began to waiver. The Israelites asked Aaron to make a sacred image of God for them so that they could have something physical to worship.

He did so by gathering golden jewelry and golden objects from the Israelites; he melted them together and made a golden calf, a symbol of abundance and an honoring of the sanctity of life.

God told Moses that the Israelites had defamed him by these actions, that any symbol of God is false, and these people should die and be replaced by new descendents of Moses. Moses prayed and pleaded for their lives and for forgiveness, and he was successful.

As Moses descended from Mt. Sinai, he brought with him the Ten Commandments. Although God had forgiven the Israelites' actions, Moses told the Israelites that those who worship this idol do not deserve the treasure of the Ten Commandments and the word of God. Then, Moses did something quite remarkable: He took the golden idol, smashed it, melted it down, ground it to dust, placed the dust in water, and forced the people to drink this water (Exodus 32).

Most biblical scholars insist that this action was Moses' way to show the Israelites the impermanence of their idol and the foolishness of worshiping false gods. Other scholars have asserted that drinking this water was akin to washing their mouths out with soap.

Another way to interpret Moses' action was that he treated them homeopathically. First, it is impressive and even amazing to note that the Bible perfectly describes how homeopathic medicines made of mineral (gold) are manufactured—ground up (the technical word is "triturated") and then diluted in water. What is also fascinating about Moses' decision to make a medicine out of the golden calf is that gold is known to cause various physical and psychological symptoms when a person is exposed to it in overdose. Physically, gold is known to cause in overdose various symptoms, including bone pain and arthritis-like symptoms. It is no coincidence, therefore, that conventional physicians for many decades have used gold salts to treat people with certain types of arthritis. Psychologically, gold has been found to cause feelings of despair and hopelessness—and, in later stages of illness, it can also cause deep and dark depression, even suicidal depression.

It seems that Moses determined that the Israelites' worshiping of false gods was the result of feelings of despair and hopelessness and that their actions in this desert represented self-destructive behaviors that were suicidal.

Whatever Moses was thinking is certainly simple conjecture, but his actions in making this "medicine" were very much like a homeopathic pharmacist and a homeopathic doctor. Although neither the Bible nor the Torah suggested that Moses diluted and succussed (shook) the medicines consecutively, as is done today to make homeopathic medicines, it is still quite provocative that the Bible highlights the fact that he ground it into powder and diluted the very substance that was a symbol of their dis-ease.

There are other references to the homeopathic principle of similars in the Bible. These examples, like many stories from the Bible, are not meant to be taken literally, but figuratively. In the following case, Moses suggested that simply looking at a symbolic representation of a snake might prevent deaths from a real snake bite.

> Numbers 21, verses 6–9:
>
> 6. And the Lord sent fiery serpents among the people, and they bit the people; and much people of Israel died.
>
> 7. Therefore, the people came to Moses, and said, We have sinned, for we have spoken against the Lord, and against thee; pray unto the Lord, that he take away the serpents from us. And Moses prayed for the people.
>
> 8. And the Lord said unto Moses, Make thee a fiery serpent, and set it upon a pole: and it shall come to pass, that every one that is bitten, when he looketh upon it, shall live.
>
> 9. And Moses made a serpent of brass, and put it upon a pole, and it came to pass, that if a serpent had bitten any man, when he beheld the serpent of brass, he lived.

Vatican Support for Homeopathy

Homeopathy arrived in Italy in 1822 with Dr. George Necker, the family physician to Austria's head army commander, Baron Francis Koller and the former doctor to Napoleon's troops. Necker was an ardent student of

Samuel Hahnemann, MD, and in 1823, he was sent by the queen of Naples to Rome to treat her sister, Maria Louisa of Bourbon, who was then the queen of Etruria (the region of central Italy). At the time, **Leo XII** (1780–1829) was the pope, and although he and his predecessor, **Pope Pius VIII** (1761–1830), were favorably inclined to homeopathy, **Pope Gregory XVI** (1765–1846) was a much stronger defender of and advocate for this new medicine (Piterà, 2001). Gregory XVI was favorably inclined enough that he allowed homeopathy to be practiced in the Vatican by a German physician, **Dr. Johann Wilhelm Wahle** (1794–1853).[126]

The Jesuits, the Christian religious order in direct service to the pope, appointed Dr. Wahle as physician to their convent and paid him twice the amount given to his allopathic predecessor (Granier, 1859).

Pope Leo XII's rule was short-lived, and with the ascendancy in 1830 by Gregory XVI, homeopathy achieved even greater support, in part because of his own personal interest in the subject and in part because of impressive successes that homeopathic doctors had in treating people exposed to the rampant cholera epidemic of that time. Gregory XVI sought to establish a homeopathic hospital; however, the conventional medical schools in Rome and Bologna worked against this effort. When the cholera epidemic subsided, the interest in creating a homeopathic hospital waned and it was never built (Negro, 2006).

Gregorio XVI also bestowed the Grand Cross, the highest honor a pope can give to a layperson, onto one of the most famous Italian doctors of the time, **Settimio Centamori**, who was known to successfully treat many cholera sufferers with homeopathic medicines. In 1837, when Dr. Centamori visited Rome, he treated the rector at St. Peter's who was dying of cholera, but he wasn't successful in this case. Several conventional physicians accused him of poisoning the prelate, though his reputation wasn't significantly affected. Later, he visited Rome again as physician to the Grand Duke of Lucca, and in 1842 he had married French royalty, Charlotte Bonaparte, the niece of Napoleon I.

In 1855, Gregory XVI conferred the Order of Saint Sylvester onto **Count des Guidi** (1769–1863), France's first homeopathic doctor, and in 1862, **Dr. Charles Ozanam** of Paris was decorated with the Order of St.

Gregory the Great. Gregory XVI showed additional significant support for homeopathy for issuing a papal bull (a special kind of charter issued by the pope) that allowed the administration of homeopathic medicines by priests in cases of emergency in the absence of any doctor.

Evidence suggests that **Pope Pius IX** (1792–1878) received homeopathic care, though more details about this treatment remain unknown (Hunt, 1863). On numerous occasions, however, this pope expressed special appreciation for the care that homeopathic physicians gave to the sick. It is confirmed that Pope Pius IX granted the Order of St. Gregory the Great[127] to **Dr. A. Charge** (1810–1890), a homeopathic doctor in Marseilles "in consideration of the services he rendered during the cholera epidemic" of 1849–1851 (Hunt, 1863). Records show that Dr. Charge treated 1,662 cases of cholera with homeopathic medicine and had only 49 deaths (2.9 percent), as compared with the usual 10–70 percent at conventional hospitals.

In 1852 Pope Pius IX granted the Order of St. Gregory the Great to **Jean-Paul Tessier, MD** (1810–1862), the French conventional physician who conducted one of the early scientific studies testing the efficacy of homeopathic treatment in patients with cholera and pneumonia (Dean, 2004). Tessier's results showed greater efficacy for homeopathic medicines, but he was ostracized from the Paris Academy of Medicine for his heretical study.[128]

The support for homeopathy from Pope Pius IX was also shown by the appointment of **Dr. Giovanni Ettore Mengozzi**, a homeopathic physician and author of a popular homeopathic book, to a Vatican professorship (Liga Medicorum). Dr. Mengozzi was also a member of numerous Italian and European academies, including La Scuola Italica, an academy of scientists. Dr. Mengozzi asked Darwin if he would accept honorary membership in this organization (November 24, 1880), and Darwin gratefully accepted it (December 15, 1880).

Father Augustus Muller (1784–1849) was a Jesuit missionary who was trained in Germany in homeopathic medicine. He moved to southern India and established a homeopathic dispensary for the poor and two hospitals (St. Joseph's Leper Hospital and the Bubonic Plague Hospital). All three entities dispensed homeopathic medicines. As a result of his work, **Pope Pius X** (1835–1914) bestowed posthumously upon Father Muller the Apostolic Benediction in 1905 (Transactions, 1908, 128).

Today, the Father Muller Charitable Institutions is sponsored by the Catholic Diocese of Mangalore; it includes a hospital complex in Mangalore that has 1,050 beds, a leprosy center, a rehabilitation center, a homeopathic medical college, a homeopathic pharmaceutical unit, a conventional college of medicine, and a college of nursing. This institution also has various undergraduate and post-graduate programs, including degree programs in physiotherapy, radiography, medical laboratory technology, and hospital management. Although most people outside of India do not recognize the name Father Muller, he has become a household name in India.

When the Father Muller Homeopathic Medical College and Hospital opened up new buildings in November 2006, the event was so important to the Catholic community that Bishop Aloysius Paul D'Souza of Mangalore chaired the inaugural ceremonies, and His Eminence Varkey Cardinal Vithayathil attended (*Indian Catholic News,* 2006).

Pope Leo XIII (1810–1903) was the only pope for whom the specifics of his ailment and his homeopathic treatment were made public (Pitera, 2001). He had suffered from a chronic tracheal infection that gravely threatened his life. Ultimately, Leo XIII led a very long life and became the oldest living pope in history.

Many of the popes in the twentieth century were as appreciative of homeopathy as those in the nineteenth century. Shortly after **Pope Pius XII** (1876–1958) received his appointment in 1939, he appointed **Dr. Riccardo Galéazzi-Lisi** as his personal physician (Homeopathic Hassle, 1956; Pitera, 2001). For the rest of the pope's life, the doctor was one of his closest confidants. Pius XII even appointed Galéazzi-Lisi to be an honorary member of the renowned Pontifical Academy of Sciences.

There is also a record of Pius XII requesting and receiving homeopathic treatment from an American homeopath, **William B. Griggs, MD,** for a recalcitrant case of hiccups. Griggs prescribed *Hyoscyamus niger* (henbane), a homeopathic medicine for spasmodic conditions, and it was effective (Yasgur, 1998, 374).

Although Pius XII lived a long life and despite the pope's longtime deep appreciation for this physician and close friend, the critics of homeopathy deemed the pope's physician to be a quack who hastened the death of the pontiff (wikipedia.com). Galéazzi-Lisi sought to clear his name and reputation after the pope's death (Galéazzi-Lisi, 1960), but the strong biases against homeopathy and other alternatives in the 1950s and 1960s were simply too strong.

Antonio Negro, MD (1907–), of Naples has been one of the leading Italian homeopathic physicians in the latter half of the twentieth century, and he was the homeopathic doctor to **Pope Paul VI** (1897–1978). Dr. Negro was granted the Order of St. Gregory for his work in homeopathy.

Antonio Negro's son, **Francesco Negro, MD** (1944–), is also a highly respected homeopathic physician, and he served as the homeopathic doctor of **Pope John Paul II** (1920–2005).

European Support from Leading Clergymen

Many of Hahnemann's earliest patients were clergymen, including **Rev. Thomas Everest** (1800–1855), who was treated successfully for asthma (see Handley, 1997, 21, 31, 130, 144). Reverend Everest was an Anglican parish priest and rector of Wickwar in Gloucestershire. He became an important lay homeopath and was even known to preach homeopathy from his pulpit. He considered homeopathic treatment the physical means to salvation that completed the spiritual means provided by biblical revelation. Everest came from a highly respected family; his brother was Colonel Sir George Everest, surveyor general of colonial India, for whom the tallest mountain in the world is named.

Father Everest's book, *A Popular View of Homeopathy* (1842), was so important that the preface to its American edition was co-authored by a stellar group of citizens, including William Cullen Bryant (famed editor of the *New York Evening Post*), Robert H. Morris (mayor of New York City), Judge Ogden P. Edwards, and three leading clergymen.

Everest wrote about one of his own experiences with homeopathy. He had experienced a chronic nasal obstruction throughout many decades of his life, and after many unsuccessful efforts at treatment from conventional physicians, Everest traveled to Paris to seek the care of Dr. Samuel Hahnemann. Shortly after he took a homeopathic medicine prescribed by Dr. Hahnemann, he experienced a profuse nasal discharge that lasted all day and continued in decreasing amounts for a month. Afterwards, he never experienced this problem again.

The priest experienced what is somewhat common in the homeopathic treatment of people with chronic diseases—a "healing crisis," that is, a temporary increase in certain symptoms that result in an externalization of the disease and that usually results in a curative process.

One could point to various homeopathic principles to find alliances to every religious tradition. However, the primary reason that so many clergymen became such strong advocates of homeopathy is that the clergy began treating their disciples and potential disciples with these medicines. Not only did the medicines work, but the efficacy of treatment led to increased numbers of church members (Kotok, 1999).

Clerical support for homeopathy also resulted in part from the homeopathic tenets that a "vital force" or life energy played an integral role in a person's health, that illness was sometimes a spiritual condition, and that the composition of medicines released a type of special energy that augmented the healing process. The fact that homeopaths use a wide variety of medicinal agents from the plant, mineral, and animal kingdoms could be understood as further evidence of divine beneficence and that God had rightfully compensated for disease by creating a natural world that provided tools for healing when used properly (Nichols, 1988, 114).

Homeopathy was first introduced into Ireland by a clergyman (Hunt, 1863). Later, in the mid-1800s, **Paul Cullen**, the **Archbishop of Dublin** (1803–1878), became an advocate for homeopathy and was a contributor to the establishment of a homeopathic hospital (Nichols, 1988, 111).

In England, the Missionary School of Medicine was established in 1903 in an effort to provide some medical knowledge, plus a good overview of homeopathy, basic surgery, and tropical medicine, and, finally, a homeopathic medicine kit to the hapless missionaries soon to be working in Africa, the Far East, or various places in the British Empire of the time. This organization's training in homeopathic medicine and primary care was handled by the teaching staff at the Royal London Homoeopathic Hospital and in association with the British Homeopathic Association. By 1934, there were more than 700 graduates from the Missionary School. Their work was a type of early "barefoot" homeopathic doctoring, and an example of the clergy teaming up successfully with homeopaths to provide health care to underserved parts of the world. The demand for this training decreased significantly in the latter half of the twentieth century, leading to the closing of the school in 1996 (Davies, 2007; Morrell, 1999).

Rev. Canon Roland Upcher (1849–1929) was initially rector at Halesworth in Suffolk. Later, he became the rural dean at Stradbroke. In addition to his involvement in the clergy and in education, his real love was for practicing homeopathy. He was known to be a great friend and student of **Dr. John Henry Clarke**, the prolific homeopathic author. Upcher was also known as a lay prescriber, and he is credited with being the first to use gunpowder as a homeopathic remedy (Morrell, 1999).[129]

Homeopathy was also very popular among Russian Orthodox clergymen. In 1880, after **Dr. Yuly Lukovsky** (1833–1912) helped in the recovery of the archimandrite, or superior, of the Irkutsk Innokenty monastery, the superior became an advocate of homeopathy. At his request, the **Archbishop of Irkutsk** ordered his clergy to buy homeopathic medicine kits and manuals and to distribute them among the missionaries. The Russian Orthodox clergy found that Buddhist priests were so impressed by the success of the missionaries' homeopathic treatments that it strongly influenced many non-Russians to become Christians (Kotok, 1999, note 52). One of the local non-Russian rulers, together with his close retainers, became Christian; the ruler himself even joined the St. Petersburg Society of Homeopathic Physicians as a correspondent member.

One of the biggest achievements of Russian homeopaths was attracting support from famous and highly respected Russian churchmen, including **Saint Ioann of Kronstadt** and the Bishop and **Saint Feofan the**

Hermit (1815–1894, also known as Georgy Govorov), both of whom who became strong advocates for homeopathy (Kotok, 1999, note 84). Saint Ioann of Kronstadt is considered one of most venerated of all Russian saints. His book, *My Life in Christ*, was translated into English and became extremely popular, though his name was spelled as St. John of Kronstadt. St. Feofan was a bishop from the town of Tambov, Russia; he was canonized in 1988.

At the opening of the new pharmacy and dispensary of the St. Petersburg Society of the Followers of Homeopathy on October 17, 1881, Father Ioann made the following speech:

> Your institution or your method of treatment of diseases is based on the motto of the ancient sages-homeopaths *Similia similibus curentur* [these famous Latin words mean "let likes cure likes," which refers to the basic homeopathic principle of similars], the most sensible and right method. Even the Divine Wisdom could not find more correct means to heal mankind plagued with sins and with numerous maladies. (Kotok, 1999, section 4.3.2)

There is a record of reports from numerous priests that it was Father Ioann's speeches on homeopathy that showed how Russian Orthodox clergymen created "miracles" in the treatment of the sick with homeopathic medicines, which led them to use homeopathic medicines to treat parishioners. Ioann's authority was so significant all over Russia that even allopaths, fiercely condemning the churchmen for their collaboration with homeopaths, could not dare to question or criticize him openly.

The growth of homeopathy among Russian clergy and the general public was particularly enhanced in 1890 when the church published a brochure entitled *Some Brief Information About Homeopathy* and printed 50,000 copies of it (in those days, a lot of copies), which were distributed free of charge to rural clergymen, teachers, and anyone wishing to read it. This homeopathic brochure was printed with personal permission of the Chief Procurator of the Holy Synod, Pobedonostsev.[130] Coincidentally, the editor of the periodical in which the brochure was inserted,

Father P. A. Smirnov, was a committed advocate of homeopathy, as was the editor of the leading church newspaper (Kotok, 1999).

The participation of the Russian Orthodox clergy in the spread of homeopathy in Russia was significant. This fact helps to explain why the Russians were able to contribute one-third of the high price (60,000 francs at the time) to secure a final resting site for homeopathy's founder, Samuel Hahnemann, in the famed Parisian cemetery, Père Lachaise.

Predictably, the reaction from conventional physicians to the involvement of clergy in medical practice was heated. In fact, the clergy's involvement in homeopathy was so threatening that physicians arranged to prosecute clergymen for practicing medicine, though they were usually not convicted because they provided treatment without charging for it. It is also interesting to note that the first lay homeopathic organization in Germany was started in 1832 after a priest had been prosecuted for his practice of homeopathy (Kotok, 1999, note 126).

In contrast with Germany, where homeopathy became widespread among Protestant clergy, in France homeopathy received active support from the Catholic Church. Among those distinguished persons who divided their time between homeopathy and church activity were the priests and physicians (father and son) **Toussaint** (1777–1852) and **Pierre-Auguste Rapous**. Their effective homeopathic treatment attracted the commitment of the Dombes convent's physician, the priest **Duquesnay** (1786–1867), to homeopathy. Duquesnay was also known to have established a homeopathic dispensary (pharmacy) in his parish. He was so well loved that he later became Archbishop of Cambrai (Rafinesque, 1876). Furthering the chain of involvement, the latter promoted the conversion of his pupil and follower, the priest **Alexis Espanet** (1811–1896), who later worked with Dr. Alexandre Charge, who Pope Pius IX awarded the Order of St. Gregory the Great for his successful treatment of people with cholera.

The clergy in Austria took a particularly active role in establishing homeopathic medicine, despite a decree in 1819 by Austria's Emperor Francis I (1792–1835) that prohibited the practice of homeopathy. This decree was initiated at the strong influence of the emperor's physician,

Dr. Stift, who, like many orthodox physicians, was offended that homeopaths so harshly criticized medical practice of that day. Despite its prohibition, homeopathy continued to spread in Austria, in large part because of clerical support.

Austrian nuns took an active role in promoting homeopathic medicines and in building homeopathic hospitals. **The Sisters of Charity**, a Catholic order, created several homeopathic hospitals in Austria, including a thirty-bed hospital in Vienna built in 1834 and later growing into a 160-bed hospital. In 1835 **Wilhelm Fleischmann, MD** (1798–1868), became head of this hospital, and helped establish it as a leading hospital providing homeopathic treatment. Dr. Fleischmann initially was a highly respected conventional physician and a member of the College of Physicians and Surgeons of Vienna.[131] However, his own case of obstinate sciatica was cured by a priest who practiced homeopathy, Father Veith (see below for his story).

When a serious cholera epidemic spread throughout Europe in 1836, this and other homeopathic hospitals exhibited substantially better results than other hospitals and clinical practices of that time. In fact, statistics show that during this severe cholera epidemic two-thirds of patients at conventional hospitals died, while only one-third of cholera patients at this Vienna homeopathic hospital died (Clarke, 1905). As a result of the obvious benefits of homeopathic treatment during this epidemic and in response to its successful treatment of other diseases, the new emperor of Austria, Ferdinand I (who ruled from 1835–1848), rescinded the prohibition against homeopathy. He later allowed homeopathic physicians to make their own medicines, which was a very important ruling because the apothecaries (pharmacists) of that day made considerably less profit making the small doses of homeopathic medicines, and thus often made fraudulent products on their own.

For a lifetime of homeopathic care for people, Dr. Fleischmann was knighted by the king of Bavaria in 1857 (Hunt, 1863). In 1860 he was decorated with the Cross of the Franz Joseph Order of Knighthood by the emperor of Austria, and from Pope Pius IX he received the Order of St. Gregory the Great.[132]

In Austria alone, at least fifty members of the clergy practiced homeopathy. Despite laws prohibiting their practice prior to 1837, many clergyman still engaged in homeopathic treatment. **Pater (Father) Maximilian** of the Franciscan order, who died in 1854, had so many remarkable cures that he was typically followed by a large crowd of patients, thereby attracting the notice of the authorities. At the encouragement of Dr. Stift, who maintained a lifelong antagonism to homeopathy, the priest's home was often searched by the police for the purpose of confiscating his remedies. They escaped detection because he kept them concealed in disguised or dummy books (History of Homeopathy in Austria, 1876).

Similarly, **Pater Faustus**, a member of a religious order called the Brothers of Charity, had cured so many patients that he developed a reputation throughout the country.

As a result of the impressive homeopathic care in Vienna, the **Bishop of Linz, Gregorius Thomas Ziegler** (1770–1852), induced the magistrate of Linz to donate land for a homeopathic hospital. Archduke Maximilian contributed 20,000 gulden toward the erection of this hospital, chapel, and funeral home. The Sisters of Charity took charge of the internal arrangement of the buildings, and it was formally opened May 30, 1842 (Huber, 1880).

The story of **Father J. M. Veith** (1787–1877) is unusual. He was born a Jew, the son an esteemed rabbi, but by the time he was 28 in 1815, he had converted to Catholicism and became a priest. In addition to his religious training, he was also educated as a doctor, a veterinary surgeon, and a botanist, and he was appointed professor of medicine. As a result of seeing great cures with homeopathic medicine, including the cure of his brother who had had severe gastric symptoms, he became an ardent advocate for homeopathic medicine (Haehl, 1922, II, 494). During the cholera epidemic of 1830, he treated 125 patients with homeopathic medicines and only three died. He also discovered an important medicine that was indicated in certain cases of advanced cholera, *Phosphoric acid,* a homeopathic remedy known to help with profuse and exhausting diarrhea.

The most common homeopathic medicine of that time for people with cholera was *Camphora* (camphor). In one of Father Veith's famous sermons, entitled "The Cholera in the Light of Providence," he asserted: "It is a remarkable provision of Providence that in the same part of the earth which was the birthplace of cholera [Asia] its most powerful remedy (Camphor) is also to be found" (Bradford, 1895, Chapter 49). Both homeopaths and clergymen were intrigued by this phenomenon.

In 1832 Father Veith became pastor at the famed St. Stephen's Cathedral, Vienna's largest church and the seat of the Roman Catholic archbishop. His sermons were so well loved that it was common for the large cathedral to be full of worshippers and appreciators of his wisdom. The archbishop instructed Father Veith to not treat humans because the archbishop didn't consider homeopathic treatment appropriate for the ministry. However, even the archbishop could not stop Father Veith from prescribing homeopathic medicines and writing about it. Father Veith ultimately played an important role in the early growth and acceptance of homeopathy in Austria for the many cures he provided to people. Father Veith's *Manual of Veterinary Science* was an important contribution to the medical literature of the day; it was used as a textbook for fifteen years. In addition to his many contributions to homeopathy, he founded the Austrian Catholic Association.

Rudolf Steiner (1861–1925) was a prominent Austrian philosopher, architect, educator, mystic, and social thinker. He founded anthroposophy, which has been called a "spiritual science." Anthroposophy was never considered a religion, but rather a way of understanding life and of using special practices to improve the quality of life. As a part of anthroposophy, Steiner developed Waldorf education (a unique educational program that integrates creative and artful thinking with academic work and spirituality),[133] biodynamic agriculture (a sophisticated form of organic farming), eurythmy (a form of "movement art" that includes dance and exercise as therapy and education), and anthroposophical medicine (which integrates many homeopathic medicines).

Steiner was greatly influenced by the German literary great, Goethe, and became an editor of Goethe's scientific writings (Treuherz, 1985).[134]

Steiner also had great admiration for Ralph Waldo Emerson. All three of these great thinkers and writers understood the dynamic, connective influence of the body to the mind and to nature.

Steiner and his followers have popularized the medicine *Iscador* ® (made from mistletoe) as part of a treatment program for people with cancer (Treuherz, 1985). Steiner's thinking was that medicines should not only be prescribed based on what they cause in overdose (as homeopaths use them) but also based on how the plant, mineral, or animal substance exists in nature. Because Steiner observed that mistletoe is a parasitic plant and had other qualities that resembled tumor growth, he suggested that it might be therapeutically useful for the treatment of tumors. Television actress Suzanne Somers used *Iscador* ® in her treatment program when she was diagnosed with breast cancer in 2001 (see Chapter 6, Stage, Film, and Television Celebrities, for more details of this story).

One European company devoted to body care based on homeopathic and Steiner's thinking and contributions is Dr. Hauschka Skin Care. Advocates of these products include Madonna, Brad Pitt, and Jade Jagger, among many others (*Vanity Fair*, 2006).

Just as clergy throughout the world have taken in refugees or citizens who were persecuted for one reason or another, European clergy were also known to take in homeopathic doctors who were being persecuted by conventional physicians and pharmacists of the day. The story of a surgeon, **Anton Fischer,** is classic. He was an early student and friend of Samuel Hahnemann, and as early as 1818, he established a homeopathic practice in what is now the Czech Republic. His clients included influential figures such as the governor of Moravia and Silesia, Karl Rudolf Count Inzaghi (1777–1856), and General Ignaz Ludwig Paul Freiherr von Lederer (1769–1849). There is even some evidence that a judge who sentenced him for violating the law prohibiting homeopathy had consulted him as a doctor (Jütte, 2006, 55). Persecution by the medical authorities forced Fischer to flee, and a Benedictine monastery in another town provided refuge for him.

American Clergy

In 1869, the American Institute of Homeopathy expressed appreciation for the important work of the clergy in spreading homeopathy: "Itinerant clergymen, observing the need and desire for homeopathy in the communities they visited, have coupled dispensing of homeopathic remedies with their religious labors" (Coulter, 1973, III, 111).

One of the co-founders of the first homeopathic medical school in the United States was **Rev. Johannes Helfrich** (1795–1852) (Knerr, 1940). Founded in 1835, the North American Academy of the Homeopathic Healing Art was established in Allentown, Pennsylvania, and it was known as the Allentown Academy.

Although Father Helfrich maintained very active pastoral duties (over his lifetime he baptized more than 4,500 children, confirmed 2,000 marriages, and presided over 1,500 funerals), he was one of the first graduates of the homeopathic school in Allentown. He typically worked two days a week as a practicing homeopath. His eldest son also became a homeopathic physician, while his youngest son followed in his ministerial footsteps.

Helfrich was a frequent participant in homeopathic experiments called provings, in which people take repeated doses of substances to discover what toxic symptoms they cause, thus illuminating the specific symptoms and syndrome that homeopathic doses of these substances will cure. He was a regular contributor to homeopathic journals, reporting on his experiments and his own clinical practice. In 1849 Mr. Helfrich authored a book on homeopathic veterinary practice—the first book on the subject published in this country.

Theodore Dwight Weld (1803–1895) was one of the evangelical antislavery advocates who was also a great appreciator of homeopathy. He moved to Boston in the 1860s to teach at Boston Normal Institute for Physical Education, a school founded by **Dr. Dioclesian Lewis** (1823–1886), a homeopathic and hydropathic practitioner and champion of physical culture and temperance. Dr. Lewis was one of many Harvard

Medical School graduates who turned to homeopathy; later he founded the first homeopathic journal for the general public, *The Homoeopathist*.

Lewis's school taught the "new gymnastics" and is credited with being the leading institution to promote physical fitness in the nineteenth century. This subject was noncontroversial enough that Lewis was able to bring together people who often disagreed on other health and medical subjects (including several who were known to be antagonistic to homeopathy). Some people who contributed to or supported this school included Amos Bronson Alcott, Edward Everett (former senator and governor of Massachusetts and former president of Harvard), and the publisher James T. Fields (publisher of Nathaniel Hawthorne's books, among others). Contributors who supported the school despite their antagonism toward homeopathy included Cornelius Felton (Harvard president) Walter Channing (former dean of Harvard Medical College), and Dr. Oliver Wendell Holmes (author and Harvard professor). Lewis's school had 420 graduates during its seven-year existence (Thomas, 1950).

Edward Everett Hale (1822–1909), the nephew of Lewis' supporter Edward Everett, was famous in his own right for being an author, Unitarian clergyman, and chaplain of the U.S. Senate. Hale also gave the opening prayer at the 1903 annual meeting of the American Institute of Homeopathy in Boston.

Theodore Parker (1810–1860) was an American minister of the Unitarian church. He has been described as a "Transcendentalist, theologian, scholar, Unitarian minister, abolitionist, and social reformer ... all of these things and more. A friend of Emerson and a foe of slavery" (www.wikipedia.org). His parishioners included Louisa May Alcott, William Lloyd Garrison, Julia Ward Howe, and Elizabeth Cady Stanton, all of whom were also advocates of homeopathy. His congregation later grew to 7,000.

Parker was the first person to use the phrase "of all the people, by all the people, for all the people," which later influenced the Gettysburg address of Abraham Lincoln. He also predicted the eventual success of the abolitionist cause and was known for a poetic statement made famous a century later by Martin Luther King, Jr.: "The arc of the universe is long but it bends toward justice."

Rev. Parker gave the eulogy at the funeral of his own homeopathic physician, Dr. William Wesselhoeft (1794–1858). Parker, however, did not take this homeopath's last advice to him. He had been suffering from an anal fistula (an abnormal opening near the anus), and Dr. Wesselhoeft specifically discouraged him from getting surgical treatment for it (homeopaths prefer to prescribe homeopathic medicines for these ailments and often avoid surgical treatment of skin symptoms because they consider them to be an important externalization of the disease process). Within two weeks after the operation, Parker developed a severe hemorrhage from the lungs and shortly afterwards, he died (Kimball, 1888).

Henry Ward Beecher (1813–1887) is still famous today as a theologically liberal Congregationalist clergyman, as well as a reformer, author, and extremely lively orator. A modern-day biographer of Henry Ward Beecher calls him "the most famous man in America" of his day (Applegate, 2006). At a time before radio, television, or even respectable theatre, preachers who were great orators drew particularly large crowds and much newspaper attention. Beecher became so popular that some people referred to him as "America's St. Paul" (Boulton, 1989).

Members of his family were homeopathic advocates, including his elder sister, **Harriet Beecher Stowe**, author of *Uncle Tom's Cabin*, and his nephew, **E. Beecher Hooker, MD**,[135] a homeopathic physician and president of the American Institute of Homeopathy. Henry Ward Beecher, like many other advocates for homeopathy, was also supportive of women's right to vote, the abolitionist movement, and temperance.

Beecher served on the board of trustees for the New York Medical College for Women, a homeopathic medical college. Beecher and two leading women's right advocates, Lucretia Mott and Elizabeth Cady Stanton, each delivered commencement speeches at the colleges' first graduation in 1864.

Until this medical college built its own hospital, the women medical students were taught clinical medicine at Bellevue Hospital, then as now a conventional hospital. However, the male conventional medical students at this hospital were extremely antagonistic to women as medical students.

Thomas Starr King (1824–1864) was a Unitarian minister who was influential in California politics during the Civil War. Before moving to California in 1860, he was one of the most famous preachers in New England. During the Civil War, he spoke zealously in favor of the Union and is credited (by Abraham Lincoln) with saving California from becoming a separate republic. Starr King has even been called "the orator who saved the nation." He was inspired by men like Ralph Waldo Emerson and Henry Ward Beecher, who, like himself, had embarked on a program of self-study for the ministry, had a love of nature, and a passion for homeopathic medicine.

Thomas Starr King's homeopath was **J. N. Eckel, MD** (1823–1901) (Wendte, 1921, 216), one of the founders of the California State Homeopathic Medical Society in 1877 as well as the Hahnemann Medical College of the Pacific in 1883.

Another well-known and respected clergyman who advocated for homeopathy was **Phillips Brooks** (1835–1893), who was the bishop of Massachusetts in the Episcopal Church (Coulter, 1973, III, 317).

Australian and Asian Clergy

Bishop Rosendo Salvado (1814–1900) was a Benedictine priest from Spain who came to Australia after a short stay in England and who may have been the first person to use and prescribe homeopathic medicines in Australia. He lived outside of Perth in Western Australia, was consecrated as a bishop of Port Victoria in 1848, and was granted the title of Lord Abbot of New Norcia for life in 1867. Salvado was reputed to have treated the aboriginals with homeopathy as early as 1857 (Treuherz, 2006). He established a monastery, a pastoral and agricultural community, and schools. A museum in New Norcia near Perth has the bishop's twenty-eight homeopathic books and his homeopathic medicine kit.

The Melbourne Homeopathic Hospital was the first homeopathic hospital in the Southern hemisphere. Its precursor, the Melbourne

Homeopathic Dispensary, was strongly supported by the heads of the Anglican and Catholic churches of Melbourne, including the Anglican dean of Melbourne, the **Very Reverend Hussey Burgh Macartney**, and the lord bishop of Melbourne, the **Right Reverend Charles Perry**. Bishop Perry was appointed the hospital's patron. His enthusiastic support for homeopathy was the direct result of having been treated in England by Australia's first homeopath, **Dr. Stephen Simpson**. In 1870 Perry reported that he had used homeopathic medicines for the thirty-three years. In 1837 he was a confirmed invalid, and yet, after treatment from Dr. Simpson, he experienced a complete cure, and he attributed these results to God's blessing and homeopathic treatment (www.homeopathyoz.org).

Baptist clergyman **Benjamin Wilson** (1823–1878) studied homeopathic medicine in England, with the goal of becoming a medical missionary. In 1858 he traveled to Brisbane, in response to a published letter seeking a clergyman to take charge of a Baptist church there. On the voyage to Australia he treated many conditions using homeopathic medicines, and apparently his treatments were more successful than those of the ship's doctor. He was Brisbane's first Baptist minister and first medical missionary. He practiced homeopathy and treated members of his congregation as well as the general population. He frequently acted as *locum tenens* (a professional who temporarily fulfills the duties of another) for Brisbane doctors.

Gladstone Clarke, a Christian missionary in China, wrote a short homeopathic manual for missionaries in 1925, which includes an introduction by a distinguished British homeopathic physician, **Dr. Edwin Neatby**, who himself wrote a manual for missionaries (Treuherz, 2006).

Jewish Support

In addition to references in the Bible, one can also find references to homeopathic healing in the Talmud, the authoritative text of Jewish traditions and a record of discussions by rabbis of Jewish law, ethics, customs, and stories. The Talmud sometimes provides medical advice, as, for example, in the treatment of people with rabies. It suggests that people who are bitten by a rabid dog eat the liver of that dog as a treatment, a treatment that is ultimately based on the homeopathic principle of similars (the Talmud, Yoma 83A, Mishnah).

The Talmud also asserts an insight that is part of the hermetic tradition: "the things above are as the things below." This dynamic between the macrocosm and the microcosm is also an integral part of homeopathic thinking and practice as it links the physical state of a person with his or her inner psychological state.

A nineteenth-century Talmudic scholar, **Rabbi Ishmael**, wrote: "Man does not heal with the same thing with which he wounds, but he wounds with a knife and heals with a plaster. The Holy One, blessed be He, however, is not so, but He heals with the very same thing with which He smites" (Lauterbach, 1976). Although this statement makes a classic reference to the homeopathic principle of similars (using small doses of whatever might cause a disease to cure it), this understanding about healing is generally a part of certain esoteric traditions in Judaism rather than its mainstream traditions. This may explain why the rabbis who were known appreciators of homeopathy, listed below, tended to be of less "mainstream" Jewish traditions.

Rabbi Menachem Mendel Schneerson (1902–1994), referred to by his followers as The Rebbe, was a prominent Orthodox Jewish rabbi who was the seventh and last rebbe (spiritual leader) of the Chabad Lubavitch branch of Hasidic Judaism. Living to a ripe old age, The Rebbe was a great appreciator of homeopathy and used it throughout the latter part of his life.

Rabbi Manis Friedman (1946–) is a biblical scholar recognized for his knowledge of Jewish mysticism. In 1971, he founded Bais Chana Institute of Jewish Studies in Minnesota, the world's first yeshiva exclusively for women, where he continues to serve as dean. During 1984–1990 he served as simultaneous translator for the Lubavitcher Rebbe's televised talks (his work here explains how The Rebbe got introduced to homeopathy). Rabbi Friedman is passionate enough about homeopathy that he speaks about it regularly in his lectures, and he considers homeopathic philosophy to be perfectly compatible with Jewish thought and practice.

Rabbi Mikhael Abuhatzeira, a scion of the famous Rabbinic Kabbalist Abuhhatzeira family (the most famous of which was **Rabbi Yisrael Abuhatzeira**, known as the Baba-Sali), was a well-known naturopath-nutritionist, who lived in the town of Netivoth, Israel. Along with diets and green clay, he often prescribed homeopathic remedies.

Rabbi Shlomo Carlebach (1925–1994) was a Jewish religious singer, composer, and self-styled rebbe who was known as "the singing rabbi." Although his original training was traditional orthodox Judaism, he created his own movement combining Hasidic-style warmth and personal interaction, public concerts, and song-filled synagogue services. In an interview published after his death, he noted the similarity in approaches between homeopathy and religion: "I once met a homeopath, and he told me the difference between conventional medicine and homeopathy is that medicine works from outside to inside, homeopathy works from inside to outside. That's the whole thing, religion has to work from inside to outside" (Carlebach, 1997).

Homeopathy was not just popular among Jews who were orthodox or interested in the Kabbalah but by many reform Jews too. **Rabbi Max Lilienthal** (1815–1882) was a highly respected German rabbi who was asked to come to Russia to start a Jewish school. He created such an impressive institution that Emperor Nicholas asked him to create more schools and showed his appreciation for his work by giving him a diamond ring. Lilienthal moved to the United States in 1844 and soon became chief rabbi at three New York congregations. He became a professor at Hebrew Union College and founded the Rabbinical Literary Association of America, which published *The Hebrew Review* (a quarterly journal). Rabbi Lilienthal and Rabbi Isaac M. Wise (1819–1900) were the leading rabbis who helped create the American reform Jewish movement (Ruben, 2003).

Rabbi Lilienthal was the brother of **Samuel Lilienthal, MD** (1815–1891), a German homeopath who also came to America. Dr. Lilienthal was editor of one of the most respected homeopathic journals, *The North American Journal of Homeopathy;* he was president of the New York Homeopathic Medical Society, a professor at the New York Homeopathic

Medical College, and chair of clinical medicine at the New York Medical College and Hospital for Women.[136]

Muslim Clerics' Support

Homeopathy also has a place, even a very important place, among certain clerics of the Muslim faith.

Mirza Tahir Ahmad (1928–2003), the most recent caliph (spiritual leader) of the Ahmadiyya movement in Islam, was a practitioner of homeopathy. The Ahmadiyya Muslim Community is a religious organization that was initially founded in India. It is international in its scope, with branches in more than 178 countries in Africa, North America, South America, Asia, Australasia, and Europe. At present, its total membership exceeds 10 million worldwide.

Mirza Tahir Ahmad embraced homeopathy early in his life and studied it in great detail. Initially, he suffered from severe migraine headaches until his father prescribed a homeopathic medicine for him. After Mirza Tahir Ahmad began studying homeopathy, he treated his wife, who had been suffering from a chronic ailment, with the homeopathic medicine *Natrum mur*. She never experienced this problem again in her life.

Mirza Tahir Ahmad treated thousands of people homeopathically, especially when the community's annual convention was held in Rabwah, Pakistan, where more than 250,000 people gathered regularly. Mirza Tahir Ahmad's contributions to homeopathy in the fifty-plus years of his practice also included lectures on homeopathy on MTA International, the global satellite channel of the Ahmadiyya Community, during 1994–1997. No other homeopath to date can claim such extensive dissemination of homeopathic thought and practice. He gave 198 lectures on homeopathy that were broadcast live to millions around the world. A compilation of the lectures was published in English and contains more than 700 pages of mostly homeopathic *materia medica* (descriptions of hundreds of homeopathic medicines and their indications); it is available online (Ahmad, 2005).

In addition to writing and speaking about homeopathy, Mirza Tahir Ahmad was instrumental in helping to establish thousands of free homeopathic clinics around the world, from the remote areas in the African continent to Pakistan's biggest cities.

One of the strict teachings of this Muslim community is that Jihad ("struggle" or "Holy war") can only be used to protect against extreme religious persecution, not as a political weapon or an excuse for rulers to invade neighboring territories. The official website (www.alislam.org) for this Muslim community highlights at their homepage "Love for all; Hatred for none." Although many mainstream Muslims consider the Ahmadiyya community to be heretical (for reasons that have nothing to do with their interest in homeopathy), it is one of the fastest growing movements in Islam.

Tuan Guru Dato' Haji Nik Abdul Aziz Nik Mat (1931–) is a Malaysian cleric and an opposition politician from the Islamic Party of Malaysia (PAS). He is perceived as an Ulema (a Muslim scholar) and is currently the PAS commissioner and the Menteri Besar (chief minister) of Kelantan state in Malaysia. Earlier, he started a homeopathic medical school and hospital, and has been known to give keynote addresses to homeopathic colleges and conferences in his country.

Sir Syed Ahmed Khan Bahadur (1817–1898) was not formally trained as a Muslim cleric, but played a seminal role in pioneering modern education for the Muslim community in India. He founded the Aligarh Muslim University, which still exists and flourishes today with 30,000 students. He was a reformer who launched a movement for science and technology and opposed violence almost a century before Gandhi did.

Khan established a homeopathic hospital in Varanasi (then called Benaras) in 1867. He also wrote numerous articles about homeopathy, including a famous one chronicling the successful use of homeopathic medicines in the treatment of cholera. In 1869, Khan traveled to England, where he was awarded the Order of the Star of India from the British government. In 1888 he was knighted by the British government.

Eastern Spiritual Leaders

The *Mahabharata* is one of the two major Sanskrit texts of ancient India (the other being the *Ramayana*). Written as early as the fifth century BC and completed by the fifth century AD, this epic text has more than 74,000 verses, plus long prose passages, or almost two million words in total, making it one of the longest poems ever published. The *Mahabharata* is also of significant religious and philosophical importance in India, in part due to its inclusion of the *Bhagavad Gita,* which is an essential text of Hinduism.

The *Mahabharata* includes references to and stories of *visa cikitsa,* the use of poisons as treatment. Lord Krishna, the heroic warrior and teacher who was worshiped by Hindus as an incarnation of God, was thought to be the originator of *visa cikitsa.* While the use of poisons, especially venoms from snakes and spiders, was common for many centuries, more recently the treatment purposes of such substances has been neglected. However, one story from the *Mahabharata* involves a member of a warring group called the Kauravas who gave poison to Bhima, a warrior who people initially declared to be dead, but after being given injections of poison, was brought back to life.

Another ancient Sanskrit text called the *Bhagwat Purana* provides additional support to homeopathic thinking and practice: "Is it not true that when a substance taken by a living being causes an ailment the same substance when prescribed in a special manner removes a similar ailment?" (Kishore, 1983).

The Hindu poet Kalidasa, believed to have lived sometime between 1 BC and the fifth century, wrote in his poem *Sringara Tilaka:* "It has been heard of old time in the world that poison is the remedy for poison."

The British brought homeopathy to India in the nineteenth century, and many German immigrants also helped to spread it there. Homeopathy is in accord with the spiritualism of India, which respects the wisdom of the body and acknowledges an energetic essence to life, and which led to widespread acceptance of homeopathy. In fact, there are more than 100 five-year homeopathic medical colleges in India today. It is therefore not surprising that many of India's most respected spiritual leaders have expressed interest in and support for homeopathic medicine.

Ramakrishna Paramahamsa (1836–1886) was one of the most

important Hindu religious leaders. The renaissance that Hinduism experienced in the nineteenth century is often attributed to Ramakrishna's important work. Sri Ramakrishna was treated by the first medical doctor in India to become a homeopath, **Mahendra Lal Sircar, MD** (1833–1904).[137] Sri Ramakrishna and Dr. Sircar later engaged in a famous dialogue on spirituality and modern science, which is still quoted today.

Belur Math is a monastery for monks of the Ramakrishna Order. One of the ways this monastery serves the community is as a charitable dispensary, providing homeopathic medicines to poor people.

One of Ramakrishna's most illustrious disciples was **Swami Vivekananda** (1863–1902), considered one of the most influential spiritual leaders of the Vedanta philosophy (Hinduism). Many people associate him with Hinduism as they associate the Buddha with Buddhism and Christ with Christianity. Swami Vivekananda spoke at the renowned 1893 World's Parliament of Religions conference in Chicago, and he was the first Hindu to address a gathering of religious leaders in America. Prior to this speech, British missionaries had considered Hinduism to be a "heathen" religion. Vivekananda's speech and visit to America is commonly considered the West's first introduction to Hinduism. Because Vivekananda held degrees in both science and philosophy, he was able to speak to the West in a way that made his different but respectable spiritual path understandable.

Swami Vivekananda once said: "An allopath comes and treats cholera patients and gives them his medicines. The homeopath comes and gives his medicines and cures perhaps more than the allopath does because the homoeopath does not disturb the patients but allows the nature to deal with them" (Vivekananda, 2003). In India today, there is a Swami Vivekananda Homeopathic Medical College and Hospital in the state of Gujarat.

When George Harrison met Ravi Shankar, Ravi taught him how to play the sitar, but he also introduced him to other important teachings, including the work of Swami Vivekananda. This is thought to have been George Harrison's introduction to Hinduism, which later became quite strong in his life. As discussed in Chapter 7, Musicians, Shankar's and Vivekananda's teachings may have provided some entree to homeopathic medicine too.

Many years after the Swami's death, the literary great Rabindranath Tagore asserted: "If you want to know India, study Vivekananda. In him everything is positive and nothing negative" (www.wikipedia.org). Swamiji was a very good singer and used to sing lots of *bhajans,* including about twelve written and composed by Tagore.

Sri Aurobindo (1872–1950) was an Indian nationalist, scholar, poet, mystic, evolutionary philosopher, yogi, guru, and advocate of homeopathy. He once said: "I have noted almost constantly that (homeopathic remedies) have a surprising effect, sometimes instantaneous, sometimes rapid.... The Mother and I have no preference for allopathy." He went on to express serious concern about conventional medicine: "Medical science has been more a curse to mankind than a blessing. It has broken the force of epidemics and unveiled a marvelous surgery, but also, it has weakened the natural health of man and multiplied individual diseases; it has implanted fear and dependence in the mind and body; it has taught our health to repose not on natural soundness but a rickety and distasteful crutch." In comparison, he said that homeopathic medicines "can strike at the psychophysical root" of disease (Aurobindo, 1969).

One of Sri Aurobindo's close disciples was a homeopath, **Bhumananda**, author of *A Few Sips of the Nectar-Ocean of Homeopathy* (published by Sri Chinmoy, undated). Sri Aurobindo is quoted as saying, "Homeopathy is nearer to yoga (than any other therapy)."

Sri Aurobindo's closest collaborator and ultimate successor was **Mirra Richard**, who became known as **The Mother** (1878–1973). The Mother was instrumental in creating a spiritual community and city in Pondicherry, India, called Aurobindo. When discussing the health care provided in Aurobindo, she said, "We have been able to work through homeopathy far better than through anything else" (Sarkar, 1968).

Meher Baba (1894–1969) was an Indian master of Persian descent who declared that he was an avatar (incarnation of God in human form). Although he maintained silence for forty-four years, Meher Baba traveled throughout the world communicating by means of an alphabet board and later through unique hand gestures. He is most commonly remembered for his quote, "Don't worry, be happy," which was made popular by a Bobby McFerrin song in 1988.[138]

From the 1920s homeopathy was practiced by several of his intimate disciples, including his brother **Adi S. Irani**, **Dr. Abdhul Ghani Munsiff**, and **Padri** (Fardoon Driver). Meher Baba stated: "Homeopathy is a perfect science. It can bring the dead back to life (meaning it may succeed even in cases considered terminal), but it requires a master of that science" (Street, 2007). In 1936, under Meher Baba's supervision, the Meher Free Dispensary was created in Meherabad India, dispensing homeopathic medicines free to all who sought treatment. Thousands of patients were successfully treated for a variety of acute and chronic diseases including typhoid, malaria, dysentery, tuberculosis, asthma, arthritis, and numerous skin problems. Meher Free Dispensary is still functioning today under the auspices of the Avatar Meher Baba Perpetual Public Charitable Trust. Presently four homeopathic practitioners treat about fifty patients each day, including an American, **Robert Street**, who received his homeopathic training under several of Meher Baba's disciples.

Madame Helena Blavatsky (1831–1891) was the founder of the Theosophical Society, one of the first and leading Western organizations to explore Eastern spirituality. She was so confident of homeopathic medicines' powerful therapeutic value that she predicted in 1882: "Homeopathy is on the eve of being demonstrated as the most potent of curative agents. Figures cannot lie" (Blavatsky, vol. IV, 71).

Madame Blavatsky maintained a high amount of respect for hypnosis (called Mesmerism at the time), along with homeopathy. She asserted:

> If in each of our [organization's] branches we were able to establish a homeopathic dispensary with the addition of mesmeric healing, such as has already been done with great success in Bombay, we might contribute towards putting the science of medicine in this country on a sounder basis, and be the means of incalculable benefit to the people at large. (Blavatsky, vol. VI, 331)

When just a teenager, **Jiddu Krishnamurti** (1895–1986) was discovered by C. W. Leadbeater (1854–1934) of the Theosophical Society, and within a couple of years, both Leadbeater and fellow leading theosophist Annie Besant (1847–1933) raised him under their tutelage, believing that he was the prophesied "world teacher." However, Krishnamurti disavowed this destiny, and typical of the teacher that he became, his message was that people should be responsible for their own teaching and guidance to spiritual awareness. In 1984, he was awarded the United Nations Peace Medal.

According to his longtime personal secretary, Krishnamurti had great respect for homeopathic medicine. However, when a well-known homeopath who was treating him at the time asked for a statement of support for homeopathy and for acknowledgment of his skills as a homeopath, Krishnamurti emphatically denied him because he simply didn't want to promote any specific health strategies nor did he want to promote individual homeopaths.

J. G. Bennett (1897–1974) was a British mathematician, scientist, technologist, industrial research director, and author. He is here, along with Eastern spiritual leaders, because he is best known for his many books on psychology and spirituality, and especially the teachings of **G. I. Gurdjieff** (1872?–1949). Although Gurdjieff was Greek and Armenian, his teachings had an Eastern orientation. Bennett was instrumental in disseminating information about the teachings and work of Gurdjieff as well as about the Sufi teachings of Idries Shah (1924–1996). Bennett was also passionate about homeopathy, even writing the foreword to a book on homeopathy by **Dr. Chandra Sharma**, the homeopath to George Harrison, Tina Turner, and other musicians. In the foreword Bennett wrote: "The study of homeopathy has greatly helped me personally to understand better the connection between living and non-living matter." He went on to say: "The claims of homeopathy do not depend upon theory, for they are reinforced by a hundred and seventy years of successful practice and by the experience of hundreds of thousands of people who owe their health and vigour to the right use of homeopathic remedies" (Sharma, 1976, 2–3).

Swami Satchidananda (1914–2000) played an important role in popularizing yoga in the West during the 1960s and 1970s. Some of his well-known students included Allen Ginsberg, Alice Coltrane, Carol King, and Jeff Goldblum. After one of his students, artist Peter Max, invited him to New York in 1966, he continued to have a significant effect on the emerging counterculture of that era. In 1969, he was the opening speaker at the Woodstock music festival. What is less known about Swami Satchidananda is that he was trained as a homeopath earlier in life and strongly believed in its efficacy.

When I once visited some friends who lived at his ashram in Buckingham, Virginia, I was asked to give a talk on homeopathy. After completing my presentation, I left the stage, at which time I was asked to go back to the microphone because the Swami had a question for me. As I walked back to the stage, I wondered what deeply spiritual question he was going to ask me. I was therefore shocked and impressed when he posed the question: "Has homeopathy been computerized?" He was quite pleased to hear that not only has homeopathy been computerized but that there are numerous expert-system software programs that help professional homeopaths prescribe more efficiently and precisely.[139]

Swami Satchidananda was one of the teachers of yoga who believed that people can and should do spiritual practice while being fully engaged in the modern cosmopolitan world. I have been told by several of his students that besides being a teacher of yoga, he also loved to do computer programming.

Swami Muktananda (1908–1982) was the first teacher of Siddha yoga in the West. Siddha yoga involves the giving of *shaktipat* initiation, a process in which a spiritually enlightened master elicits a powerful spiritual experience by transmission of a sacred word or mantra, a look, a thought, or by touch. Muktananda was known to give his students a touch of his right hand or from a peacock feather held in his right hand, and there are innumerable accounts of people having profound experiences from his shaktipat.

A *New Yorker* story (Harris, 1994) described the numerous well-known admirers of Muktananda, including John Denver, Andre Gregory, Diana

Ross, Isabella Rossellini, Phylicia Rashad, Don Johnson, Melanie Griffith, Marsha Mason, and former California governor Jerry Brown.

In the late 1970s one of his senior students was a physician who was studying homeopathy with me. When the Swami experienced an acute respiratory infection, I was called to treat the guru. After interviewing him about his physical symptoms, I sought to assess his psychological state, which is often important in the selection of the most appropriate homeopathic medicine for him. It was, however, challenging for me as a homeopath to ask questions of a psychological nature to a guru of Muktananda's stature in a way that he could acknowledge emotional states through his translator, who was one of his students.

I was later told that the Swami got over this respiratory infection shortly after he took the remedy I prescribed for him.

Swami Rama (1925–1996), a teacher of yoga and meditation, was one of the first yogis to be examined by scientists at the Menninger Clinic. Swami Rama showed that he could control specific physiological processes in his body, including his heartbeat, blood pressure, and body temperature.

Swami Rama was formally trained in homeopathic and Ayurvedic medicine, and it is no surprise that the medical school and hospital he established in India and the clinics he started in the U.S. include homeopathic medicine as a primary treatment modality.

Yogi Bhajan (1929–2004) was another spiritual leader from India who had a special appreciation for homeopathy. Yogi Bhajan was the head of the Sikh Dharma in the western hemisphere, and he was widely known as a master and leading teacher of Kundalini yoga. Besides being very knowledgeable about homeopathy, he encouraged many of his students to become homeopaths and literally hundreds of them have done so.

Sri Chinmoy (1931–) is an Indian philosopher and spiritual teacher. Besides teaching meditation, he is also a promoter of physical fitness, having participated in and encouraged others to run marathons and ultramarathons. In the mid-1980s he began weightlifting, and one of his distinctive practices is to lift followers, celebrities, and public figures as a sign of his respect for their work. He has lifted musician Carlos Santana, jazzman John McLaughlin, South African leaders Desmond Tutu and Nelson Mandela, and Olympic gold medalist Carl Lewis. In 2003, he lifted several homeopaths, including Roger Morrison, MD, Nancy Herrick, PA, Jacquelyn Wilson, MD, and me.

His organization sponsors various marathons and ultramarathons, including the world's longest certified road race (over 3,000 miles). These ultra-long-distance road races are famous in the running community for how well they take care of participants, including trackside medical tents where most of the medicines dispensed are homeopathic.

Sri Chinmoy has authored hundreds of books, including one about Sri Ramakrishna's homeopath-disciple, and a short story called "The Kind-Hearted Homeopath."

Colleges and Hospitals

In the United States, some clergymen and churches were such advocates of homeopathic medicine that they created medical schools to teach it. Between 1851 and 1854, a future U.S. President **James Garfield** (1831–1881) and his wife Lucretia were both students at the Western Reserve Eclectic Institute.[140] The Disciples of Christ (today, called the Christian Church) founded this college in Hiram, Ohio, in 1850. Garfield and his wife became lifelong advocates of homeopathy and natural medicine.

Garfield ultimately graduated from Williams College in 1856, but he returned to the Eclectic Institute to teach. A classical scholar, Garfield taught Greek and Latin, as well as mathematics and geology. He became the college's president, and significantly expanded the curriculum, which helped make the college successful. He changed its name to Hiram College, the name it still carries today.

Garfield was also a minister and an elder for the Church of Christ, making him the first preacher and only member of the Church of Christ to serve as president. When he became president of the United States, he was forced to relinquish his eldership. He did so, saying, "I resign the highest office in the land to become President of the United States."

Chicago Baptist Hospital, the largest denominational hospital in Chicago in the late 1800s, had an entirely homeopathic staff (Karst, 1988,

18). Also, the pastor of Pittsburgh's Presbyterian Church commented on the important work of his city's homeopathic hospital, noting that it provided more effective treatment and at a cheaper price:

> This hospital not only expresses in its work Christian thought and feeling and belief, but expresses it effectively —economically, because it has maintained its patients at a cost per week of less than the average estimate set down by competent judges of first-class city hospitals—effectively, because, again, out of every one hundred treated, the number of those that have died, as shown by figures, is not only within, but actually below the average. (Rosenberg, 1987, 266)

The Good Samaritan Hospital, the first Protestant hospital in St. Louis, was founded in 1856 and staffed entirely by homeopathic doctors. The forty-room building had space for 120 patients, though at times during the Civil War as many as 250 soldiers were hospitalized there. **Edward C. Franklin, MD** (1822–1885), the esteemed surgeon and homeopath, was on staff at this hospital in its early years.[141] In 1902 the staff was completely reorganized with the appointment of allopathic (conventional) physicians.

In 1865 St. Luke's Infirmary was established in St. Louis as a Protestant hospital through the initiative of the Young Men's Christian Association (YMCA). Its founders determined that a large number of the "most upright, wealthy, and influential members of the Protestant Episcopal Church" were advocates of homeopathy. The executive committee resolved that a portion of the hospital should be established for patients who preferred homeopathic treatment (Proceedings, 1866, 47).

At that time, there were two other hospitals in St. Louis: City Hospital (allopathic) and Post Hospital (homeopathic). In order for the Good Samaritan Hospital to determine whether to provide homeopathic or allopathic care, the hospital's board sought to evaluate the death rates in the two other larger hospitals in St. Louis. Statistics from these hospitals uncovered a death rate of 37.2 percent for those who sought conventional/

allopathic treatment and a 1.1 percent death rate for those who sought homeopathic treatment (Proceedings, 1866, 48). These statistics included the four leading causes of death at that time (dysentery, typhoid, diarrhea, and pneumonia), and there were substantially better results for all four conditions for homeopathic patients.

When conventional physicians in St. Louis heard that the new St. Luke's Infirmary might have a homeopathic ward, they decided that they would not participate in this hospital, and they insisted that the executive committee choose either conventional or homeopathic approaches. The power of the majority number of physicians was able to influence the committee to rescind its offer to the homeopaths.

Mary Baker Eddy

The story of Mary Baker Eddy (1821–1910) is highlighted here because of the influence she had and continues to have on health and spirituality and because of her longtime use of and appreciation for homeopathic medicines.

Eddy was chronically ill as a child until reaching middle age. She was married at 22, though her first husband died within a year of marriage. As a strong-minded single woman, Mary apparently attended the famous First Woman's Rights Convention at Seneca Falls in 1848, organized by feminists Elizabeth Cady Stanton and Susan B. Anthony (Miller, 2000). Whether Mary herself was a feminist isn't clear, but she didn't accept her frail physical health and actively sought to overcome it. She was sharply critical of the orthodox medicine of her day and instead studied and used homeopathic medicines, hydrotherapy, and nutrition. She even became a homeopath, though there is no record of her attending a homeopathic college, even though the New England Female Medical College had opened in Boston in 1848.

In 1853 she married Daniel Patterson, a dentist and homeopath (Watchman Fellowship, no date), and although there is no record of him graduating from a homeopathic medical school, there is a record of them practicing and traveling together in small towns in New England. Patterson deserted her in 1866, and they ultimately divorced in 1873.

In the 1860s she began to explore faith-healing and to study with Phineas Quimby (1902–1866), who used theological ideas and mental healing. She was even known to lecture on the "Quimby method." Although there is an obvious similarity between his ideas and the ideas that Mary Baker Eddy developed into Christian Science healing, advocates for Christian Science disavow any connection, saying that Quimby's work was more Mesmerism-based (hypnotic) than Christian.

In 1866, she suffered a spinal injury when she fell on an icy street. She was able to heal herself by relying on the Bible as a source of inspiration and guidance. She recovered fully, and went forward to teach and heal this new method, which she called Christian Science healing.

In 1888, Mary Baker Eddy and her third husband (Asa G. Eddy) legally adopted Ebenezer J. Foster-Eddy, MD, an 1869 graduate of the famed homeopathic school, Hahnemann Medical College of Philadelphia. Initially, he followed her Christian Science teachings until 1897 when they broke all ties to each other.

Mary Baker Eddy's major book on her work was *Science and Health with Key to the Scriptures* (1875, updated in 1910), and it was the culmination of her own lifelong search for a spiritual system of healing.

Eddy made numerous references to homeopathic medicine in her famous book. Vehemently antagonistic to conventional medicine (as she was earlier in life too), she noted homeopathy's considerable differences:

> Evidences of progress and of spiritualization greet us on every hand. Drug-systems are quitting their hold on matter and so letting in matter's higher stratum, mortal mind. Homeopathy, a step in advance of allopathy, is doing this. Matter is going out of medicine; and mortal mind, of a higher attenuation than the drug, is governing the pellet. (Eddy, 1875, 158:24)

She felt that she had discovered a rule to healing in an understanding of God as the divine principle above the limitations of a material sense of reality she termed "error." She wrote: "Error produces error, sin and sickness, for both are errors of belief, and what causes disease cannot cure it, unless it be the homeopathic dose where matter is destroyed and mind says this" (Eddy, 1891, 375).

Eddy assumed that homeopathic medicines must work through the mind because her nontechnical mind had no other explanation for how it could work.

> Homeopathy diminishes the drug, but the potency of the medicine increases as the drug disappears. Metaphysics, as taught in Christian Science, is the next stately step beyond homeopathy. In metaphysics, matter disappears from the remedy entirely, and Mind takes its rightful and supreme place. Homeopathy takes mental symptoms largely into consideration in its diagnosis of disease. Christian Science deals wholly with the mental cause in judging and destroying disease. (Eddy, 1875, 155:25)

In explaining the homeopathic principle of similars, Eddy wrote:

> Homeopathy furnishes the evidence to the senses, that symptoms, which might be produced by a certain drug, are removed by using the same drug which might cause the symptoms. This confirms my theory that faith in the drug is the sole factor in the cure. The effect, which mortal mind produces through one belief, it removes through an opposite belief, but it uses the same medicine in both cases. (Eddy, 1875, 370:12)

Ultimately, she never explained how homeopathic medicine can be effective in treating different animals as well as babies, let alone how it can cure those who didn't initially believe in it (or in the healing power of the Bible).

While Mary Baker Eddy discouraged the use of all medicines and advocated the placement of one's complete faith in God, she was known to receive homeopathic treatment secretly from **Frederick S. Keith, MD**, a respected classical homeopath who had studied with **James Tyler Kent, MD**, one of America's leading homeopaths at that time (Winston, 1999, 344).[142]

She founded Massachusetts Metaphysical College in Boston in 1882 to provide formal training in her teachings. The college closed in 1889 and was replaced by her church's board of education. Because so many women became Christian Science practitioners, Eddy's movement provided independence and a self-sufficient income for many women during a time when most were dependent on the men around them. This fact in part explains why so many suffragists were supportive of her work.

In 1908, at the age of 87, she founded *The Christian Science Monitor*, a daily newspaper devoted to balanced reporting, as distinct from the sensational, "yellow" journalism that was common at that time (and today too).

Mother Teresa

Mother Teresa (1910–1997) studied homeopathic medicine with **Dr. Diwan Jai Chand** (1887–1961), a highly respected Indian homeopath whose two sons and grandson are also leaders of Indian homeopathy. Mother Teresa told others that she would not do a "physician's prescribing" (that is, she would not treat people with chronic or potentially fatal illnesses) but instead would use homeopathy in many first aid situations.

According to a report from a conventional physician who worked closely with Mother Teresa from 1945 through at least 1988, the Mother "believes that homeopathic treatment is indispensable for the poor and distressed people of India in particular, [and] all other countries of the world in general, for its easy approach, effectiveness, and low cost" (Gomes, 1988). Mother Teresa's mission opened a charitable homeopathic dispensary in Calcutta in 1950 and it is reported that the Mother prescribed homeopathic medicines herself and assisted homeopathic physicians.

Emanuel Swedenborg

Emanuel Swedenborg (1688–1772) was a Swedish scientist, philosopher, mystic, and theologian. He had a prolific career as an inventor and scientist. Among the famous people who were inspired by Swedenborg are: Tennyson, Goethe, Thoreau, Blake, Emerson, James, Baudelaire, de Balzac, Dostoyevsky, Pound, Strindberg, and Jorge Luis Borges (Treuherz, 1984). Further, the American transcendentalism movement in the nineteenth century, a spiritual movement that drew many of the great writers in America's New England, was profoundly influenced by Swedenborg's philosophy. Some of the New England transcendentalists who became "Swedenborgians" included Thoreau, Longfellow, William Lloyd Garrison, Elizabeth Peabody, Theodore Parker, Bronson Alcott, and Louisa May Alcott. More recently, Helen Keller was a Swedenborgian. Very few people in history have influenced so many and such diverse cultural heroes.

Swedenborg was one of the few intellectuals who was well-schooled in the sciences and in theology. Swedenborg's concept of God was that of a spiritual essence that flowed through all things. He believed there was a fundamental and mystical correspondence that existed between the spiritual world and our material world. He taught that the human's form and function (microcosm) had been modeled on the spiritual higher reality (macrocosm). Everything that existed and happened in this higher world was reflected by its counterpart existing in the worldly reality on earth. This concept of "correspondences" (also more popularly referred to as the concept "as above, so below, and as below, so above") is ancient and is a part of the alchemical tradition.

It didn't take long for the followers of Swedenborg to discover that homeopathy was a new scientific medicine that embodied the vitalistic tradition,[143] which was an integral part of Swedenborgian thought. Also, homeopaths prescribed a medicine from the natural world for its correspondence in causing the similar symptoms that the sick person was having.

Well-known followers of both Swedenborg and homeopathy included Hans B. Gram, MD (America's first homeopath), Constantine Hering, MD ("father of American homeopathy"), the Boericke and Tafel families (owners of the largest manufacturer of homeopathic medicines, a company still alive today under different ownership), Mary Florence Taft, MD (respected homeopath and cousin of President William Taft), and James Tyler Kent, MD (leading American teacher of homeopathy).

John James Garth Wilkinson, MD (1812–1899), a homeopathic physician who trained at the Hahnemann Medical College of Philadelphia, was introduced to the work of Swedenborg by his friend Henry James, Sr., the influential publisher of a newspaper of utopian ideas and father of the American writers William James and Henry James, Jr. Wilkinson, who was also a widely knowledgeable scholar, began translating Swedenborg's work (which Henry James, Sr. financed), and Wilkinson's work is known to have helped create the Swedenborg movement (Treuherz, 1984).

Emerson lectured on Swedenborg for several years, and in 1850 he published his lecture "Swedenborg the Mystic" in *Representative Men*, which also included biographies of Plato, Montaigne, Shakespeare, Napoleon, and Goethe. In another book, Emerson eloquently wrote:

> Wilkinson, the editor of Swedenborg, the annotator of Fourier [the French utopianist], and the champion of Hahnemann, has brought to metaphysics and to physiology a native vigor, with a catholic perception of relations, equal to the highest attempts, and a rhetoric like the armory of the invincible knights of old. There is in the action of his mind a long Atlantic roll not known except in deepest waters, and only lacking what ought to accompany such powers, a manifest centrality. If his mind does not rest in immovable biases, perhaps the orbit is larger, and the return is not yet: but a master should inspire a confidence that he will adhere to his convictions, and give his present studies always the same high place. (Emerson, 1856)

Later, Emerson wrote that Swedenborg "saw and showed the connections between nature and the affections of the soul. He pierced the emblematic or spiritual character of the visible, audible, tangible world. ... The importance of the Swedenborgian attraction lay in its thrust ... towards an ordered and predictable universe, towards a synthesis of matter and spirit" (Emerson, 1903, 113).

Homeopathic and Swedenborgian thought maintained a similar critique of orthodox medicine. Both viewpoints saw orthodox medicine as treating the external effect of the disease process, not the deeper internal sources (Treuherz, 1984).

Constantine Hering, MD, a homeopath and a Swedenborgian, was the type of person and teacher who didn't like to mix his understanding of medicine and science with his spirituality. This may explain why Hering once said, "While there is good reason why Swedenborgians might prefer homeopathic treatment, there is none at all that all homeopaths be Swedenborgians" (Peebles, 1988, 468–472).

James Tyler Kent, MD (1849–1916), may have had the greatest influence on homeopathic practice in America, second only to Samuel Hahnemann. Kent was also strongly influenced by Swedenborg. One homeopath asserted that Kent's homeopathic thinking was a mixture of Hahnemann's and Swedenborg's ideas. Swedenborg recognized different levels or degrees of the human experience, and he considered the spiral to be the connecting structure that links the various levels of experience. Swedenborg's idea that became a part of Kentian homeopathics was the recognition that the deepest part of a person is the soul, which manifests in a person's will. Outward from a person's will, according to Swedenborg, is human reason, intellect, and intention. Farther outward is a person's memory and desires, and still farther is the human body, each part with varying degrees of depth.

Kent utilized these ideas by his pronunciations that a person's "will and understanding" is the deepest part of a person's health and that the various emotions represent the next layer outward from the deepest part of the person's being, both of which have a dynamic interaction back and forth into the physical body.

References

Ahmad, M. T. *Homoeopathy: Like Cures Like.* Tilford, UK: Islam International Publications, 2005. Available at www.alislam.org

Applegate, D. *The Most Famous Man in America: The Biography of Henry Ward Beecher.* New York: Doubleday, 2006.

Aurobindo, S. Sri Aurobindo on Medical Science, *Orissa State Homoeopathy Board Journal,* August 1969, 2(3).

Blavatsky, Madame H. *Complete Works,* vol IV, Another Orthodox Prosecution, 1882–1883. Available at http://collectedwritings.net/

Blavatsky, Madame H. *Complete Works,* vol. VI, Spiritual Progress, 1883–1885. Available at http://collectedwritings.net/

Boulton, A. O. The Gothic Awakening, *American Heritage Magazine,* November 1989, 40(7).

Bradford, T. L. *The Life and Letters of Samuel Hahnemann.* Philadelphia: Boericke and Tafel, 1895.

Carlebach, S. Practical Wisdom from Shlomo Carlebach, *Tikkun Magazine,* Fall 1997, 5758 (Jewish year).

Clarke, J. *Homoeopathy Explained.* London: Homoeopathic Publishing Company, 1905. Available at http://homeoint.org/books5/clarkehomeo/statistics.htm

Coulter, H. L. *Divided Legacy: A History of the Schism in Medical Thought.* Vol. III: The Conflict Between Homeopathy and the AMA. Berkeley: North Atlantic Books, 1973.

Davies, A. History of MSM—Homeopathy and Natural Medicines, *Homeopathy,* 2007, 96:52–59.

Dean, M. E. *The Trials of Homeopathy.* Essen, Germany: KVC, 2004.

Eddy, M. B. *Science and Health with Key to the Scriptures.* Boston: First Church of Christ, Scientist, 1875 (updated 1910).

Eddy, M. B. *Retrospection and Introspection.* Boston: First Church of Christ, Scientist, 1891.

Emerson, R. W. *Representative Men.* 1850. Available at http://www.rwe.org/comm/index.php?option=com_content&task=view&id=145&Itemid=145

Emerson, R. W. *English Traits,* Chapter XIV, 1856. Available at www.rwe.org/works/English_Traits_Chapter_XIV_Literature.htm

Emerson, R. W. *The American Scholar, Complete Works.* 1903, Vol. 1.

Everest, Rev. T. R. *A Popular View of Homeopathy.* New York: William Radde, 1842.

Frass, M., Dielacher, C., Linkesch, M., Endler, C., Muchitsch, I., Schuster, E., and Kaye, A. Influence of Potassium Dichromate on Tracheal Secretions in Critically Ill Patients, *Chest,* March 2005a.

Frass, M., Linkesch, M., Banjya, S., et al. Adjunctive Homeopathic Treatment in Patients with Severe Sepsis: A Randomized, Double-Blind, Placebo-Controlled Trial in an Intensive Care Unit, *Homeopathy,* 2005b, vol. 94, pp. 75–80.

Galéazzi-Lisi, R. *Dans l'ombre et dans la Lumiere de Pie XII.* Paris: Flammarion, 1960.

Gomes, Dr. (Sister). Personal communication, October 14, 1988. (Dr. Gomes was a conventional physician whose mother's life was saved by homeopathic medicine, and thereafter, she has prescribed it to her family and patients.)

Granier, M. *Conferences upon Homeopathy.* London: Leath and Ross, 1859.

Haehl, R. *Samuel Hahnemann: His Life and Letters.* London: Homeopathic Publishing Company, 1922 (two volumes). (Reprint New Delhi: B. Jain, no date.)

Handley, R. *In Search of the Later Hahnemann.* Beaconsfield, UK: Beaconsfield Publishers, 1997.

Harris, L. O Guru, Guru, Guru, *New Yorker,* November 14, 1994.

Henderson, W. *Homoeopathy Fairly Represented.* Philadelphia: Lindsay and Blakiston, 1854.

Huber, E. History of Homeopathy in Austria, *Transactions of the American Institute of Homeopathy,* 1880, Vol. II, Part I.

Homeopathic Hassle, *Time,* August 20, 1956.

Hunt, W. F. The Condition of Homeopathy in Europe, *Transactions of the New York State Homeopathic Medical Society,* 1863, pp. 118–123.

Indian Catholic News, Muller's Adds New Homeopathic Facility, Nov 8, 2006. Available at www.theindiancatholic.com/newsread.asp?nid=4362

Jütte, R. *The Hidden Roots: A History of Homeopathy in Northern, Central and Eastern Europe.* Stuttgart: Institute for the History of Medicine, 2006.

Karst, F. Homeopathy in Illinois, *Caduceus,* Summer 1988, pp. 1–33.

Kimball, S. A. The Organon Society of Boston, *Homeopathic Physician,* vol. 2, 1888.

Kishore, J. Homeopathy: The Indian Experience, *World Health Forum,* 1983, issue 4, pp. 105–107.

Knerr, C. *Life of Hering.* Philadelphia: Magee Press, 1940.

Kotok, A. The history of homeopathy in the Russian Empire until World War I, as compared with other European countries and the USA: Similarities and discrepancies. PhD thesis submitted to the Senate of the Hebrew University of Jerusalem, November 1999. Available at http://homeoint.org/books4/kotok/index.htm

Lauterbach, J. Z. Mekilta de-Rabbi Ishmael I-III. Translated by J. Z. Lauterbach. Philadelphia: JPS (Jewish Publication Society, 1933–1936. (Reprint Philadelphia: JPS, 1976.)

Liga Medicorum Homeopathica Internationalis (LMHI). www.lmhint.net/his_italy.html

Miller, R. L. *150 Years of Healing: America's Great New Thought Healers.* Portland: Abib Publishing Company, 2000. Available at http://website.lineone.net/~newthought/150.3.htm

Morrell, P. *British Homeopathy during Two Centuries* (1999). http://homeoint.org/morrell/british/index.htm

Negro, F. *Grandi a Piccole Dosi.* Milan: Franco Angeli, 2006.

Nichols, P. A. *Homoeopathy and the Medical Profession.* London: Croom Helm, 1988.

Peebles, E. Homeopathy and the New Church, in *Emanuel Swedenborg : A Continuing Vision* (ed. R. Larsen). New York: Swedenborg Foundation, 1988.

Piterà, F. Divina omeopatia: Le falsità di Quark e la disinformazione su Vaticano e omeopatia, *Athropos & Iatria,* January–March 2001. Also available at www.mclink.it/personal/MH0077/Therapeutike/therapeutike%201/pitera%20%20divina_omeopatia.htm

Proceedings of the 19th Session of the American Institute of Homeopathy, June 6–7, 1866.

Rafinesque, C. General Report on the Rise and Progress of Homoeopathy in France, *Transactions of the American Institute of Homeopathy,* 1876, Vol II, Part I.

Rosenberg, C. E. *The Care of Strangers: The Rise of America's Hospital System.* New York: Basic Books, 1987.

Ruben, B. L. Max Lilienthal and Isaac M. Wise: Architects of American Reform Judaism, *The American Jewish Archives Journal,* 2003, 55(2):1–29.

Rutkow, L. W., and Rutkow, I. M. Homeopaths, Surgery, and the Civil War, *Archives in Surgery,* July 2004, 139:785–791.

St. John of Kronstadt. *My Life in Christ.* New York: Holy Trinity Monastery, 1911.

Sarkar. B. K. *Essays on Homeopathy.* Calcutta: Hahnemann Publishing, 1968.

Sharma, C. H. *A Manual of Homoeopathy and Natural Medicine.* New York: Dutton, 1976.

Street, R. Personal correspondence, February 22, 2007.

Thomas, B. P. *Theodore Weld: Crusader for Freedom* (1950). Available at www.gospel-truth.net/Weld/weldbioch18.htm.

Transactions of the American Institute of Homeopathy, Minutes of the AIH Meeting, Kansas City, Mo., 1908, p. 128.

Treuherz, F. The Origins of Kent's Homeopathy, *Journal of the American Institute of Homeopathy,* December 1984, 77(4):130–149.

Treuherz, F. Steiner and the Simillimum: Homeopathic and Anthroposophic Medicine: The Relationship of the Ideas of Hahnemann, Goethe and Steiner, *Journal of the American Institute of Homeopathy,* June 1985, 78(2):66–82.

Treuherz, F. Strange, Rare and Peculiar: Aborigines, Benedictines and Homeopathy. *Homeopathy,* 2006, 95(3):182–186.

Vanity Fair, May 2006, p. 90.

Vivekananda, Swami. *The Complete Works of Swami Vivekananda,* Vol. I: Raja-Yoga/Prana. Hollywood: Vedanta Press, 2003 (reprint).

Watchman Fellowship. Christian Science Profile. Available at http://www.watchman.org/profile/ChrSciProfile.htm

Wendte, C. W. *Thomas Starr King: Patriot and Preacher.* Boston: Beacon, 1921.

Winston, J. *The Faces of Homoeopathy.* Tawa, New Zealand: Great Auk, 1999.

www.wikipedia.org, Swami Vivekananda.

Yasgur, J. *Homeopathic Dictionary.* Greenville, Penn.: Van Hoy, 1998.

Homeopathic Resources

Homeopathic Organizations

National Center for Homeopathy
801 N. Fairfax #306
Alexandria, VA 22314 (703)548-7790
www.homeopathic.org

American Institute of Homeopathy
801 N. Fairfax #306
Alexandria, VA 22314 (703)548-7790
www.homeopathyusa.org

North American Society of Homeopaths
PO Box 450039
Sunrise, FL 33345-0039 (206)720-7000
www.homeopathy.org

Homeopathic Internet Sites

The following listing of sites dealing with homeopathic medicine is not meant to be complete. The sites listed were selected due to the significant amount of free information on homeopathy that each provides.

Homeopathy Home Page: www.homeopathyhome.com
This website provides a linking to various homeopathic resources and websites throughout the Internet. You can also subscribe, without cost, to a homeopathic discussion group, or access various past discussion topics by searching the table of contents. You can also find links to commercial and noncommercial sites in homeopathy (and in various languages).

The National Center for Homeopathy: www.homeopathic.org
The NCH is the leading homeopathic organization in the United States. This site includes several dozen articles plus a searchable directory for homeopaths in the U.S. It also includes information on the organization's magazine and various educational programs.

Homeopathic Educational Services: www.homeopathic.com
At this site are more than 100 articles by Dana Ullman, MPH, on homeopathic principles, self-care, professional care, clinical and laboratory research, how to use homeopathic medicines for home care of various acute ailments, and other interesting stuff. This site also contains an extensive catalogue of homeopathic books, tapes, medicines, software, and correspondence courses. They will send you a free list of homeopathic practitioners in your U.S. state upon request with any book order.

Homeopathe International: www.homeoint.org
This website has many articles in various languages. It also has a rich archives of photos of homeopaths, past and present.

Liga Medicorum Homeopathica Internationalis (LMHI):
www.lmhint.net
LMHI is an international homeopathic medical society established in 1925.

Homeopathic Online Discussion Groups
One of the good online discussion groups that primarily focus on homeopathy is called homeolist. There are 10–40 postings each day. You can subscribe it in two ways, either with each individual posting or as one long "digest" (with an initial and invaluable table of contents). I recommend the digest verson. Go to www.homeolist.com.

Also, there is some discussion at www.homeopathyhome.com.

Another online discussion on homeopathy is at minutus@yahoogroups.com.

Homeopathic History Archives: www.julianwinston.com
This site has links to an archive of information about the history of homeopathic pharmacies and their pharmacological processes. It also has

links to articles from the International Hahnemannian Association, the *Homeopathic Recorder,* and other resources.

European Council for Classical Homeopathy(ECCH):
www.homeopathy-ecch.org
If you need to find a homeopath in a European country or wish to find out about the work of the European Council for Classical Homeopathy (ECCH), which represents homeopathic professionals and their patients in Europe, please visit this website.

Suggested Reading

Introductory and Family Guidebooks
Chernin, Dennis. *The Complete Homeopathic Resource.* Berkeley: North Atlantic Books, 2006.
Cicchetti, Jane. *Dreams, Symbols, and Homeopathy: Archetypal Dimensions of Homeopathy.* Berkeley: North Atlantic Books, 2003.
Grossinger, Richard. *Homeopathy: The Great Riddle.* Berkeley: North Atlantic Books, 1998.
Kruzel, Thomas. *Homeopathic Emergency Guide.* Berkeley: North Atlantic Books, 1992.
Lansky, Amy. *Impossible Cure: The Promise of Homeopathy.* Portola Valley: RL Ranch, 2004.
Ullman, Dana. *Discovering Homeopathy: Medicine for the 21st Century.* Berkeley: North Atlantic Books, 1991.
Ullman, Dana. *The Consumer's Guide to Homeopathy.* New York: Jeremy Tarcher/Putnam, 1995.
Ullman, Dana. *Homeopathy A-Z.* Carlsbad: Hay House, 1999.
Ullman, Dana. *Essential Homeopathy.* Novato: New World Library, 2002.
Ullman, Dana. *Homeopathic Family Medicine* (an ebook that integrates practical information with updated clinical research). www.homeopathic.com
Whitmont, Edward C. *The Alchemy of Healing.* Berkeley: North Atlantic Books, 1993.

Specialized Self-Care Books
Bailey, Philip. *Homeopathic Psychology.* Berkeley: North Atlantic Books, 1995.
Castro, Miranda. *Homeopathy for Pregnancy, Birth and Your Baby's First Year.* New York: St. Martin's, 1993.
Chappell, Peter. *Emotional Healing with Homeopathy.* Berkeley: North Atlantic Books, 2003.
Hamilton, Don. *Homeopathic Care for Cats and Dogs.* Berkeley: North Atlantic Books, 1999.

Hershoff, Asa. *Homeopathy for Musculoskeletal Healing.* Berkeley: North Atlantic Books, 1996.

Lalor, Liz. *A Homeopathic Guide to Partnership and Compatibility.* Berkeley: North Atlantic Books, 2004.

Moskowitz, Richard. *Homeopathic Medicine for Pregnancy and Childbirth.* Berkeley: North Atlantic Books, 1992.

Reichenberg-Ullman, Judyth. *Whole Women Homeopathy.* Edmonds: Picnic Point, 2000.

Reichenberg-Ullman, Judyth, and Robert Ullman. *Ritalin-Free Kids.* New York: Three Rivers, 1996.

Reichenberg-Ullman, Judyth, and Robert Ullman. *The Quick and Simple Guide to Homeopathic Self-Care.* New York: Three Rivers, 1998.

Reichenberg-Ullman, Judyth, and Robert Ullman. *Prozac Free: Homeopathic Medicines for Depression, Anxiety, and Other Mental and Emotional Problems.* Berkeley: North Atlantic Books, 2002.

Subotnick, Steven. *Sports and Exercise Injuries: Conventional, Homeopathic, and Alternative Treatments.* Berkeley: North Atlantic Books, 1991.

Ullman, Dana. *Homeopathic Medicine for Children and Infants.* New York: Jeremy Tarcher/Putnam, 1992.

Homeopathic Research Texts

Bellavite, Paolo, and Signorini, Andrea. *The Emerging Science of Homeopathy: Biodynamics, Complexity, and Nanopharmacology.* Berkeley: North Atlantic Books, 2002.

Dean, Michael Emmans. *The Trials of Homeopathy.* Essen, Germany: KVC, 2004.

Ullman, Dana. *Homeopathic Family Medicine* (an ebook that integrates practical information with updated clinical research). www.homeopathic.com

Notes

Introduction

1. This fact is extremely startling, but the source is reputable: Marcia Angell, MD, is former editor of the *New England Journal of Medicine*.

2. Double-blind and placebo-controlled studies are those clinical trials in which some patients are given a medicine or treatment and others are given a fake medicine that resembles the medicine. Neither the subject nor the experimenter knows who was given which treatment until after the results are completed.

CHAPTER 1. Why Homeopathy Makes Sense and Works: Nanopharmacology at Its Best

3. Samuel Hahnemann, MD (1755–1843), a renowned German physician and chemist, was the founder of homeopathy.

4. For a historical discussion of various homeopathic drugs that have been incorporated into conventional medicine, see Dr. Harris Coulter's *Homoeopathic Influences in Nineteenth Century Allopathic Therapeutics* (1973), as well as his more detailed book on homeopathy's history, *Divided Legacy: The Conflict Between Homeopathy and the American Medical Association* (1975).

5. The Greek word *homoios* means similar, and the Greek word *pathos* means suffering; thus, homeopathy means similar suffering, through the use of very small doses of medicines to treat those specific disease syndromes that they are known to cause. The Greek word *allo* means other or different from. Therefore allopathy refers to a system of medicine that may use similars, opposites, or whatever could possibly diminish symptoms at least temporarily. Hahnemann's use of the word *allopathy* was actually derogatory because he considered it a mongrel system that was not based on any principle in nature. From the nineteenth century until today, many conventional physicians used this word to describe themselves (the Association of American Medical Colleges describes the type of medicine they teach as allopathic, and the American Medical Association refers to MD students as allopathic medical students), even though the general public has little knowledge of what it actually means.

6. There are also more simple software programs for nonprofessionals, though the expert system programs are not hard to learn. When any of these software programs are used with some basic knowledge of homeopathic methodology, they help make more precise the prescribing of homeopathic medicines.

7. For an excellent review of many substances that have significant biological activity in extremely small doses, see Bellavite and Signorini's *Emerging Science of Homeopathy: Complexity, Biodynamics, and Nanopharmacology* (2002); see also Eskinazi, 1999.

8. According to statistics taken from the states of Illinois and Michigan's penitentiaries which had separate prisons for which homeopathic and conventional medical treatment was provided, it was discovered that the death rates in the prison population under conventional medical care were more than twice as high, the number of days lost due to illness were more than twice as high, and the cost per prisoner was more than three times as high. The death rates in the conventional mental health hospitals (called insane asylums at that time) in New York in the 1880s were ten times the death rate in the homeopathic mental health hospitals.

9. The pre-1900 research testing homeopathic medicines had a similar pattern of results as homeopathic research conducted today. Whenever skeptics of homeopathy sought to test it, they specifically designed their experiments to disprove it and homeopathic guidelines on how to prescribe accurately were rarely followed. In contrast, whenever research was conducted that following homeopathic guidelines, the research usually, though not always, successfully showed the healing benefits of homeopathic medicines.

10. When reviewing only the highest-quality studies and when adjusting for publication bias, the researchers found that subjects given a homeopathic medicine were still 1.86 times more likely to experience improved health as compared with those given a placebo. The researchers also noted that it is extremely common in conventional medical research for more rigorous trials to yield less positive results than less rigorous trials.

11. The P expressions in parentheses refer to the probability of these results occurring simply by chance. Thus, the lower the number, the greater the likelihood that the treatment used is effective. When P equals 0.05, this means that there are 5 chances out of 100 (5 percent) that the effective use of a specific treatment happened by chance, and scientists today consider a 5 percent or less chance as adequate evidence of a treatment's effectiveness. In this study, however, there was an extremely high likelihood that the treatment was effective because there were only seven chances out of 10,000 that this result happened by chance. In the study referenced here, there was "substancial significance" between the treated and the placebo groups.

12. A BBC television series called *Horizon* produced a one-hour documentary on homeopathy in 2002 in which they sought to integrate "science" and "reality television" by replicating the Ennis study and then revealing the results to advocates and skeptics of homeopathy on live TV. Although this type of television may be a great idea, TV science and real science are not always the same thing. When Professor Ennis was finally shown the specific protocol used for this study in 2004, she was horrified to note that this study had very little resemblance to her study. Ennis also learned that the researcher that *Horizon* used was a low-ranking medical technologist who had no graduate degree, that this person had never published any research on basophils in the past, and that this protocol included the use of a chemical known to kill basophils even before the homeopathic medicines were used in the study. It

was literally impossible for this badly designed study to evaluate properly the effects of homeopathic medicines. I uncovered the evidence of this flawed experiment after I was interviewed for the American television series *20/20*. The producer of this *20/20* show promised to use Professor Ennis as a consultant, and when he was informed before the study was conducted that this research design was ill-conceived and flawed, he told me that he simply promised to consult Professor Ennis but was not required to take her advice. For more details about this "junk science/junk journalism" on network television, go to http://homeopathic.com/articles/media/index.php.

13. The authors of this review of research include Rustom Roy, PhD (head of a materials science lab at Penn State University, considered one of the best labs in this field in the world), William Tiller, PhD (professor emeritus and former head of the materials science department at Stanford University), and Iris Bell, MD, PhD (head of research for Dr. Andrew Weil's program in integrative medicine at the University of Arizona). These researchers assert that anyone who says or suggests that there is nothing of value in homeopathic water is simply wrong.

CHAPTER 2. Why Homeopathy Is Hated and Vilified

14. As many as 41 million leeches were imported into France in 1833. In the United States, one company imported 500,000 leeches in 1856, and one of its competitors imported 300,000 leeches (Ullman, 1991).

15. Some of the fictitious names that were used for fake homeopathic drugs were *Madaroma fraudulentum, Urticaria rubra,* and *Tuber cinereum.*

16. See the chapter Politicians and Peacemakers for an incredible story about U.S. President Abraham Lincoln and his Secretary of State William Seward.

17. The AMA also had specific rules for patients of conventional physicians. Rothstein noted these obligations included blind acceptance of their doctor's prescriptions and a critique of the homeopath's interview that seeks to understand a patient in his or her complete family and life context: "The patient was instructed to confide in his physician freely without, however, wearying the physician 'with a tedious detail of events or matters not appertaining to his disease' nor 'the details of his business nor the history of his family concerns.' Furthermore, the patient was warned that his 'obedience ... to the prescriptions of his physician should be prompt and implicit. He should never permit his own crude opinions as to their fitness to influence his attention to them'" (Rothstein, 1985, 173).

18. One other leader of the effort to change the code of ethics to allow consultation with homeopaths was Daniel Bennett St. John Roosa (1838–1908), a founder of Manhattan Eye, Ear and Throat Hospital and the president of the faculty of the prestigious New York Post-Graduate Medical School, which later became New York University School of Medicine.

19. In 1850 John Epps, a British homeopathic pharmacist, produced a comprehensive justification of homeopathy for the lay and medical public. Fully one-fourth of the 320 pages are devoted to an examination of coroners' inquests, including details of a manslaughter trial of 1840, and analysis of medical and other witnesses' evidence, and press comment (Treuherz, 1984).

20. Many Americans know this name, but they confuse it with his son, Oliver Wendell Holmes, Jr., who was the famous Supreme Court Chief Justice. The father was not the same gentleman scholar as was his son.

21. One great characteristic of Rush was his commitment to individual freedoms for citizens. Besides being anti-slavery, Rush was an advocate of "medical freedom." He has been reported to have argued: "Unless we put Medical Freedom into the Constitution, the time will come when medicine will organize into an undercover dictatorship ... to restrict the art of healing to one class of men, and deny equal privilege to others, will be to constitute the Bastille of Medical Science. All such laws are un-American and despotic and have no place in a Republic. ... The Constitution of this Republic should make special privilege for Medical Freedom as well as Religious Freedom."

22. Homeopaths use various snake venoms, though they use them in extremely small and safe doses, based on the specific syndrome that each venom is known to cause.

23. Zoe Mullan, senior editor at *The Lancet*, acknowledged, "Professor Egger stated at the onset that he expected to find that homeopathy had no effect other than that of placebo. His 'conflict' was therefore transparent. We saw this as sufficient" (EHM News Bureau, 2005). The editors chose not to inform readers of this bias.

24. Skeptics of homeopathy often assert that homeopathic research is not high-quality science, and yet, this study confirms that more than twice as many homeopathic studies were of a high caliber when compared with conventional medical studies. The researchers did not comment on this obvious fact.

25. Ultimately, the vast majority of MDs who practice homeopathic and/or various alternative therapies prefer to practice integrative medicine, taking the best from all medical worlds.

CHAPTER 3. **Literary Greats: Write On, Homeopathy!**

26. A discussion of the factors that led to the closing of the homeopathic medical schools is provided in Chapter 11, Corporate Leaders and Philanthropists' Support for Homeopathy.

27. Henry Wadsworth Longfellow and Nathaniel Hawthorne both graduated from Bowdoin College in the so-called Bowdoin Banner Class of 1825, which also included Franklin Pierce (who would become the fourteenth U.S. president), John S. C. Abbott (a highly respected biographer), Jonathan Cilley (state senator and general), and Richmond Bradford (initially trained as a conventional physician who then became a leading homeopathic doctor in Maine).

28. Transcendentalism in America began as a protest against the general state of culture and society at the time and especially against the intellectualism at Harvard. Transcendentalism was rooted in the personal and social utopianism derived from the German idealism of Immanuel Kant, English romanticism, and Vedic thought. Transcendentalists believed that an ideal spiritual state "transcends" the physical and empirical and is only known through the individual's intuition, rather than through the doctrines of established religions.

29. Elizabeth and many of her family members were also appreciators of phrenology, a system of determining a person's character and personality by evaluating the shape of his or her head. Although this system is harshly ridiculed and ignored today, it was the most widely credited system of the mind in the 1830s. At that time phrenology was taught at Harvard and was accepted as "gospel" by the Boston Medical Society. When Johann Gaspar Spurzheim (1776–1832), phrenology's leading proponent, died in Boston, his funeral procession included the entire Boston Medical Society and 400 Harvard students (Marshall, 2005).

30. William Wesselhoeft, MD (1794–1858), discussed later in this chapter as the homeopath who treated Emily Dickinson, was one of the people who helped get Peabody's pharmacy started.

31. Other appreciators of Swedenborg who are not referenced in this chapter include: Walt Whitman, Robert and Elizabeth Barrett Browning, Carl Jung, William Blake, Immanuel Kant, D. T. Suzuki, and Helen Keller.

32. William Wesselhoeft, MD, was an eminent physician and homeopath. It wasn't unusual for his patients to experience relief from their physical complaints along with improvement in their emotional and mental state. In fact, in his last address before the Homeopathic Society of Boston, he described the goal of a physician to do more than improve physical health: "The art of awakening and increasing the vitality of the human body, *that* is our highest aim" (Bingham, 1955, 175). Wesselhoeft was not the only member of his family involved in homeopathy. His brother Robert Wesselhoeft was also a leading homeopath, and Robert had two sons, Conrad and Walter, who were professors at the homeopathic medical school at Boston University. Conrad Wesselhoeft, MD, was Louisa May Alcott's homeopath.

33. One randomized, double-blind study published in a major AMA medical journal showed that a homeopathic formula product (called *Vertigoheel* or *Cocculus compositum*) was as effective as a leading conventional drug in the treatment of vertigo (dizziness) (Weiser, 1998). *Vertigoheel* is a prescription drug in the United States marketed for the treatment of vertigo, while *Cocculus compositum* is considered an over-the-counter drug that does not require a doctor's prescription because it is marketed for motion sickness, which is, according to the FDA, a less serious medical condition. These products have identical ingredients.

34. Holmes wrote *Homeopathy and Its Kindred Delusions* just six years after he graduated medical school. Even though his book was full of misinformation about homeopathy, Holmes had a certain brilliance and respectability such that this book was taken seriously by people antagonistic to homeopathy. For a more detailed story about Dr. Holmes, see Chapter 2, Why Homeopathy Is Hated and Vilified.

35. The fact that Dr. Holmes chose to prescribe medicated cigarettes for Irving's asthma and cough is but one more example of bad medicine, and yet, he and other orthodox physicians had the nerve to attack homeopathy as quackery.

36. Various kings and queens of England since the 1830s have sought care from homeopathic physicians. For details, see Chapter 12, The Royal Medicine.

37. Critics of Abrams have asserted that he never got a medical degree from the University of Heidelberg, but according to the AMA, he did graduate, and in fact,

was the youngest person to graduate from this school in 100 years (Scholten, 1999; Abrams, 1922). Some critics of Abrams have excessive venom for him, asserting that he was one of the greatest quacks of all time (www.wikipedia.org; Wilson, 1998). Various present and past professors from Stanford have led attacks against Abrams in their effort to distance their school's good reputation from him. However, ironically enough, Leland Stanford (1824–1893) may have gone to a homeopathic doctor himself. One homeopathic journal posted an announcement that Charles W. Breyfogle, MD, a respected San Jose, Calif. homeopathic physician and former mayor of this city (1886–1887) traveled to Washington, D.C. to serve as the physician to Stanford while he was the U.S. Senator representing California (Sayings and Doings, 1893). However, modern-day biographers insist that there is no solid evidence that Stanford sought or received homeopathic treatment, though there is ample evidence that his wife, Jane, had a longtime interest in various paranormal phenomena (Tutorow, 2004, 2006). What is also verified is that this homeopathic physician was one of eight people who served as pallbearers at the funeral of Leland Stanford. Stanford obviously had some type of exceptionally close relationship with Breyfogle for this to occur, though it is possible that Breyfogle's role as mayor of San Jose and as the founding president of a local bank may have given them business reasons for their relationship rather than medical reasons.

38. Skeptics rarely, if ever, make reference to the support that Albert Abrams, MD, received from the former president of the British Medical Association. Further, they rarely make reference to the formal investigation of Abrams's work led by Sir Thomas Horder (noted cancer expert and physician to the Prince of Wales). The Horder committee included experts in physics, clinical medicine, electro-therapeutics, and psychology. Morris Fishbein, president of the American Medical Association between 1924 and 1950, who was extremely antagonistic to homeopathy and Albert Abrams, reluctantly admitted: "The whole Committee was satisfied, and drew the conclusion that these experiments establish to a very high degree of probability the fundamental proposition underlying the apparatus designed for eliciting the electronic reactions of Abrams" (Fishbein, 1926, 112–116).

39. It is interesting and significant that Chekhov chose a woman to be the homeopathic doctor in this story. In the 1880s women represented a very small minority of physicians, though the few that existed tended to be homeopathic doctors (see Chapter 10, Women's Rights Leaders and Suffragists). The fact that Chekhov chose this woman to be a widow of a general makes sense because homeopathy was especially popular among the Russian elite, including the royalty, clergy, and the military.

40. Alpine Pharmaceuticals (San Rafael, Calif.) sponsored a double-blind, placebo-controlled study using two potencies of *Arnica* in the treatment of patients who underwent facial plastic surgery (Seeley, et al., 2006). This study, conducted by the head of the Facial Plastic Surgery Department at the University of California, San Francisco, was published in a respected AMA surgical journal.

41. Although mercury is a well-known toxic substance, the doses used in homeopathic medicine are known to be safe and have a 200-year history of safety and efficacy. In the United States, the Food and Drug Administration has regulated the sales

of homeopathic medicines since 1938, and has determined the safe dosage levels of the 1,000-plus legally recognized homeopathic medicines.

CHAPTER 4. Sports Superstars: Scoring with Homeopathy

42. This information refers to the homeopathic medicine *Arnica* in the form of pills or external applications (there are various external applications of it, including gel form, ointment, or spray).

43. Although there has been a tremendous amount of clinical success using *Arnica* and although there have been several well-controlled clinical trials to further verify its efficacy, it is important to acknowledge that not all research testing *Arnica* has shown positive results. There are good and simple reasons for negative results: (1) *Arnica* was sometimes tested for conditions for which it is not indicated; (2) some of the studies testing *Arnica* used too small a number of subjects to determine its efficacy. ; and (3) some of the research was not well-controlled or well-designed.

CHAPTER 5. Physicians and Scientists: Coming Out of the Medicine Closet

44. For a more detailed discussion about the strong animosity against homeopathy and homeopaths, see Chapter 2, Why Homeopathy is Hated and Vilified.

45. Recently, some scientists have speculated that Darwin suffered from systemic lactose intolerance (Campbell and Matthews, 2005), but this remains speculation and may at best represent only one aspect of a more complex disease syndrome.

46. Homeopaths have consistently observed a similar phenomenon, called "Hering's Law of Cure," whereby patients experience an "externalization" of an internal illness. Externalizations are an important part of the healing process. Sadly, however, some patients who seek conventional medical care receive treatment to suppress these skin symptoms, pushing them back into the body and worsening the person's overall health.

47. In reference to clairvoyance, the woman who Gully used was thought to be able to look directly into a person's body.

48. The additional drama to the lives of Gully and Hastings is that their sons were also antagonists to each other. Gully's son, William Court Gully, became speaker of the British House of Lords (1895–1905), while Hastings' son, George Woodyatt Hastings, became a lawyer and politician. Like his father, George Hastings was actively antagonistic to unconventional medical treatments. Ultimately, the younger Hastings's reputation was severely tarnished when he was sent to prison for stealing money from a client whose will he executed.

49. One additional story about Dr. James Gully has nothing to do with homeopathy. Dr. Gully became a part of what was the most sensational British legal drama and murder mystery of the nineteenth century. In 1871, when Dr. Gully was 63 years old, he began an affair with Florence Ricardo, a woman in her early twenties who was in a very troubled marriage. Florence's husband died just a couple of months after the affair started. In 1872, although Florence was a widow and Dr. Gully was long separated from his wife, their affair became public and created great embarrassment for them both. It later became public that Dr. Gully performed an abortion

on Florence Ricardo. In order to recoup some of her lost dignity, Florence quickly married a distinguished lawyer, Charles Bravo. However, shortly after the wedding, Mr. Bravo became extremely abusive toward Florence. Within five months of their wedding, he was found dead due to poisoning. His wife was a possible murderer, but there was also the possibility that the head housekeeper was the culprit due to evidence suggesting that she was soon to be fired. There was also evidence that a recently fired employee might have been the murderer because he bragged at a bar that he was going to kill Mr. Bravo. Although there was no significant evidence that Dr. Gully killed Mr. Bravo, he too was implicated. This murder mystery has remained unsolved, though a recent book on this subject more strongly suggests that Florence Bravo did the deed herself (Ruddick, 2001).

50. Harvey Williams Cushing, MD (1869–1939), was considered by many the greatest neurosurgeon of the first half of the twentieth century. In his biography of Osler, he said, "His [Osler's] belief that over-treatment with drugs was one of the medical errors of the day has been hinted at, and it was always one of his favorite axioms that no one individual had done more good to the medical profession than Hahnemann, whose therapeutic methods had demonstrated that the natural tendency of disease was toward recovery, provided that the patient was decently care for, properly nursed, and not over-dosed" (Cushing, 1940, p. 171).

51. For further information about James Compton-Burnett, see the story in Chapter 4, Literary Greats, of his famous daughter, Dame Ivy Compton-Burnett.

52. To read an interesting story about Rev. Thomas Everest, see Chapter 13, Clergy and Spiritual Leaders.

53. It should be noted that the doses that Bier tested were not in the extreme high dilutions often used by homeopaths, though it is also common for homeopaths to use so-called low potencies for select cases (and when individualized homeopathic treatment is not possible or chosen).

54. "Medical superintendent" means that he was chief of medical care at the hospital.

55. The contributions to the field of anesthesia from homeopaths and homeopathic medical schools have been quite significant. Thomas Drysdale Buchanan, MD (1876–1940), graduated from the New York Homeopathic Medical College in 1897 and became professor of anesthesia there in 1904. He later became the first president of the American Board of Anesthesiology and holder of Certificate #1, which means that he was the first board-certified anesthetist in history.

56. Flower Homeopathic Hospital with its 200 beds, Hahnemann Hospital with its 132 beds, New York Homeopathic Medical College and Hospital with its 55 beds, New York Ophthalmic Hospital with its 80 beds, and Laura Franklin Free Hospital for Children with its 75 beds.

57. Pat Hardy, MD, formally known as Eugene A. P. Hardy, MD, was a graduate of Hering Medical College. Dr. Hardy was a longtime member of the International Hahnemannian Association, an elite organization of physicians who specialized in classical homeopathy.

58. The correct spelling of his name is Justus Gaige Wright. He graduated from a conventional medical school, Long Island Hospital, but shortly after his graduation,

became a homeopath. He was a member of the American Institute of Homeopathy as early as 1905, and was listed in this organization's directory in 1925, 1931, and 1941.

CHAPTER 6. Stage, Film, and Television Celebrities: Starring in Homeopathy

59. Booth's uncle, Algernon Sydney Booth, was the great-great-great-grandfather of Cherie Blair (née Booth), wife of former British Prime Minister Tony Blair.

60. James Ward, MD, was a highly respected homeopathic doctor who was a professor at the Hahnemann Hospital College of San Francisco. He was also president of the San Francisco Board of Health during 1902–1907. During his tenure the famous 1906 earthquake rocked San Francisco.

61. *Arnica* is an herb that is commonly prescribed for sprains and strains from injury or overexertion. This herb is typically prescribed in internal doses in pill form after undergoing the homeopathic potentization process, or it is prescribed in an ointment or gels and is applied externally. In the John Wayne movies, it was not made clear which form of *Arnica* he was recommending.

CHAPTER 7. Musicians: Singing Out for Homeopathy

62. Beethoven was showing a fine sense of humor when he made reference to "notes save from distress" because the German word for notes, like the English word, refers to both musical notes as well as money.

63. Otto von Bismarck (1815–1898), minister-president of Prussia in 1862–1890 and the first chancellor of the various states of Germany during 1871–1890, was another advocate for natural medicine.

64. Ignaz Schuppanzigh (1776–1830) was the leader of Count Razumovsky's private string quartet, which was considered to be the first professional string quartet. Schuppanzigh and his group premiered many of Beethoven's string quartets, in particular, the later pieces.

65. For more details about this story, see Chapter 12, The Royal Medicine. For more details about Father Veith and his homeopathic practice, see Chapter 13, Clergy and Spiritual Leaders.

66. An entire book, *Beethoven's Hair: An Extraordinary Historical Odyssey and a Scientific Mystery Solved*, was written about this subject. Although recent analysis has determined a high concentration of lead in Beethoven's hair, the deafness associated with it seldom takes the form that Beethoven exhibited. However, it is also possible that the homeopathic treatment that Beethoven received may have reduced some but not all of the symptoms of typical lead poisoning. One review of 105 studies investigating the use of homeopathic medicines to reduce the toxic effects of heavy metal poisoning found beneficial results, especially among the highest-quality scientific studies in this field (Linde, et al., 1994). More recent studies have also confirmed these results (Ullman, 2007; Khuda-Bukhsh, et al., 2005; Belon, et al., 2006).

67. Each homeopathic medicine is known to treat a certain body-mind syndrome, and people who benefit from *Sulphur* are typically artist-philosopher types who wear tattered clothing, develop a personal attachment to whatever possessions they

have, and have a thin body frame and gaunt face. For more details about the constitutional types of various homeopathic medicines, see select books called "homeopathic *materia medica.*"

68. Dr. Schwenninger was also the medical adviser of Prince Otto von Bismarck, the minister-president of Prussia who engineered the unification of the numerous states of Germany and who was a longtime advocate of natural medicines.

CHAPTER 8. Artists and Fashionistas: Homeopathy in Style

69. Although Dr. Gachet identified himself primarily as a homeopathic physician and even likened himself to homeopathy's founder, Samuel Hahnemann (Negro, 2005), Gachet had interests in other natural therapies also, including hydrotherapy, physical exercise, nutrition, metal therapy (the use of minerals), and climatology (the influence of climate on health).

70. It is also known that Dr. Gachet provided treatment to Juliette Dranet, Victor Hugo's headmistress, though there is no evidence that Hugo sought his treatment (Negro, 2005).

71. For the story about Chopin and his experiences with homeopathy, see Chapter 7, Musicians. Gachet was also a student of homeopathy with Dr. Léon Simon (1798–1867), one of the earliest and most respected French homeopaths.

72. In Auvers today, Dr. Gachet's home still stands and is a historical site of note (Roe, 2006).

CHAPTER 9. Politicians and Peacemakers: Voting with Their Lives and Health

73. A correspondent for the *Courier Journal* (Louisville, Kentucky) reported that the man who attacked Seward was given entrance into his home by pretending to have a homeopathic medicine for Seward from his homeopath, Dr. T. Verdi. This reporter also stated something that this author has not yet fully confirmed: "It is not generally known that Lincoln and his entire Cabinet were homoeopathists." (Other Days, 1887). This reporter also listed Jefferson Davis as a known advocate for homeopathy, though this fact is not yet verified.

74. William H. Mussey, vice president of the AMA, sought to censure Surgeon General Barnes, but the AMA's convention delegates did not take his advice.

75. Trustees of the college included Thomas Hoyne, Joseph B. Doggett, John H. Dunham, Norman B, Judd, George A. Gibbs, Orrington Lunt, William H. Brown, George E. Shipman, MD, and David S. Smith, MD.

76. McClellan's father was a prominent surgeon, author, and educator, and his uncle and older brother were highly respected members of the regular medical profession. McClellan's use of homeopathic treatments can be attributed to his wife, Ellen Marcy McClellan. One of the doctors who treated the general was her uncle, Erastus E. Marcy, who was founder and editor of the prestigious *North American Homeopathic Journal*, and had been one of homeopathy's leading advocates during the 1840s and 1850s.

77. Some appointments of homeopathic physicians and surgeons were made surreptitiously, as in the case of G. S. Walker (1820–?). He graduated from an allopathic medical school, Jefferson Medical College, in 1852, and immediately moved to St.

Louis. In 1860 he formally declared his interest in homeopathic medicine, and was summarily kicked out of his local medical society for professional heresy. During the Civil War, he initially entered the Union army as surgeon of volunteers and later was appointed brigade surgeon under General Sherman (King, 1905, II, 388–389).

78. In addition to Dr. Alfred Hughes working as a homeopathic doctor in the Confederate army, Samuel Hunt, MD, of Georgia also practiced openly as a homeopath. The story of Hughes, however, is a very interesting one because he practiced in Richmond, Virginia, where many leading Union officers were his patients, including General Peter Michie, the federal quartermaster general who was in charge of all the supplies for the army.

79. Willis Danforth, MD (1826–1891), received his medical training in conventional medicine, though after being cured of sciatica by a homeopath, he began studying and practicing homeopathy. He became a professor of surgery at Hahnemann Medical College in Chicago.

80. "Eclectic" institutes and medical schools taught homeopathic and natural medicine as well as conventional medical treatments, thus their being called eclectic.

81. Burke Hinsdale took over the presidency of Hiram College shortly after Garfield held that position. Burke was the son of distinguished Ohio homeopath Wilbur Hinsdale. Garfield always had a special place in his heart for his alma mater, and even during the time that Garfield was U.S. president, he visited the school on a regular basis.

82. H. J. Heinz also showed his support for homeopathy by contributing $10,000 toward a dormitory at Kansas City University (which had a Hahnemann Medical College affiliated with it), as a memorial to his wife.

83. The Western College of Homeopathy was founded in 1850, and in 1855 changed its name to Cleveland Homeopathic Hospital. It was one of the early medical schools that had a teaching hospital associated with it. Many amazing stories are associated with this medical school and hospital's history; one started when a prominent citizen discovered that his daughter's tomb had been raided and her body stolen, presumably by the Cleveland Homeopathic Hospital College. A mob of citizens broke into the school, and although no body was found, they burned and gutted the college and hospital. Due to so much support from Cleveland's wealthiest citizens, the college and hospital moved to new and larger quarters, but as it turns out, ten years later, a physician at the rival allopathic medical college in Cleveland acknowledged that they had stolen the body and quickly shipped it out of the city once a public disturbance started (Murphy, 1974).

84. Chapter 5, Physicians and Scientists, includes statements made about homeopathy by William J. Mayo, MD, Charles's older brother and co-founder of the Mayo Clinic.

85. Some recent research has tested *Kali bichromicum* for treating people with chronic bronchitis or emphysema who had a thick and sticky bronchial discharge, and double-blind, placebo-controlled study has found very impressive results (Frass, et al., 2005). In this study, conducted by a respected professor from the University of Vienna and published in a respected journal in internal medicine, fifty patients received either *Kali bichromicum* 30C globules or a placebo. The amount of tracheal

(throat) secretions was reduced significantly in those given the homeopathic medicine, and none of them required reintubation (technological intervention to help them breathe), while 16 percent of those who took the placebo required this intervention.

86. C. R. Das and Pandit Motilal Nehru were two co-founders of the Swaraj Party, which was an important political effort to create an India independent from British rule. Motilal Nehru was the father of Jawaharlal Nehru, the first prime minister of a free India.

87. In addition to other politicians from India who have expressed support for homeopathy, the present deputy prime minister of Nepal, who is also the minister of health, Amik Sherchan, recently asserted that his government should promote homoeopathy, as it is the most accessible, affordable, and appropriate treatment for the general public in the country: "If we promote homeopathy, we can deliver service to a large section of the population in the country" (Health Minister, 2006).

88. Dowsing is the use of a pendulum in order to tune into one's own subconscious mind to find information not easily accessible through normal means. Like water witching, dowsing uses a pendulum to diagnose people or to find appropriate treatments for them. Although dowsing sounds like the epitome of quackery, the use of a pendulum in the right hands can discover startling information. Albert Abrams, MD (1863–1924), chief pathologist at Cooper Medical School (later, Stanford Medical School), was a well-known user of dowsing instruments. The authors Upton Sinclair and Sir Arthur Conan Doyle, of Sherlock Holmes fame, were great admirers of Abrams's work. Upton Sinclair referred to Abrams's laboratory as the "House of Wonders." Even Sir James Barr, a past president of the British Medical Association, described Abrams as the "greatest medical genius that the medical profession has produced for half a century" (Russell, 1973, 17). For further information about Abrams, see the information on Upton Sinclair in Chapter 4, Literary Greats.

CHAPTER 10. Women's Rights Leaders and Suffragists: Pro-Homeopathy

89. Woodhull, Claflin & Company opened in 1870 with the assistance of a wealthy benefactor, her admirer, Cornelius Vanderbilt.

90. A truly fascinating book about Samuel and Melanie Hahnemann is *A Homeopathic Love Story* by Rima Handley (Berkeley: North Atlantic Books, 1990).

91. Clemence Lozier's support for temperance arose out of her personal life. She divorced her first husband due to his drunkenness.

92. See Chapter 13, Clergy and Spiritual Leaders, for a discussion of Swedenborg and his followers.

93. To clarify some misconceptions, homeopaths do not oppose surgery; they oppose unnecessary surgery, especially since homeopathic medicines sometimes are effective enough to prevent the need for surgical procedures. And once surgery is found to be necessary, homeopaths prescribe certain remedies to help reduce surgical shock and promote healing.

94. The New York Homeopathic Medical College is today known as New York Medical College, and sadly, it no longer teaches homeopathy.

CHAPTER 11. Corporate Leaders' and Philanthropists' Support for Homeopathy: A Rich Tradition

95. The homeopathic clinic at Montgomery Ward and Company (in Chicago) treated 49,034 employees in 1915 alone. The company prided itself on a significant reduction in drug costs due to the use of homeopathic medicines and a considerably reduced number of days of illness for employees (American Institute of Homeopathy, 1916). During the notorious flu epidemic of 1918, the Montgomery Ward homeopathic clinic experienced only eight deaths instead of the hundreds experienced at clinics of Marshall Field and Sears Roebuck operated by orthodox physicians (Suits, 1985, 79). As a result of these impressive statistics, the United Cigar Company placed homeopathic physicians in charge of all of the medical clinics serving their employees in Chicago.

96. The National Cash Register Company in Dayton, Ohio, was known for its progressive management. The medical department at NCR started officially in 1903 with H. H. Herman, MD. Dr. Herman was trained as a conventional physician and became a homeopath shortly before working at the NCR clinic. He was officially a member of the Dayton Homeopathic Medical Society before 1903, and in 1908 joined the Ohio State Homeopathic Medical Society. In 1915, this clinic was exclusively run by homeopathic physicians and oversaw the care of 25,025 patients (American Institute of Homeopathy, 1916, 96). Shortly after Dr. Herman got involved in NCR, the company's newsletter to its employees highlighted various natural treatments.

97. The Chalmers Motor Company was an extremely popular car manufacturer in the 1910s and 1920s. They also created the Chalmers Award in professional baseball that later became the Most Valuable Player Award.

98. Another leading member of the American medical establishment who graduated from a homeopathic medical school (Chicago Homeopathic Medical College, 1883) was George H. Simmons, MD, who was general secretary of the AMA (1899–1911) and editor of *JAMA* (until 1924). Also, at the time the Flexner Report was published, Eugene H. Porter, MD, was the commissioner of health for the state of New York; he was a graduate of New York Homeopathic Medical College in 1885 and an active member of the American Institute of Homeopathy.

99. Flexner and Gates also strongly contended that only the larger medical schools should continue to exist, and yet, statistics from 1912 medical students who took the state licensing examination found that the larger medical schools did not have a higher percentage of students who passed (Our Colleges, 1913). Further, Boston University (a homeopathic school) had a failure rate of only 3.3 percent, while Harvard's failure rate was 11.8 percent.

100. "Scientific medicine" should more accurately be called "reductionistic medicine," whereby a person is not looked at or understood as a total complex of body and mind characteristics, but instead, problems are reduced to individual symptoms or diseases that are biochemical in nature.

101. Dr. McCann's statistics have been frequently misquoted. One modern-day popular book on the flu epidemic of 1918 (Barry, 2004) erroneously criticized the

"absurd" statements from homeopaths because he asserted that 28.2 percent of people with the flu could not have died from it or there would have been millions of deaths in the U.S. alone (and there weren't). McCann was specific in his statistics, and he clearly stated that he was comparing the death rates in homeopathic hospitals to those in conventional hospitals. Sadly, as has been historically repeated by critics of homeopathy, they tend to report misinformation to try to substantiate their case against homeopathy.

102. W. B. Hinsdale's son, Albert E. Hinsdale, was also a homeopathic doctor, and he became professor of materia medica at OSU. One of Albert's scientific studies was on the action of *Kali bichromicum* (potassium dichromate), a very important homeopathic medicine that was recently found to be extraordinarily effective in the treatment of patients suffering from chronic bronchitis or emphysema. Called Chronic Obstructive Pulmonary Disease (COPD), this is the number four reason that people die in the U.S. This study was conducted at the University of Vienna hospital and was published in the highly respected medical journal, *Chest* (Frass, et al., 2005).

103. In homeopathy, as in any medical specialty, there are varied opinions on how to best treat patients. Some significant infighting in homeopathy occurred between those homeopaths who use high-potency doses (diluted 1:10 or 1:100 thirty or more times) and those who used low-potency doses (usually 3X to 30X). There were also conflicting opinions on how to best conduct research. Some homeopaths wanted to emulate conventional medical care and test one drug against a specific disease, while other homeopaths insisted that homeopathy required more individualized prescriptions. One of the more significant conflicts arose from those homeopaths who believed that no conventional drugs should be used at all, and those who were eclectic and used homeopathic, herbal, and conventional medications. Kettering's homeopath, T. A. McCann, MD, was a classical homeopath who used high potencies and insisted upon individualizing their application to the totality of the patient, not just the disease.

104. See Chapter 12, The Royal Medicine, for more details about Queen Olga's support for homeopathy.

105. Ironically, George Simmons actually graduated from a Chicago homeopathic medical college in 1882. He also obtained a conventional medical degree from Rush Medical College in 1892, though there is no evidence that he attended any classes more than a couple of days nor did he take formal examinations there. A respected physician-urologist who was an alumni of Rush uncovered death certificates and prescriptions that Simmons wrote in Nebraska during every week over the six-month period that Simmons was supposedly attending classes in Chicago, more than 500 miles away (Lydston, 1909). Simmons also asserted that he had received a diploma from Rotunda Hospital in Dublin, Ireland, and yet that hospital never issued diplomas. He further advertised himself as having spent a year and a half working in the largest hospitals in London and Vienna, facts that were in dispute. Simmons even declared himself a specialist in skin diseases, genito-urinary diseases, and rectal diseases (he did seem to be "imbued" in this latter subject but not medically speaking).

When confronted with these charges, Simmons asserted that his errors in advertisements were not regarded as unethical in Nebraska, where he practiced (Ausubel, 2000; Mullins, 1988). It seems that Simmons was the epitome of the quack-charlatan to which he was so vehemently antagonistic. Even more startling is the fact that he openly had a mistress and attempted to get rid of his wife. In those days one technique to do this was to have her committed to an insane asylum. Simmons heavily drugged her and then tried convincing her that she was going insane. However, this strategy backfired. Mrs. Simmons took her husband to court in 1924, and the sensational trial ruined his image. This trial inspired numerous books, plays, and movies, the most famous of which was *Gaslight*, starring Charles Boyer and Ingrid Bergman.

106. Historians of homeopathy assert that the homeopathic medical colleges experienced so much pressure to provide training in conventional medical sciences that they were not providing adequate training in homeopathy itself (Winston, 1999). In fact, it was estimated that 92 percent of the homeopathic medical school's curriculum was required for conventional medical subjects (Roberts, 1938). In this light, it may be more accurate to say that conventional medical colleges taught "an exclusive dogma," because they never taught homeopathic medicine while the homeopathic colleges taught a much broader range of subjects.

107. Even Henry Pritchett, head of the Carnegie Foundation, came to view the council's power "in much the way Dr. Frankenstein viewed his own creation" (Brown, 1979, Chapter 4).

108. Some states didn't recognize graduates of medical schools with a "B" or "C" rating, giving additional power to the AMA's educational standards (Roberts, 1938).

109. One of the earliest pre-paid health insurance plans was the Group Health Association. When Mario Scandiffio, MD, agreed to become one of the doctors to provide care on a pre-paid basis, his membership in the District of Columbia Medical Society was terminated. A similar situation happened to Charles R. Wiley, MD, who was chairman of the Medical Civic Center of Chicago. When he and eighteen members of his medical staff agreed to provide care for the Group Health Association, they were all suddenly expelled from the Chicago Medical Society, and they lost whatever professorial appointments they had.

110. One of Fishbein's other obsessions was his strong resistance to admitting black physicians into local medical societies. Fishbein and the AMA's technique for keeping black physicians out of local medical societies was simply by allowing local societies to establish their own membership criteria. Shockingly, this was not changed until 1964.

CHAPTER 12. **The Royal Medicine: Monarchs' Longtime Love for Homeopathy**

111. The classical British spelling is "homoeopathic," and thus the hospital is officially called the Royal London Homoeopathic Hospital. However, most people in the U.S., Britain, and Europe use the modern-day spelling, "homeopathic."

112. In 1939, King Haakon VII of Norway bestowed upon Sir John Weir the Knight Grand Cross of St. Olav, the highest honor granted by his country (*Homoeopathy*, 1939).

113. For an interesting story about the homeopathic treatment of Disraeli (Britain's prime minister during Queen Victoria's reign), see Chapter 9, Politicians and Peacemakers.

114. Many of Dr. Quin's close friends were conventional physicians. There is one story of a conventional physician, Sir Charles Lococke, telling Dr. Quin that he had seen one of his patients, and he chose to use Quin's homeopathic approach. When Quin asked him which medicine he gave the patient, Sir Charles replied, "Nothing!" In response, Quin said that he happened to see one of Sir Charles's patients, and he chose to prescribe with conventional drugs. When Quin was asked what the result was, he replied, "Dead!"

115. It is interesting to note Hahnemann's skepticism of this report of Napoleon's use of and appreciation for homeopathy. Hahnemann's remarks about the authenticity of the report show that he was not a zealot—he would accept positive reports about his discoveries only if they were fully verified. I have chosen to discuss this controversy in hopes that other researchers might further clarify what really was said (or not). Based on the evidence to date, I agree with Hahnemann's skepticism about Napoleon's interest in homeopathy.

116. In the last year of his life, Napoleon told his doctor Francesco Antommarchi: "The smell of your drugs alone suffices to make [my stomach] contract. Apply to my exterior all the medicaments you please, I consent to it, but you shall not introduce into my body a concoction of preparations, made of ingredients capable of destroying the most robust constitution—never. I do not wish to have two diseases, one due to nature and the other to medicine" (Young, 1915, 201).

117. Despite the more significant evidence showing the interest in and support for homeopathy from Napoleon III and his wife, a review of numerous biographies of their lives do not mention these facts. Recorded history is strongly influenced by the recorder as well as by the dominant worldview at the time.

118. Dr. von Böenninghausen was not trained as a doctor but as a lawyer. Born in the Netherlands, he was respected enough to become auditor to King Louis Napoleon of Holland. After contracting tuberculosis in 1827 and being cured of it by a homeopath, von Böenninghausen took up the serious study of homeopathy. He authored numerous important textbooks, including homeopathy's first repertory.

119. "Grand Duke" is a title equivalent to Prince.

120. A letter from Duke Ferdinand and his duchess to Dr. Hahnemann has survived:

> While expressing to you my thanks for your medical help this year, and for the past two years, and assuring you of my complete satisfaction, I wish you to accept the enclosed trifle as a slight recompense for your medicines and for your services. May heaven preserve you in good health for many years to the benefit of suffering humanity.
>
> – [Signed] Ferdinand, Duke

My best thanks, my dear Hofrath, for your kind wishes for my birthday. I owe to your exertions one of the pleasantest gifts on entering on a new year, improved health. I hope to preserve this to your praise and credit.

– With sincere pleasure,
Yours very affectionately,
[Signed] Julie, Duchess of Anhalt
(Bradford, 1895, Chapter 27)

121. Professor Friedrich Jaeger was the protégé and son-in-law of Georg Joseph Beer, who in 1815 became chairman of the first university eye department in the world. Jaeger informed the emperor and allegedly told Radetzky to "trust Hartung." Conventional medical colleagues harshly ridiculed Jaeger for expressing any positive regard for homeopaths, even if improvement resulted. A modern-day ophthalmologist re-examined these records and determined that the proper diagnosis was an orbital abscess (Blodi, 1989), though modern textbooks assert that this ailment, especially a severe case such as that experienced by Radetzky, tends to be resistant to treatment and usually leads to vision loss.

122. After Dr. Necker's death in 1848, the Duke of Lucca asked Joseph Attomyr (1807–1856), a respected Hungarian homeopath, to become his personal physician.

123. Dr. Nichols also was respected as the editor of the homeopathic journal *New England Medical Gazette*. He combined his literary skills with his interest in natural science by contributing articles on tropical climate, ferns, and Polynesian life to a variety of respected magazines, including *Harper's Magazine, New England Magazine, Overland Monthly, Science, Popular Science Monthly,* and *Review of Reviews*. In 1891 and 1892 he was a member of the editorial staff of *Science* (Mamiya Medical Heritage Center, 2005).

124. Prince Charles prefers to use the words "complementary medicine" rather than "alternative medicine." While "complementary" is a more familiar term in Britain than in other places, some advocates of this field consider its use demeaning because it suggests a secondary status to conventional medicine.

125. I wish to extend special thanks for help on this chapter to:
Peter Morrell, and his writing on British homeopathy across two centuries (cited in the References),
Dianna Medea, CCH, MA, for her editing, and
Dr. Robert Mathai of the British Homeopathic Association for helping to correct some details about the British royal family.

CHAPTER 13. Clergy and Spiritual Leaders: More than Prayer for Homeopathy

126. Foreign physicians required official permission to practice, and Dr. J. W. Wahle was a highly respected student and colleague of Dr. Samuel Hahnemann and the personal doctor in Rome to the ambassador of Prussia. Besides studying with Hahnemann in Leipzig, Wahle conducted several well-known provings of homeopathic medicines, including those for *Lycopodium, Sepia, Silica, Mezereum, Dulcarama, Carbo animalis,* and *Parafinnum*.

127. The Order of St. Gregory the Great is the highest honor that a layman (or woman) can receive.

128. Jean-Paul Tessier, MD, was a highly respected conventional physician of his day who worked in the St. Marguerite Hospital in Paris. He chose to study the homeopathic treatment of pneumonia because his mentor, well-known physiologist Francois Magendie, asked him to do so. Pneumonia was good for evaluation because it was a common, well-known, and unambiguous disease with a clear diagnosis and prognosis.

Tessier learned how to individualize homeopathic treatment, and he prescribed remedies in various potencies, from 6C to 30C. To reduce bias, he arranged for analysis of the results of treatment by two allopathic interns. Based on results from other studies of his day in the treatment of pneumonia, he expected a mortality rate of 33 percent. However, Tessier found that the patients in this study experienced a 7.5 percent mortality rate.

Rather than being honored for his study, Tessier was attacked by his medical colleagues and passed over for promotion at the hospital. The conventional physicians were so crazed against Tessier and the results of his study that all of his clinical assistants were also ostracized and never granted admission into the Academy of Medicine.

129. Gunpowder is an important homeopathic medicine for blood poisoning (sepsis), boils, poison ivy or poison oak rashes, and for wounds that are slow to heal.

130. The "Chief Procurator" is the highest Russian government official connected to the Russian Orthodox Church.

131. Despite the longtime opposition to homeopathy from various professors at the University of Vienna, today a small group of physicians have conducted high-quality clinical research evaluating the efficacy of homeopathy as treatment for people suffering from serious diseases. One study on patients with chronic obstructive pulmonary disease (emphysema and chronic bronchitis) showed that those given a homeopathic medicine experienced significantly more improvement in their breathing and health than those given a placebo (Frass, et al., 2005a). A similar group of researchers at this university conducted a study of patients with severe sepsis (a hospital-borne infection that typically leads to death in 50 percent of patients), and this study showed that those patients who were given individually chosen homeopathic medicines had a 50 percent greater chance of survival than those given a placebo (Frass, et al, 2005b).

132. Sir John Forbes, a highly respected conventional physician who was physician to Queen Victoria of England, was one of the few critics of homeopathy who spoke well of certain homeopaths and certain contributions from homeopathic medicine. He described Dr. Fleischmann as a "regular, well educated physician, as capable of forming a true diagnosis as other practitioners, and he is considered by those who know him as a man of honor and respectability, and incapable of attesting a falsehood" (Henderson, 1854, 65). Fleischmann's reputation even extended to

America, where he was granted honorary membership in the Massachusetts Homeopathic Medical Society in 1864.

133. Some well-known graduates of Waldorf schools include actresses Jennifer Aniston and Julianna Margulies, and American Express president and chairman Kenneth Chenault.

134. Goethe (1749–1832) was also a strong advocate for homeopathy. For further information, see Chapter 3, Literary Greats.

135. E. Beecher Hooker was the son of Isabelle Beecher Hooker, a leader of the women's suffrage movement and author.

136. Samuel Lilienthal's son was James Lilienthal, MD, who was also a homeopath. He established a free dispensary for the poor on Mission Street in San Francisco, and he served as professor of children's diseases at the Hahnemann College of the Pacific. One of Samuel's grandchildren, also named Samuel, married Alice Haas, whose family owned the Levi Strauss clothing company. Samuel and Alice Lilienthal donated their beautiful Queen Ann-style Victorian home to the City of San Francisco, and it is now a historical monument.

137. A wealthy businessman, Rajendra Lall Dutt, who is considered the father of Indian homeopathy, became interested in homeopathy in 1850, and he convinced Mahendra Lal Sircar, a dedicated scientist and allopathic doctor, to investigate the system. Sircar's conversion to homeopathy led to a crisis at the University of Calcutta, which actually sought to rescind his medical degree. This drama was ultimately averted when he resigned from the university. In 1861, Dr. Sircar successfully treated patients during a virulent epidemic of malaria fever in southern Bengal. In 1868, he started the *Calcutta Journal of Medicine*. His objective was not simply the cause of homeopathy but to encourage unbiased thinking and cultivate the scientific spirit, which found expression in his establishment of the Indian Association for the Cultivation of Science (IACS) in 1876, an organization that still flourishes today.

138. Actually, the entire quote is: "Do your best, then don't worry, be happy. Leave the rest to me."

139. For more details about software programs for both professional homeopaths and the general public, go to www.homeopathic.com.

140. As described earlier, "eclectic" institutes and medical schools taught homeopathic and natural medicine as well as conventional medical treatments, and thus were called eclectic.

141. Edward C. Franklin, a direct descendent of Benjamin Franklin, was a private pupil of Valentine Mott, MD (1785–1865), one of America's leading surgeons during the first half of the nineteenth century. Franklin became a homeopath after he was cured of a condition that conventional medicine could not successfully treat. During the Civil War, conventional physicians of the Union army would not let homeopathic doctors treat soldiers, but because Franklin was so respected as a conventional surgeon, he was able to use his homeopathic medicines in secrecy (Rutkow and Rutkow, 2004). Later, Franklin authored several books on homeopathy and surgery.

142. Elinore Peebles (1897–1992), daughter of a Boston homeopath, tells the story of how Dr. Keith showed her the back gate in which he entered the home of Mary Baker Eddy to provide homeopathic treatment to her in times of need.

143. Vitalism is an ancient and modern-day tradition that recognizes the energetic essence of all things and respects the wisdom of the body in its power and ability to defend and heal itself.

Index

A

Abbott, George, 256–257
Abrams, Albert, 73–74
Abuhatzeira, Rabbi Mikhael, 323
accreditation, medical school, 257
actors and actresses, support for homeopathy, 5, 137–151
Adams, Victoria, 89
Adelaide, Queen (Great Britain), 271, 272, 293
Adlerberg, Count Nikolai (Finland), 281
Aegidi, Julius, 290
African American education, 261
Ahmad, Mirza Tahir, 324–325
Alcott, Amos Bronson, 68
Alcott, Louisa May, 6, 67–68
Alexander II, Czar, 281
Alexandra, Empress, 280
Alexandrine Marie, Queen (Germany), 282
allergies
   principle of treatments for, 21
   scientific studies on, 30–31
   Selfridge, Grant L., work of, 126
allopathic medicine
   coining of term, 22
   cure vs. symptomatic relief, 2–3
   healing, assumptions about, 41–42
   limitations of, 6–13
   science vs. business of, 8
   treatments, nineteenth century, 40, 213
alternative medicine, 18
AMA
   attacks on homeopathy, 255, 257–258
   and the Council on Medical Education, 257
   early history of, 43–45
   and the Medical Society of New York, 9
   relationship to the Carnegie Foundation, 233–236
   seal of approval, 256–257, 259
   suppression of homeopathy, 4
   suppression of OSU College of Homeopathic Medicine, 242
   and the tobacco companies, 259
American Institute of Homeopathy, 43, 217, 219
American Medical Association. *See* AMA
Amies, Hardy, 178
Anderson, Pamela, 141–142
Andral, Gabriel, 52–53
Andrés Marino, Don, 288
Andrew, Prince, 296
anesthesia, 122–123
Angell, Marcia, 8, 11
Anglesey, Marquess of, 271

Aniston, Jennifer, 150
Anthony, Susan B., 4–5, 215, 221
anxiety, 11
apothecaries, 41, 289
Argentum nitricum, 167
Arndt-schulz law, the, 27
Arnica, 5, 79, 95, 139–140
Arthur, Chester A., 190–191
artists, support for homeopathy, 5, 173–181
aspirin, 10, 264
athletes, support for homeopathy, 6, 89–97
Attomyr, Joseph, 290
Auersberg, Princess Wilhelmina (Austria), 284
Auric, Georges, 170
Aurobindo, Sri, 328
Austin, Alonzo, 239
avian flu, 127
Avogadro's number, 32
Ayerst, James Smith, 109

B

Bacillinum, 118–119
Baehr, Bernhard, 282
Bahadur, Sir Syed Ahmed Khan, 325
Balzac, Honoré de, 252
Barber, Samuel LeRoy, 160
Barr, Sir James, 73
Bates, Alan, 148
Batthyany, Duke of, of Stein-am-anger (Hungary), 291
Baxter, Jedediah Hyde, 190
Beck, Alfons, 280
Becker, Boris, 6, 91
Beckham, David, 6, 89–90
Beckham, Victoria, 170
Beckwith, D. H., 260

Beckwith, Seth R., 260
Beecher, Henry Ward, 4, 319
Beethoven, Ludwig van, 5, 154–156
Behring, Emil Adolph von, 21, 116–118
Belfast, Lady, 253
Bell, Alexander Graham, 189
Belladonna, 204–205
Bennett, J. G., 330
Bernhardt, Sarah, 5, 137–138
Best, Charles, 129–130
Bhagwat Purana (Sanskrit text), 326
Bhajan, Yogi, 332
Bhumananda, 328
Bible, the, 302–304
Biddle family, 247
Bier, August, 120–121, 206–207
Bigel, Jean, 279
Biggar, Hamilton Fiske, 192, 194, 230–231, 237, 262–263
Billings, Frank, 232
biomimicry, 20–21
birth control, 216
Blackie, Margery, 81–82
Blackwell, Elizabeth, 217, 220–221
Blair, Cherie, 209
Blair, Tony, 209
Blavatsky, Madame Helena, 329
Bliss, D. W., 189, 190
bloodletting, 40, 48
Bloom, Orlando, 150
Bocco, Jules, 277, 279
Boden, Margarete, 206
Böenninghausen, Clemens Maria Franz von, 277, 278
Bonaparte, Bathilde, 278
Bonaparte, Charles Louis Napolean, III, 277–279
Bonaparte, Napoleon, 275–277

Index

Bonington, Chris, 94–95
Boole, Mary Everest, 119–120
Boone, Joel T., 4, 196, 197–198
Booth, Edwin, 137
Booth, Lyndsey, 209
Bosch, Robert, 254–255
Bouton, Jim, 93
Boyd, Patti, 164
Boynton, Silas, 189, 190
Braunhofer, Anton, 154–156
Brooks, Phillips, 320
Brown, William H., 248
Bryant, William Cullen, 69–70, 71

C

Cadbury family, 253
Caine, Michael, 146
Camphora, 315
cancer therapies
    Iscador, 143, 316
    radiation, 122
    Vinca minor, 291
Capel, Lord, 253
Capen, Robert, 218
Carlebach, Rabbi Shlomo, 323
Carnegie, Andrew, 233–234, 250
Carnegie Foundation for the Advancement of Teaching, 233–234, 242, 250
Carstens, Karl, 207–208
Carstens, Veronica, 207–208
Carstens Foundation, 207–208
Cartland, Dame Barbara, 84
Cattrall, Kim, 149
Centamori, Settimio, 287, 305
Chand, Diwan Jai, 338
Charge, Alexandre, 277, 306
Charles, Prince of Wales, 295–296
Chekhov, Anton, 76–77
Cher, 5, 165–166
Chinmoy, Sri, 332–333
Chiranjeevi, 149
cholera
    epidemic of 1854, 46
    homeopathic *vs.* conventional medicines, 48–49, 277
    medicines used for curing, 314–315
    and support for homeopathy, 305
    understanding of cause, 103
Chopin, Frédéric, 5, 157, 158
Christian Science healing, 336–337
chronic obstructive pulmonary disease (COPD), 29–30
Cierach, Lindka, 180
Cinchona officinalis, 156
Civil War, 184–185
Clarke, Gladstone, 321
Clarke, John Henry, 310
Claude, Jacques, comte de Beugnot, 252
Clemons, Samuel. *See* Twain, Mark
clergy, support for homeopathy, 273, 301–344
clinical studies. *See* scientific studies
clinical training in homeopathic education, 235–236
clinics, 329. *See also* hospitals, homeopathic
Clinton, Hillary Rodham, 208
Clinton, William Jefferson, 208
Clisby, Harriet, 222–223
Clothier family, 247
Codman, Charles R., 247
colleges of homeopathic medicine
    AMA Council on Medical Education report, 257
    Cleveland Homeopathic Hospital College, 230, 237–238
    curriculums, 237–238

colleges of homeopathic medicine *(continued)*
  decline of, 237–238
  the Flexner Report, 233–237, 257
  Hahnemann Medical College, 261
  Missionary School of Medicine, 309–310
  New York Homeopathic Medical College, 225
  New York Medical College and Hospital for Women, 219–220
  nineteenth century, 18, 63
  North American Academy of the Homeopathic Healing Art, 317
  Ohio State University College of Homeopathic Medicine, 4, 241–243
  Post-Graduate School of Homeotherapeutics, 249
  twentieth century, early, 18
  Western Reserve Eclectic Institute, 333
  for women, 234, 237
  women's experiences of, 221
  The Women's Medical College, 220–221
Compton-Burnett, Dame Ivy, 81
Compton-Burnett, James, 118–119
constitutional homeopathy, 85
consultation clause, the, 43
Coolidge, Calvin, 197
Cooper, Peter Fennimore, 250–251
COPD (chronic obstructive pulmonary disease), 29–30
Copeland, Royal S., 126–128
corporate leaders, support for homeopathy, 4, 229–270
coughing, 19
Cousins, Norman, 82–84
Crawford, Cindy, 180
Crump, Walter Gray, 225
Crumpler, Rebecca Lee, 223

Cullen, Paul, Archbishop of Dublin, 309
cure *vs.* symptomatic relief, 2–3, 19–21
Curie, Paul Francois, 199
curriculums in homeopathic education, 237, 238
Czaky, Count, of Zips (Hungary), 290

D

Danforth, Willis, 186
Darwin, Charles, 3, 104–114, 306
Davet, A. J., 277
David, Pierre-Jean, 252
Davis, Carl, CBE, 169
Davis, Nancy, 266–267
Dean, Michael Emmans, 29
Degas, Edgar, 5
Delphic Oracle, 21
Dennett, Mary Coffin Ware, 216–217, 263–264
depression, 11
Depression, the, 261
dermatological conditions, 120–121
detective work, homeopathic, 78–79
d'Hervilly, Melanie, 217–218, 252
diagnosis
  in conventional medicine, 22–23
  in homeopathy, 23–24, 78–79
Diana, Princess of Wales, 296
diarrhea, 19, 31
Diaz, Portifio, 201
Dickens, Charles, 6, 81
Dickenson, Emily, 68–69
Dietrich, Marlene, 138–139
dilution, serial
  Behring's experiments with, 117
  Darwin's experiments with, 111
  Hahnemann's experiments with, 102
  in preparing homeopathic medicines, 25
  vs. potential toxicity, 205

Index

Dinnet, Marcel, 165
discharges, 19
discrimination against homeopathy. *See* AMA; persecution of homeopaths
Disraeli, Benjamin, 199–200
distilled water, double, 24–26
doctors, eclectic, 236
Doggett, Joseph B., 248
dosages, homeopathic
    Darwin's experiments with, 110–111
    Hahnemann's development of, 102
    hypersensitivity response, 22
    nanodosage, 24–28
    nineteenth century view of, 42
Dostoevsky, Fyodor, 6, 75–76
Dows, David, 245
Doyle, Sir Arthur Conan, 6, 73, 78–80
Drexel, Anthony Joseph, 247
Drosera rotundifolia, 110–111
drug companies, 7–8, 10, 256
drug treatments. *See also* specific drugs; specific symptoms
    discoveries, important, 264
    efficacy of, *vs.* symptomatic relief, 10–13
    historical patterns of use, 7, 42
    symptomatic relief, 2–3
    symptoms, suppression of, 20
    warnings about, 232–233
Drummond, Lady, 253
Dunsford, Harris, 272
Dupin, Amandine-Aurore-Lucile. *See* Sand, George
Duquesnay, Archbishop, of Cambrai, 312

E

Eastman, George, 240
Eastman, Linda, 163
Eckel, J. N., 320
eclectic medicine, 236
economic factors, in attacks on homeopathy, 45, 47, 214
Eddy, Mary Baker, 5, 335–338
Edison, Thomas, 57
Edson, Susan, 190
education, homeopathic. *See also* colleges of homeopathic medicine
    Carnegie Foundation survey of, 233–234
    decline of, 237–238
    eclectic, 236
    the Flexner Report, 233–237, 257
    laboratory science *vs.* clinical training, 235–236
    orthodox, 99–100
    self-teaching of homeopathy, 214
education, medical, AMA council on, 257
education, medical, and minorities, 225, 261
Edward, Prince, Duke of Windsor, 272
Edward VII, King (Great Britain), 272
Edward VIII, King (Prince Edward, Duke of Windsor), 272
Egger, M., 54
Elgin, Lord, 253
Eliot, Charles W., 99–100
Elizabeth II, Queen, 271, 273, 294–295
Emerson, Ralph Waldo, 6, 63, 66
Emmanuel, King Vittorio (Sardinia), 287
Englis, John, 245
Ennis, Madeleine, 32
epidemics
    1918 influenza, 241
    cholera, 46, 48–49, 277, 305, 314–315
    nineteenth century, 213
    typhoid fever, 184, 185
    typhus, 275
    understanding causes of, 103

Espanet, Alexis, 312
Eugenie, Empress (France), 277–278
Everest, Thomas, 308–309
Evia, Edgar de, 178

F

Faddis, Jon, 168–169
Fairbanks, Douglas, Jr., 138
families, homeopathic care of, 214
fashionistas, support for homeopathy, 178–180
Father Muller Charitable Institutions, 307
Faustus, Pater, 314
FDA (U.S. Food and Drug Administration), 11, 73, 127
Federal Food, Drug, and Cosmetics Act of 1938, 127–128
Feodorovna, Alexandra (Empress of Russia), 280
Feofan the Hermit, Saint, 310–311
Ferdinand, Duke of Anhalt (Germany), 282
Ferdinand VII (Spain), 288
Ferguson, Sarah, Duchess of York, 296
Ferret, Jean-Marcel, 89–90
fever, 10
fibromyalgia, 31
Field, Cyrus West, 245
financial motives
  of the AMA, 256, 259
  of drug companies, 7–10
  of nineteenth century apothecaries, 41, 289
  stifling of homeopathic medical education, 233–237, 239, 242–243
financial support for homeopathy. *See* philanthropists
Fischer, Anton, 316
Fishbein, Morris, 103, 256, 257–259

Fisher, Peter, 294–295
Fleischmann, Wilhelm, 313
Flexner, Abraham, 232, 233, 234–237
Flexner Report, 233–237, 257
Flint, Austin, 44–45
Flower, Roswell P., 245
flu. *See* influenza
Food and Drug Administration, U.S. *See* FDA
Forbes, John Murray, 245–246
Forbes, Sir John, 114–115
Fowler, Lydia Folger, 217
Franklin, Benjamin, 57
Franklin, Edward C., 334
fraud
  and the AMA, 258–259
  amongst apothecaries, 41
Friedman, Rabbi Manis, 322
Friedrich Wilhelm IV, King (Prussia), 289–290
Friedricka, Princess (Prussia), 290
Furtado, Nelly, 168

G

Gabriel, Infante Don Sebastian (Spain), 288
Gachet, Paul, 173–174, 175, 176
Galeazzi-Lisi, Riccardo, 307
Galilei, Galileo, 1
Gallinger, Jacob H., 191–192
Gandhi, Indira, 203
Gandhi, Mahatma, 4, 10, 202
García Márquez, Gabriel, 85–86
Gardner, A. K., 44
Gardner, Franklin A., 191
Garfield, James, 188–190, 333
Garrison, William Lloyd, 4, 187–188
Gates, Frederick T., 231–232, 237, 239
Gaudi, Antoni, 177–178

Gauguin, Eugène Henri Paul, 176
gender, and statistics in medicine, 225
George V, King (Great Britain), 272
George V, King (of Hanover), 282
George VI, King (Great Britain), 272–273
Gillespie, Dizzy, 5, 161–162
glass, role of, in making homeopathic medicines, 25, 33
Goehrum, Heinrich, 254
Goethe, Johann Wolfgang von, 6, 75, 284
Gogh, Vincent Willem van, 5, 173–175
gold, 303
Gram, Hans Burch, 43
Grauvogl, Eduard von, 281–282
Gray, Asa, 112
Greenwood, Will, 91
Gregory XVI, Pope, 305, 306
Griffith, Alexander Randall, 123
Griffith, Harold Randall, 122–124
Griggs, John William, 192–193
Griggs, William B., 307–308
Grouse Lodge recording studio, 169–170
Grubbe, Emil, 122
Guess, George, 56–57
Guidi, Count Sebastiano de, 277–278, 287, 305
Gully, James, 3, 80, 105–109, 215–216
Gurdjieff, G. I., 330

H

Haehl, Richard, 276
Hahnemann, Melanie, 217–218, 252, 278, 279
Hahnemann, Samuel
   allopathy, coining of term, 22
   allopathy, early criticism of, 40
   August Bier on, 121
   biographical information, 251–252
   burial site, 312
   homeopathy, development of, 101–104
   monument to, 104, 192–193, 249
   refinement of his work, 35
   and the royalty, 275
   second wife, 217–218, 252, 278, 279
   Sir John Forbes on, 114–115
   tombstone of, 39
Haldar, Indrani, 148
Hale, Edward Everett, 318
Hall, A. Oakey, 245
Hall, Jerry, 179
Hall, Sir Benjamin, 46–47
Hampshire, Susan, Lady Kulukundis, OBE, 148
hangover, 147
Hanna, Mark A., 194
Harding, Florence, 915
Harding, Phoebe, 194–195
Harding, Tyron, 194–195
Harding, Warren G., 194–197
Harrach, Countess (Austria), 284–285
Harrison, Benjamin, 191
Harrison, George, 5, 163–164, 327–328
Harrison, Olivia, 164
Hartmann, Franz, 156, 158
Hartung, J. Christophe, 286
Harvey, William, 57
Hastings, Charles, 109
Hawthorne, Nathaniel, 6
Hayes, Rutherford B., 188
healing, assumptions about, 41–42
healing crisis, 309
health histories, 24
health insurance, 258
Hearst, Phoebe, 250
heilpraktikers, 206

Heinz, H. J., 249
Helfrich, Rev. Johannes, 317
Henderson, Sir William, 292
Hering, Constantine, 276
Herrick, Myron T., 251
Hess, Rudolf, 206
Higgins, Van H., 249
high blood pressure, 19
Hippocrates, 2, 21
Hitler, Adolf, 203–207
Hoffman, Heinrich, 204
Hoffman, Nicholas Von, 103
Holmes, Oliver Wendell, 50–53, 70–71
homeopathy
  advocates
    actors and actresses, 5, 137–151
    artists and fashionistas, 5, 173–181
    athletes, 6, 89–97
    corporate leaders, 4, 229–270
    literary figures, 6, 63–87
    musicians, 5, 153–172
    physicians and scientists, 3, 99–135
    politicians and peacemakers, 4–5, 183–212
    religious leaders, 5, 301–344
    royalty, 6, 271–299
    women's rights leaders and suffragists, 4, 213–227
  American Institute of Homeopathy, 43, 217, 219
  antagonism towards
    AMA, 4, 9, 43–45, 257–259
    persecution, 43–57, 293–294
    physicians, 1–2
    reasons for, 39–42, 99
  colleges of homeopathic medicine
    AMA Council on Medical Education report, 257
    Cleveland Homeopathic Hospital College, 230, 237–238
    decline of, 237–238
    the Flexner Report, 233–237, 257
    Hahnemann Medical College, 261
    Missionary School of Medicine, 309–310
    New York Homeopathic Medical College, 225
    New York Medical College and Hospital for Women, 219–220
    nineteenth century, 18, 63
    North American Academy of the Homeopathic Healing Art, 317
    Ohio State University College of Homeopathic Medicine, 4
    Post-Graduate School of Homeotherapeutics, 249
    twentieth century, early, 18
    Western Reserve Eclectic Institute, 333
    women's experiences of, 221
    The Women's Medical College, 220–221
  constitutional, 85
  diagnosis, method of, 22, 23–24, 78–79
  dosage of medicines
    Darwin's experiments with, 110–111
    Hahnemann's development of, 102
    hypersensitivity response, 22
    nanodosage, 24–28
    nineteenth century view of, 42
  earliest evidence of, 17
  healing, assumptions about, 42
  hospitals, homeopathic
    Chicago Baptist Hospital, 333–334
    Cleveland Protestant Homeopathic Hospital, 260
    Fabiola Homeopathic Hospital and Free Dispensary, 261
    Good Samaritan Hospital, 334
    Rochester Homeopathic Hospital, 240
    Royal London Homoeopathic Hospital, 273

liberalism, political, and, 214
medicines (*See also* specific medicines)
   criticism and defense of, 14
   dilution, serial, 25, 102, 111, 117, 205
   dosages, 22, 24–28, 42, 102, 110–111
   nanopharmacology, 24–28
  notoriety, first, 275
  organizations, 345
  principles (*See* principles of homeopathy)
  scientific studies
   Arnica, 95
   confirming efficacy of, 10–12, 29–32
   efforts to discredit homeopathy, 54–55
   on homeopathy, 29–32
   on horses, 27
  symptoms, treatment of (*See also* specific symptoms)
   drug treatments, 2–3
   relief of *vs.* efficacy, 10–13
   similars, principle of, and, 17–18
   wisdom of, 19–21, 42, 302
Hooker, E. Beecher, 319
Hoover, Herbert A., 198
Hopetoun, Countess of (Scotland), 253
Horatiis, Cosmo Maria de, 287
hormesis, 27
hospitals, homeopathic
  Chicago Baptist Hospital, 333–334
  Cleveland Protestant Homeopathic Hospital, 260
  Fabiola Homeopathic Hospital and Free Dispensary, 261
  Good Samaritan Hospital, 334
  Rochester Homeopathic Hospital, 240
  Royal London Homoeopathic Hospital, 273

hot flashes, 145
Houdret, Jean-Claude, 179
Howe, Julia Ward, 222
Hoyle, E. Petrie, 95
Hoyne, Thomas, 248
Hubbard, Elizabeth Wright, 139, 170, 177
Hufeland, Christoph Wilhelm, 103
Hughes, Alfred, 185
human testing of homeopathic substances, 23
Hunt, J. G., 186
Hyman, Misty, 94
hypersensitivity response
  Darwin's experiments with *Drosera*, 111–112
  to homeopathic medicines, 26, 34

I

Ikense, Ifeoma, 166
immunization, principle of, 21
immunotherapy, homeopathic, 31
income, physician's, 221
India, support for homeopathy, 201–202
Indian Association for the Cultivation of Science, 49
individualization of homeopathic treatments, 14, 23–24, 273
infant mortality rates, 1
infectious diseases, 127, 213
inflammation, 19
influenza
  1918 epidemic, 241
  Oscillococcinum, clinical trials, 29
  Oscillococcinum, origins of, 127
insomnia, 11
insulin, 264
insurance
  health, 258
  life, homeopathic, 244

International Homeopathic Medical
    League, 206
Internet resources
  Boiron (homeopathic medicines), 94
  Carstens Foundation, 207
  Homéopathe International, 278
  homeopathic organizations and web
    sites, 345–347
  *The Hospitals and Sanatoriums of the
    Homeopathic School of Medicine*,
    229
  Indian Association for the
    Cultivation of Science, 49
  International Homeopathic Medical
    League, 206
  Iscador, 143
  National Center for Homeopathy,
    144
  New Scientist magazine, 32
  New York Medical College for
    Women, 225
  Samueli Institute of Information
    Biology, 29, 265
interviews, patient, 14
Ioann of Kronstadt, Saint, 310, 311
Irani, Adi S., 329
Irving, Washington, 6, 70–71
Isabelle II, Queen (Spain), 288
Iscador, 143, 316
Ishmael, Rabbi, 322

J

Jackson, Mercy B., 218–219
Jacobi, Abraham, 44
Jagger, Jade, 179–180
Jagland, Thorbjørn, 208–209
Jahr, George Heinrich Gottlieb, 290
James, Henry, 6, 64–65
James, William, 67
Jameson, Louise, 147
Jeanes, Anna T., 261–262

Jeanes, Jacob, 261
jet lag, 168
John Paul II, Pope, 308
Johnson, Virginia, 128
Joseph, Viceroy, 291
Josephson, Brian, 130–132
Judd, Ashley, 149
Jütte, Robert, 112–113

K

Kalakaua, King (Hawaii), 291
Kali bichromicum, 30
Kander, Arnie, 92
Keep, Henry, 245
Keith, Edson, 248
Keith, Frederick S., 337–338
Kent, James Tyler, 249, 338, 341
Kepler, Johannes, 58, 154
Kettering, Charles F., 4, 240–243
Khan, Muhammad Ayub, 207
Kidd, Joseph, 199–200
King, Coretta Scott, 226
King, Thomas Starr, 320
Kinnaird, Lady (Scotland), 253
Koch, Augustus Wilhelm, 113
Koller, Baron Francis (Austria), 286
Koop, C. Everett, 130
Kramer, Gustav, 282
Krishnamurti, Jiddu, 330
Kumar, Ashok, 148

L

laboratory science in homeopathic
    education, 235–236
Ladies Physiological Societies, 214
Lagerfeld, Karl (Otto), 178–179
Lancaster, John, 224
Lancet, The, 53–54
law of spirality, 112, 113

Index

Lawson, Victor, 248–249
Leaf, William, 253
Lee, Robert E., 185
Lennox, Annie, 167
Leo XII, Pope, 305
Leo XIII, Pope, 307
Leopold I, King (Belgium), 275
Lewis, Dioclesian, 317–318
liberalism, political, and homeopathy, 214
life expectancy rates, 13
life insurance companies, homeopathic, 244
Lilienthal, Rabbi Max, 323
Lilienthal, Samuel, 323–324
Liliuokalani, Queen (Hawaii), 292
Lincoln, Abraham, 58, 183–184, 186
Lincoln, Mary, 186
literary figures, support for homeopathy, 6, 63–87
Lombard, Benjamin, 248
Longfellow, Henry Wadsworth, 6
Lopez-Knight, Nancy, 91
Louis Philippe, King, 279
Lozier, Clemence Sophia, 219–222
Lukovsky, Yuly, 310
Lunt, Orrington, 248
Lyszcynski, A., 158

M

Mabit, J., 278
Macartney, Very Reverend Hussey Burgh, 321
Madero, Francisco I., 201
Madero, Raúl, 201
Maguire, Tobey, 150
Mahabharata (Sanskrit text), 325–326
Maier, Hermann, 93–94
Manet, Édouard, 176

Maragnot, J. P., 276
Marenzeller, Matthias, 156, 289–290
Maria Olazábal, José, 6, 91
marketing, and prescription drugs, 8, 10, 11
Márquez, Gabriel García, 85–86
Martin, George Henry, 291–292
Mary, Queen (Great Britain), 272
Mathai, Isaac, 296
Mauro, Giuseppe, 287
Maximilian, Pater, 314
Maynard, Joyce, 84–85
Mayo, Charles H., 128–129
Mayo, William J., 128–129
McCann, Thomas Addison (T. A.), 4, 241
McCartney, Linda Eastman, 163
McCartney, Paul, 5, 163
McClellan, George Brinton, 184–185
McCormick, Robert Sanderson, 249
McGraw, Phillip, 145
McGraw, Robin, 145
McKinley, William, 192–193
McKinney, Susan Smith, 223
medical board examinations, 238–239
medical insurance. *See* health insurance
medical schools
    Carnegie Foundation survey of, 233–234
    eclectic, 236
    the Flexner Report, 233–237, 257
    homeopathic (*See* colleges of homeopathic medicine)
    and minorities, 225, 261
    orthodox, 99–100
medical-industrial complex, 7–9, 10
medicine, conventional
    allopathy, 22
    criticism of, by homeopaths, 39–42
    drugs, 7–8

medicine, conventional *(continued)*
  efficacy, 2–3, 10–13, 11
  healing, assumptions about, 41–42
  homeopathic principles, use of, 21–22
  limitations of, 6–13
  nineteenth century, 40, 213
  science *vs.* business of, 8
medicine, modern, 10–13
medicines, homeopathic. *See also* specific medicines
  criticism and defense of, 14
  dilution, serial, 25, 102, 111, 117, 205
  dosages, 22, 24–28, 42, 102, 110–111
  glass, role of, 25, 33
  human testing of, 23
  hypersensitivity response, 26, 34, 111–112
  individualization of, 14, 273
  nanopharmacology, 24–28
  and polypharmacy, 40
  provings, 23, 317
Meher Baba, 328–329
Melford, Duchess of, 253
Mengozzi, Giovanni Ettore, 306
Menninger, Charles Frederick, 124–125
menopausal symptoms, 145
mental illness, 20
Menuhin, Sir Yehudi, 5, 169–170
Merrick, Myra King, 230, 231
Milhaud, Darius, 170
Milton, John, 74
minorities and medical education, 225, 261
Moby, 167–168
Molin, Jean Jacques, 157
monarchs, support for homeopathy, 271–299
Moncoutié, David, 93
Monet, Claude, 5

monument to Hahnemann, 104, 249
Morell, Theodor, 204–206
Morrill, Alpheus, 188
Morse, Samuel F. B., 250
Moses, 302–304
Mother, The (Mirra Richard), 328
Mother Teresa, 338
Mott, Lucretia, 4–5
Muhlenbein, G. A. H., 282–283
Muktananda, Swami, 331–332
Muller, Father Augustus, 306–307
Muller, Wolfgang, 158
Muller-Wohlfahrt, Hans-Wilhelm, 91
multiple sclerosis, 266–267
Munsiff, Abdhul Ghani, 329
Musard, Philippe, 252–253
music of the spheres, 153
musicians, support for homeopathy, 5, 153–172

N

name-calling, in conventional medicine, 13–14
nanodosage
  of homeopathic medicines, 14, 24–28
  nature, examples from, 32–33
nanopharmacology, 24–28
Napoleon I, 275–277
Napoleon III, 277–279
Narayanan, Shri K. R., 203
Navratilova, Martina, 6, 90–91
Neatby, Edwin, 321
Necker, George
Negro, Antonio, 308
Negro, Francesco, 308
Nehru, Jawaharlal, 203
Nehru, Pandit Motilal, 202
Newton, Wayne, 170

Nicholas I, Czar (Russia), 279
Nichols, Charles F., 292
Nightingale, Florence, 215–216
Nik Mat, Tuan Guru Dato' Haji Nik Abdul Aziz, 325
NoJetLag (homeopathic medicine), 168
Nua, Russell, 92
Nuñez, José, 288
Nux vomica, 92, 147, 204–205

O

Ohio State University College of Homeopathic Medicine, 241–243
Olazábal, José Maria. *See* Maria Olazábal, José
Olga, Queen, of Württemberg, 254, 280
Oliver, Henry, 251
O'Neill, Paul, 92
online resources. *See* Internet resources
Oracle, Delphic, 21
organizations, homeopathic, 345
Ornish, Dean, 208
Oscillococcinum, 29, 127, 267
Osler, Sir William, 116, 235
Ozanam, Charles, 305–306

P

Padri (Fardoon Driver), 329
Paganini, Nicolo, 5, 156–157, 252
Paget, Henry William, 253
painkillers, 10–11
panic attacks, 11
Paracelsus, 21
Parker, Theodore, 318–319
Pasteur, Louis, 117
patrons, royal, 274
Patterson, John H., 251

Paul VI, Pope, 308
Peabody, Elizabeth Palmer, 64–65
Pellicer, Joaquin, Jr., 289
Pellicer, Tomás, Sr., 288
penicillin, 206, 264
Perry, Right Reverend Charles, 321
persecution of homeopaths
  AMA, 4, 9, 43–45, 257–259
  the Flexner Report, 233–237, 257
  in medical journals, 293
  modern day attacks, 53–57
  in nineteenth century Europe, 45–48
  in nineteenth century India, 48–49
  by Oliver Wendell Holmes, 50–53
  physicians, conventional, 1–2
Peters, John C., 70–71
pharmaceutical industry. *See* drug companies
Phelps, Elizabeth Stuart, 68
philanthropists, support for homeopathy, 229–270
Phosphoric acid, 314
physical fitness, 318, 332–333
physiology, modern, 19
Pissarro, Camille, 5, 175–176
Pitcairn, John, 249
Pitcairn, Robert, 249
Pius VIII, Pope, 305
Pius IX, Pope, 306
Pius X, Pope, 307
Pius XII, Pope, 307
politicians and peacemakers, support for homeopathy, 4–5, 183–212
Pollock, Jackson, 176–177
polypharmacy, 40
Pons, Lily, 170
Pope, Sarah A., 247
Pope, William, 246
potentization. *See* dilution, serial

Prémont, Marie-Hélène, 94
prescription drugs
   discoveries, important, 264
   efficacy, long-term, 2–3
   efficacy *vs.* symptomatic relief, 10–13
   historical patterns of use, 7, 42
   symptoms, suppression of, 20
   warnings about, 232–233
prescriptions, homeopathic. *See* medicines, homeopathic
Presley, Lisa Marie, 149
Presley, Priscilla, 149
principles of homeopathy
   healing crisis, 309
   hypersensitivity, 26, 34, 111–112
   individualization of treatment, 14, 273
   resonance, 26
   similars
      ancient understanding of, 74
      Biblical examples, 303–304
      in conventional medicine, 21–22
      explanation of, 17–18
      Hahnemann's development of, 101–102
      in Hindu texts, 325–326
      Mary Baker Eddy on, 337
      nanodosage, 34
      Talmudic references, 322
   symptoms, wisdom of, 19–21, 42, 302
   syndromes as basis of treatment, 22–24, 34, 118
Pritchett, Henry S., 233–234, 242
profits, of drug companies, 7, 8, 10
proof, scientific, controversies over, 13
provings, homeopathic, 23, 317
psychiatric conditions, 11
Pulsatilla, 219
Pure Food and Drug Act of 1906, 73
Pythagoras, 153

Q

quackery, medical, and the AMA, 258–259
Quain, Richard, 200
quantum medicine, 35
Quarin, Freiherr Von, 251
Queen Elizabeth II, 271, 273, 294–295
Quin, Frederick Hervey Foster, 80–81, 272, 273, 275

R

Radetzky, Joseph von, 285–286
Radhakrishnan, Sarvepalli, 203
radiation therapy, 122
Rama, Swami, 332
Ramakrishna Paramahamsa, 326–327
Rapous, Pierre-Auguste, 312
Reece, Gabrielle, 93
reforms, medical school, 233–237
religious leaders, support for homeopathy, 5, 301–344
remedies, homeopathic. *See* medicines, homeopathic
Remson, Ira, 236
Renner, John, 243
Renoir, Pierre-Auguste, 5
Republican politics and homeopathy, 214
resonance, as basis of homeopathy, 26
Richand, Pierre, 179
Richard, Mirra (The Mother), 328
RIMR (Rockefeller, Institute for Medical Research), 231, 232
Ringer, Sydney, 119
Robbins, Royal E., 246
Rockefeller, Institute for Medical Research (RIMR), 231, 232
Rockefeller, J. D., 4, 71

Index

Rockefeller, John D., Sr., 230–233, 237–238, 239
Rodgers, Paul, 166–167
Romani, Francesco, 271–272, 286–287
Romanov, Constantine Pavlovich, Grand Duke, 279
Rose, Axl, 167
Rosenberg, H., 291
Roses, Allen, 13
Rothschild, Baron Mayer Amschel de, 253
Rothstein, William, 63–64
Rowntree family, 253
royalty, support for homeopathy, 6, 252, 253, 271–299
Rush, Benjamin, 50–51
Russell, Henry Sturgis, 246
Russian Orthodox Church, 5
Ruth, Henry, 123

S

safety of drug treatments, 7, 232–233
Salinger, J. D., 84–85
Salvado, Bishop Rosendo, 320
Samueli, Henry, 265
Samueli, Susan, 265–266
Samueli Institute of Information Biology, 29, 265
San Martín, José Francisco de, 4, 199
Sand, George, 157
Sarkar, Mahendra Lal, 48–49
Sassoon, Vidal, 179
Satchidananda, Swami, 331
Sawalha, Julia, 146
Sawalha, Nadia, 146–147
Sawyer, Charles, 195, 196–197
Schenck, Ernst-Günther, 205
Schmit, Anton, 282

Schneerson, Rabbi Menachem Mendel, 322
schools of homeopathy. *See* colleges of homeopathic medicine
Schumann, Clara Wieck, 158–159
Schumann, Robert, 158
Schwarzenberg, Prince Karl Phillip von (Austria), 283–284
Schwenninger, Ernst, 160
scientific method, 10–12, 132, 264
scientific studies
    Arnica, for trauma and healing, 95
    effectiveness of, 10–12, 29–32
    efforts to discredit homeopathy, 54–55
    on homeopathy, 29–32
    on hormesis, 27
scientists, support for homeopathy, 3, 99–135
seal of approval, AMA, 256–257, 259
Segura y Pesado, Joaquin, 201
Selfridge, Grant L., 126
self-teaching of homeopathy, 214
Sepia, 145
Seward, William, 183–184
Seymour, Jane, 142–143
Shakespeare, William, 74
shaking of homeopathic preparations. *See* succussion
Shankar, Ravi, 162, 327–328
Sharma, Chandra, 162, 164, 330
Shaw, George Bernard, 6, 77–78
Shrewsbury, Earl of, 271
Sibley, Hiram, 240
side effects of drug treatments, 7, 20
similars, homeopathic principle of
    ancient understanding of, 74
    in conventional medicine, 21–22
    examples from the Bible, 303–304
    explanation of, 17–18

similars, homeopathic principle of (*continued*)
   Hahnemann's development of, 101–102
   in Hindu texts, 325–326
   Mary Baker Eddy on, 337
   nanodosage, 34
   Talmudic references, 322
Simmons, George H., 256–258
Simms, Harry, 237–238
Simon, Leon, 289
Simpson, Stephen, 321
Sinclair, Upton, 73–74
Singh, Manmohan, 203
Sircar, Mahendra Lal, 327
Sisters of Charity, 313
skin conditions, 120–121
Slater, Kelly, 91–92
sleep-inducing drugs, 11
Sloan-Kettering Institute, 243
Smith, Julia Holmes, 222
smoking, 260
socioeconomic classes, 248
Somers, Suzanne, 143, 316
Spencer, Carleton, 216
sports figures, support for homeopathy, 6, 89–97
Stanton, Elizabeth Cady, 4–5, 214–215, 221
Stanton, Henry, 215
Stapf, Johann Ernst, 272
Starr, Paul, 18, 257
statistics in medicine, and gender, 225, 226
Stearn, R. H., 246
Stearns, Guy Beckley, 178
Stebbins, Henry G., 244
Steiner, Rudolf, 315–316
Stephanopoulos, George, 208
Stetson, John Batterson, 247

Stewart, Alexander Turney, 245
Stirling, Jane, 157–158
Stojko, Elvis, 94
Stowe, Emily Jennings, 224
Stowe, Harriet Beecher, 6, 319
Strawbridge family, 247
Strawn, Julia Clark, 263
Street, Robert, 329
studies, scientific. *See* scientific studies
succussion, 25, 33
suffrage, women's, 222–223, 224
Sulphur iodatum, 121, 157
suppression of symptoms, 20
survey of U.S. medical schools, 233–234
Swedenborg, Emanuel, 65–66, 249, 339–340
symptoms. *See also* specific symptoms
   drug treatments, 2–3
   relief of *vs*. efficacy, 10–13
   similars, principle of, and, 17–18
   suppression of, 20
   wisdom of, 19–21, 42, 302
syndromes as basis of treatment, 22–24, 34, 118
syphilis, 205–206

T

Taft, Cincinnatus, 72
Tagore, Rabindranath, 82
Talmud, 321–322
Tate family, 253
Temple, Jack, 179, 296
Tennyson, Alfred, Lord, 6, 80
Teresa, Mother, 338
Tessier, Jean-Paul, 45–46, 306
Thomas, George C., 247
Thompson, Mary Harris, 223–224
Thoreau, Henry David, 6, 63
tobacco companies and the AMA, 259

Index

Toussaint, 312
Townshend, Pete, 164–165
toxicology, homeopathic study of, 23, 118
Transcendentalism, 64–65
treatments, conventional. *See* medicine, conventional
trials, clinical. *See scientific studies*
Trinius, C. Bernhard, 282
Trinks, Karl Frederick, 48
tuberculosis, 118
Turner, Tina, 5, 162–163
Twain, Mark, 6, 71–72
Tyler, John, 188
Tyler, Margaret, 274
typhoid fever, 184–185
typhus, 275

U

U.S. Homeopathic Pharmacopeia, 127–128
Upcher, Rev. Canon Roland, 310

V

vaccination, 117
van Gogh, Vincent, 5
Varlez, L. J., 290
Vatican support for homeopathy, 304–308
Veith, Father J. M., 156, 314–315
Verdi, Tullio S., 188
Vereen, Ben, 149
Verrett, Shirley, 169
Vinca minor, 291
Vivekananda, Swami, 327–328

W

Wagner, Lindsay, 144–145
Wagner, Richard, 5, 159–160
Wahle, Johann Wilhelm, 305
Ward, Florence Nightingale, 224–225
Ward, James, 225
Warren, Lesley Ann, 140–141
water
  body content, 34
  imprinting of homeopathic properties, 33
  role in making homeopathic medicines, 24–26
  structure of, and homeopathy, 131–132
Watts, Naomi, 149–150
Wayne, John, 139
Web resources. *See* Internet resources
web sites, homeopathic. *See* Internet resources
Webb, E. Cook, 291
Weber, G. A., 282
Webster, Daniel, 4
Webster, Horace, 245
Weir, Bob, 166
Weir, Sir John, 273
WEIU (Women's Educational and Industrial Union), 222–223
Weld, Theodore Dwight, 317
Wesselhoeft, Conrad, 68
Wesselhoeft, Karl, 75
Wesselhoeft, William, 69
Wesson, Daniel B., 250
Westinghouse, George, 249
Wharton, Joseph, 247
Widener family, 247
Wilkinson, John James Garth, 65–66, 340–341
William I, King (the Netherlands), 290
William III, King (the Netherlands), 290
Williams, Vanessa, 145
Wills family, 253
Wilson, Benjamin, 321

Women's Educational and Industrial Union (WEIU), 222–223
women's homeopathic colleges, 234, 237
Women's Homeopathic Fraternity, 225
women's rights leaders, support for homeopathy, 4, 213–227
Woodhull, Victoria Claflin, 215
World War I, 186, 196
Worthington, George, 243–244
Wright, Sir Almroth, 78
Wrigley, William, 248, 263

X
Xanax, 11

Y
Yeats, William Butler, 81
York, Michael, 143–144

Z
Zeta-Jones, Catherine, 5, 139–140
Ziegler, Gregorius Thomas, Bishop of Linz, 314

About the Author

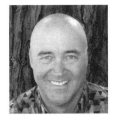

Dana Ullman received his master's degree in public health from the University of California at Berkeley. He is the founder of Homeopathic Educational Services, America's largest publisher and distributor of homeopathic books, tapes, software, and medicine kits, and is widely recognized as the foremost spokesperson for homeopathic medicine in the United States.

In addition to authoring nine other books, Ullman has written chapters on homeopathic medicine for several leading medical textbooks for practicing physicians and has served as a consultant for or on the advisory board to alternative medicine institutes at Harvard, Columbia, and University of Arizona schools of medicine. From 1993 to 1995 (and again in 1998), he co-taught a ten-week course on homeopathy at the University of California at San Francisco School of Medicine. He also developed the curriculum in homeopathy for physician associate fellows at Dr. Andrew Weil's Program in Integrative Medicine at the University of Arizona.

Ullman has been particularly effective in working with major institutions to change policies toward natural health care. He has organized successful conferences that were sponsored by the federal Department of Health and Human Services (Holistic Health: Policies in Action, May 1980) and UC Berkeley (Conceptualizing Energy Medicine, March 1981). Ullman authored the San Francisco Foundation's Health Report, which changed the funding priorities of this major philanthropic institution, consulted on a research project sponsored by the Medical Board of California, which ultimately recommended many of his proposals, and served as a consultant to the World Health Organization. He lives in Berkeley, California.